A Treatise on Topical C
in Dermatology

Koushik Lahiri

Editor

A Treatise on Topical Corticosteroids in Dermatology

Use, Misuse and Abuse

Springer

Editor
Koushik Lahiri
Department of Dermatology
Apollo Gleneagles Hospitals and WIZDERM
Kolkata
India

ISBN 978-981-13-5180-8   ISBN 978-981-10-4609-4   (eBook)
DOI 10.1007/978-981-10-4609-4

This Springer imprint is published by Springer Nature
The registered company is Springer Nature Singapore Pte Ltd.
The registered company address is: 152 Beach Road, #21-01/04 Gateway East, Singapore
189721, Singapore

To,

My
Parents,
Professors,
Partner,
Progenies,
Peers,
Patients,

And everyone else from whom I have learned something

Foreword

Topical Corticosteroids: The Boon and the Bane

We have been blessed with the use of topical corticosteroids. And we have been cursed by the use of topical corticosteroids.

For more than 60 years, first by dermatologists, then by general medical practitioners, and then by pharmaceutical companies and pharmacists, these creams, lotions, ointments, solutions, gels, sprays, and pastes have been prescribed and promoted for a variety of cutaneous disorders and ailments, mainly pruritus, atopic dermatitis, psoriasis, and other corticosteroid-responsive cutaneous afflictions, and used by the general public, indiscriminately, for itching, redness, swelling, hyperpigmentation, and lately as a panacea for all their skin woes. This has been reinforced by all the publicity that we see on television and read in ladies' magazines and supported, advertised, promoted, and endorsed by the pharmaceutical industry. It is egregious and unconscionable to advertise these ever-increasing potent and damaging products to an unsuspecting, gullible public.

The first reported use of a topical corticosteroid, hydrocortisone, was by Sulzberger and Witten in 1952 in the *Journal of Investigative Dermatology* (J Invest Dermatol. 1952 Aug; 19(2):101–2). Since then, a plethora of warnings has been launched on a trusting but ignorant public, to no avail. Some of these corticosteroids are powerful enough to cause irreparable damage not only to the skin but to internal organs as well. These steroidal ointments, creams, lotions, gels, solutions, aerosols, sprays, shampoos, foams, drops, and other vehicles can be found in drugstores and pharmacies and can often be purchased without a doctor's prescription.

There are myriad side effects to many of the stronger, more potent, varieties of topical corticosteroids, some of which are serious and hazardous and can lead to permanent damage. Fluorinated steroids, particularly the ointment varieties, when used under occlusion, should be used cautiously and not for any length of time.

Steroid atrophy is a serious side effect of protracted applications of topical corticosteroids. Steroids are absorbed at different rates depending on the thickness of the stratum corneum. The eyelids and the genital areas absorb about 25%, the palms and soles about 0.1%, the upper and lower extremities about 2%, and the face about 7%. The absorption rate is much greater when the steroid is used in an ointment base.

It is almost criminal to recommend or to prescribe corticosteroids, particularly the high potency varieties, for mild to moderate dermatoses, for long periods of time, for infants and children and for the elderly where the ravages of time coupled with prolonged exposure of the sun have already caused some skin impairment.

The present obsession with fairness!

Did you ever consider that skin color did not determine the social status in ancient Greece and Rome? The preferred skin color has varied by culture and time. The Maasai people of Kenya have associated pale skin with being cursed by evil spirits. Many cultures have historically favored lighter skin in women. Before the Industrial Revolution in Europe, pale skin was a sign of high social status. The poor classes worked outdoors and got dark from exposure to the sun. The idle rich stayed indoors and had lighter skin. Slavery and colonization in Europe inspired racism and led to the belief that darker-skinned people were inferior and uncivilized; the lighter-skinned black people were more beautiful and more intelligent. These people were often preferred to be house slaves and given an education; the darker people worked in the fields in the sun. The preference for fairer skin among blacks was noteworthy and still is. A light skin signifies a higher social status in some countries and suggests that person is wealthier.

Like other Asian countries, in India, fairness mania is very much evident. Steroid containing bleaching creams are misused by many to get fair, resulting in devastating consequences. Suggestion: stop all sales of these OTC products!

Population in India as of today is on the order of 1,400,000,000. (No. I did not get the number of zeroes wrong!) In the United States, there are roughly 330,000,000 people. Both countries have almost the same number of dermatologists: 9000… Go figure!

"Fairness" and whitening are major problems. They must be dealt with as we speak.

Jerome Z. Litt, MD

Author of Litt's Drug Eruption and Reaction Manual, updated yearly for 23 years. CRC Press. Also the website: Litt's DRUG ERUPTION and REACTION DATABASE

Preface

When the proposal of publishing a book with one of the leading publishing houses reached me, spontaneously, this topic came to my mind.

Over almost the last seven decades, topical corticosteroids have significantly influenced the dermatologist's capability to effectively treat several difficult dermatoses. During this period, they have completely changed the face of therapy of dermatological disorders. The available range of formulations and potency gives flexibility to treat all groups of patients, different phases of disease, and different anatomic sites and made it almost inseparable from the practice of dermatology anywhere in the globe. But, these are supposed to be used in various dermatological disorders based on evidence-based knowledge and expertise.

It was indeed surprising that in spite such important locus in the practice of dermatology, a complete discourse dedicated only to this subject of topical corticosteroids in its entirety has never been attempted in an exhaustive manner.

Most of the time, at least initially, dermatological disorders are largely managed by family physicians and general practitioners. Inadequate awareness about the potency-based classification and insufficient acquaintance about the mechanism of action, indications, and contraindications of topical corticosteroids have given rise to the rapid incidence of the improper use of these drugs which threatens to bring disrepute to the entire group of these remarkable drugs.

As we had to deal with an extremely specialized topic and as this was the first book entirely dedicated to a single topic, topical corticosteroids, we had to select experts from all over the world for this ambitious project.

They are all working on specific topics assigned to them for many years, and some have contributed articles in journals.

The benefits of rational and ethical use and the harm of overuse and misuse for nonmedical, especially for cosmetic, purposes should be clearly conveyed before penning a prescription involving topical corticosteroids. Despite being the most useful drug for such treatment, they are known to produce serious local, systemic, and psychological side effects when overused or misused.

A separate book dedicated to topical corticosteroids has never been planned or executed.

This treatise aims to fill up that lacuna and to contribute significantly to the dissemination of knowledge about the indication/contraindication, mechanism of action, ethical use, side effects, and various other facets related to topical corticosteroids.

In order to give shape to this ambitious vision, we tried to rope in the best global experts on this topic.

Knowing some of the authors helped us draw on their personal experience as well as scientific evidence in these chapters.

The final result is a never before compilation on this subject authored by fifty top thought leaders in the field.

This is an astonishing treatise, a collective wisdom of key academic opinion leaders bejeweled with rich illustration from the extensive and priceless clinical arsenal of the authors.

We hope this comprehensive compendium will be of value to all dermatologists whether postgraduate students, senior practitioners, or academicians in India, Asia, and the globe. General practitioners/family physicians would also immensely benefit from this book.

This is our sincere and humble effort to bridge gaps in the subject while presenting the latest advances to our fellow dermatologists. We know the road ahead is still long, but a beginning was necessary.

We look forward to your feedback.

Kolkata, India   Koushik Lahiri

Acknowledgments

Even after working closely on the nuances of topical steroid use and misuse for well over an entire decade, I was a little apprehensive when I first agreed to take-up the project.

My apprehension was partly for the fact that I did not have a charted track before me and partly because of such overwhelming importance of topical corticosteroids in the practice of dermatology. It was intriguing that a complete discourse dedicated only to this subject of topical corticosteroids in its entirety has never been attempted in an exhaustive manner.

These initial concern and consternation turned into pleasure and enthusiasm when all esteemed contributors whom we approached responded in a very positive way. They are virtually the topmost key opinion leaders in the field. I would like to personally thank each author who contributed for the project. No words of appreciation are enough for them. In spite of their very busy schedule, they have done a stupendous job in writing so meticulously.

All the credit of the book goes to the brilliant contributors only.

Astonishing polymath Professor (Dr.) S Premalatha, Dermamom, as she is fondly known in India, helped me to divide the chapters and topics. I sincerely appreciate her invaluable contribution.

JoAnne VanDyke, the volunteer president and executive director of International Topical Steroid Awareness Network (ITSAN), was a source of constant encouragement behind this project.

I must thank Springer, the world's leading publisher of scientific, technical, and medical e-Books, for inviting me to publish with them.

Eti Dinesh, senior editor, Medicine Books and Journals, Springer India, took personal care of this project. I owe a lot to her.

Kumar Athiappan, the assigned project coordinator for this project, was there with us with his sincere and professional competence.

Rajesh Sekar, the project manager, worked tirelessly during the last lap of this journey who oversaw the production from manuscript to final print and online files.

The icing on the cake was the foreword from a real living legend, Professor Jerome Z. Litt. His priceless foreword has certainly enhanced the credibility and definitely added value and recognition to our humble effort.

Contents

About the Editor

Biography

Dr. Koushik Lahiri is the editor of the *Indian Journal of Dermatology*, Vice President of the *International Society of Dermatology*, and the immediate past president of the *Association of Cutaneous Surgeons of India*.

Dr. Lahiri is a foundation fellow of the Asian Academy of Dermatology--Venerology, fellow of IADVL Academy of Dermatology, International fellow of American Academy of Dermatology, and founder council member of the Asian Skin Foundation and Asian Society for Pigment Cell Research (ASPCR).

He is a fellow of all the three Royal Colleges of Physician of England, FRCP (London, Edinburgh and Glasgow), and a member of the Royal College of Physicians and Surgeons, MRCPS (Glasgow).

Dr. Lahiri is an editorial board member or reviewer for the *British Journal of Dermatology*, *International Journal of Dermatology*, *Dermatology Online Journal*, *Egyptian Dermatology Online Journal*, *IJDVL*, *IJSTD*, etc.

Dr. Lahiri has published more than *100 articles* in several indexed journals in the last two decades and contributed several chapters in different textbooks. He has compiled an extremely popular megaproject *100 Interesting Cases in Dermatology* and edited a highly acclaimed exhaustive compendium *Pigmentary Disorders* and the first *Textbook of Lasers in Dermatology.*

He has received various national and international awards, including the two highest oration awards for Indian dermatologists, the *Dr. B M Ambady memorial oration* and *Dr. P N Behl oration.*

As the former honorary national general secretary of IADVL, Dr. Lahiri conceptualized and proposed the *IADVL Academy of Dermatology*, which has now become the academic lifeline for Indian dermatologists. *ACSI Academy of Dermatosurgery* was also his brain child.

Today his name is inseparable with an extremely familiar entity among the dermatologist community in India, *TSDF* or Topical Steroid-Dependent/Damaged Face—a term he coined.

As a tireless protagonist in the fight against the misuse of topical corticosteroids in India, Dr. Lahiri has worked relentlessly to sensitize other doctors (even dermatologists), government agencies, chemists, media, and the common people regarding this shameful practice. As the founder chairperson of the countrywide *IADVL Taskforce Against Topical Steroid Abuse (ITATSA)*, he became the face of a historic and epoch-making movement of Indian dermatologists.

He is the sixth Indian who has received the *International League of Dermatological Societies (ILDS) prestigious Certification of Appreciation (CoA)* award. He was the first Indian to be honored for *outstanding leadership, with special recognition from the Rutgers State University of New Jersey and New Jersey Medical School Chapter of Sigma Xi, the Scientific Research Society.*

Contributors

Anil Abraham Department of Dermatology, St. John's Medical College, Bangalore, India

Shyamanta Barua Assistant Professor, Department of Dermatology, Assam Medical College and Hospital, Dibrugarh, Assam, India

Manas Chatterjee Department of Dermatology, Institute of Naval Medicine, INHS Asvini, Colaba, Mumbai, India

M.U. Kabir Chowdhury Principal, Samorita Medical College Hospital, Dhaka, Bangladesh

Professor of Dermatology, Holy Family Medical College, Dhaka, Bangladesh

Director, Kabir National Skin Centre, Dhaka, Bangladesh

Ex Visiting Professor, Faculty of medicine, University of Ottawa, Ottawa, Canada

Arijit Coondoo Department of Dermatology, K.P.C Medical College and Hospital, Kolkata, West Bengal, India

Paschal D'Souza Department of Dermatology, ESIC-PGIMSR, New Delhi, India

Rajetha Damisetty Consultant dermatologist and additional medical director, Oliva Chain of Skin and Hair Clinics, Hyderabad, Telangana, India

Anupam Das Department of Dermatology, KPC Medical College and Hospital, Kolkata, India

Sandipan Dhar Department of Pediatric Dermatology, Institute of Child Health, Kolkata, India

Nejib Doss Department of Dermatology, Military Hospital of Tunis, Tunis, Tunisia

Mototsugu Fukaya Tsurumai Kouen Clinic, Nagoya, Japan

Hassan Galadari College of Medicine and Health Sciences, United Arab Emirates University, Al Ain, United Arab Emirates

Aparajita Ghosh Department of Dermatology, KPC Medical College and Hospital, Kolkata, West Bengal, India

Evangeline B. Handog Department of Dermatology, Asian Hospital and Medical Center, Muntinlupa City, Philippines

Swaranjali V. Jain Department of Dermatology, St. George Hospital, and Faculty of Medicine, University of New South Wales, Sydney, NSW, Australia

Maria Juliet Enriquez-Macarayo Department of Dermatology, AUF Medical Center, Pampanga, Philippines

Subekcha Karki Di Skin Health and Referral Centre, Kathmandu, Nepal

Niti Khunger Department of Dermatology and STD, Vardhman Mahavir Medical College, Safdarjang Hospital, New Delhi, India

Rishi Kumar Pharmacovigilance Division, Indian Pharmacopoeia Commission, National Coordination Centre, Pharmacovigilance Programme of India, Ministry of Health and Family Welfare, Government of India, Ghaziabad, Uttar Pradesh, India

Anil Kumar Jha DI Skin Health and Referral Centre, Maharajgunj, Kathmandu, Nepal

Nepal Medical College, Jorpati, Kathmandu, Nepal

Gagandeep Kwatra Department of Pharmacology, Christian Medical College-Ludhiana, Ludhiana, Punjab, India

Koushik Lahiri Department of Dermatology, Apollo Gleneagles Hospitals and WIZDERM, Kolkata, West Bengal, India

Sagar Mani Jha DI Skin Health and Referral Centre, Maharajgunj, Kathmandu, Nepal

Shree Birendra Army Hospital, Kathmandu, Nepal

Yogesh S. Marfatia Department of Skin-VD, Medical College Baroda, Vadodara, Gujarat, India

Sharad Mehta Department of Dermatology, RNT Medical College, Udaipur, Rajasthan, India

Devi S. Menon Department of Skin-VD, Medical College Baroda, Vadodara, Gujarat, India

Asit Mittal Department of Dermatology, RNT Medical College, Udaipur, Rajasthan, India

Sandip Mukhopadhyay Department of Pharmacology, Burdwan Medical College, Burdwan, West Bengal, India

Dedee F. Murrell Department of Dermatology, St. George Hospital, and Faculty of Medicine, University of New South Wales, Sydney, New South Wales, Australia

Venkataram Mysore Venkat Charmalaya, Centre for Advanced Dermatology and Postgraduate Training, Bangalore, India

T.S. Nagesh Department of Dermatology, Venereology and Leprosy, Sapthagiri Institute of Medical Sciences and Research Center, Bangalore, India

Saumya Panda Department of Dermatology, KPC Medical College and Hospital, Kolkata, India

Deepak Parikh Department of Pediatric Dermatology, Wadia Hospital for Children, Mumbai, India

Kumar Parimalam Professor and Head of Dermatology, Sree Balaji Medical College & Hospital, Chromepet, Chennai, India

Nisha V. Parmar Aster Medical Centre, Dubai, United Arab Emirates

Meghana Phiske Dr. Meghana's Skin Clinic, Navi Mumbai, India

Sanjay K. Rathi In Private Practice, Consultant Dermatologist, Siliguri, West Bengal, India

Abir Saraswat Indushree Skin Clinic, Lucknow, India
Indushree Skin Clinic, Lucknow, India

Rashmi Sarkar Department of Dermatology, Maulana Azad Medical College and Lok Nayak Hospital, New Delhi, India

Sujata Sengupta Department of Dermatology, K.P.C. Medical College and Hospital, Kolkata, West Bengal, India

Nidhi R. Sharma Department of Dermatology, Venereology and Leprosy, Shaheed Hasan Khan Mewati Government Medical College, Nuh, Haryana, India

Rajeev Sharma Bishen Skin Centre, Aligarh, India

Belinda Sheary Royal Randwick Medical Centre, Belmore Road, Randwick Australia

Gousia Sheikh Venkat Charmalaya, Centre for Advanced Dermatology and Postgraduate Training, Bangalore, India

G.N. Singh Secretary-cum-Scientific Director, Indian Pharmacopoeia Commission, National Coordination Centre- Pharmacovigilance Programme of India, Ministry of Health and Family Welfare, Government of India, Ghaziabad, Uttar Pradesh, India

Sahana M. Srinivas Department of Pediatric Dermatology, Indira Gandhi Institute of Child Health, Bangalore, India

Jayakar Thomas Professor and Head of Dermatology, Sree Balaji Medical College & Hospital, Chromepet, Chennai, India

Kathryn Z. Tullos ITSAN, Palm Beach Gardens, FL, USA

JoAnne VanDyke ITSAN, Palm Beach Gardens, FL, USA

Shyam Verma Nirvan Skin Clinic, Vadodara, India

Omid Zargari Consultant Dermatologist, DANA Clinic, Rasht, Iran

Evolution and Development of Topical Corticosteroids

1

Sandip Mukhopadhyay and Gagandeep Kwatra

Abstract

Corticosteroids are the steroidal compounds derived from the adrenal gland or prepared synthetically. Topical corticosteroids are mainly glucocorticoids. The first use of corticosteroids was in the form of adrenal extracts which was reported in 1930 by Swingle et al. In the same year, Tadeus Reichstein in Zurich; Edward Kendall at the Mayo Clinic, USA; and Oskar Wintersteiner at Columbia had been able to isolate small amount of active steroid from the adrenal gland. Systemically it was used successfully to treat rheumatoid arthritis in 1948. Reichstein, Kendall and Hench received a 'Nobel Prize' for their work with adrenal steroids. The first successful use of topical hydrocortisone in human dermatoses was reported in 1952 by Sulzberger and Witten. This landmark event opened up the avenue for the search of newer molecules with more potency and desirable properties. Gradually, the fluorinated compounds like flumethasone, flurandrenolone and triamcinolone were developed by early 1960. All these preparations were more potent than cortisone and hydrocortisone. The third generation of topical corticosteroids, betamethasone, beclomethasone or fluocinolone, found their places in the early 1960s which gradually extended their presence from systemic to topical therapy. Betamethasone, a remarkable one, after primarily systemic use, was placed successfully in the topical world in 1964. Betamethasone valerate was prepared by 1967 by esterification which further added to the potency of the parent

S. Mukhopadhyay (✉)
Department of Pharmacology, Burdwan Medical
College, Burdwan, West Bengal, India
e-mail: sandipcmcl@gmail.com

G. Kwatra
Department of Pharmacology, Christian Medical
College-Ludhiana, Ludhiana, Punjab, India
e-mail: kwatragagandeep@gmail.com

© Springer Nature Singapore Pte Ltd. 2018
K. Lahiri (ed.), *A Treatise on Topical Corticosteroids in Dermatology*,
DOI 10.1007/978-981-10-4609-4_1

compound. With the increase in the number of topical corticosteroid preparations, the World Health Organization classified such agents into seven groups. Several assay methods were developed for assessment of potency and activity of topical corticosteroids. Human vasoconstrictor assay, described by McKenzie and Stoughton in 1962, was one of the methods which has been very common for years.

Keywords

Topical steroids • Adrenal extracts • Hydrocortisone • Betamethasone • Dermatoses • Sulzberger and Witten

Learning Points

1. First systemic corticosteroid use was reported by Swingle et al in 1930 and it was in the form of adrenal extract. In the same year some small amount of corticosteroid were isolated from the adrenal gland by Tadeus Reichstein, Edward Kendall and Oscar Wintersteiner.

2. Evolution of topical corticosteroids was sincere efforts by the scientists during the World War ravaged world.

3. First successful use of topical corticosteroid in dermatoses was reported by Sulzberger and Witten in 1952 in the form of hydrocortisone.

4. Though first fluorinated compound was 9- α-fluorohydrocortisone acetate and it was successfully used in topically in 1954, the real success came with the flumethasone, flurandrenolone and triamcinolone in 1960s which were much more potent than hydrocortisone.

5. Betamethasone was a significant discovery and the first topical use was reported in 1964. Betamethasone valerate was prepared by 1967 which was more potent than the parent compound.

6. Human vasoconstrictor assay was successfully used for screening of the compounds with topical activities.

1.1 Introduction

Corticosteroids are steroid hormones produced either from the cortex of the adrenal gland or synthetically derived from it. These are subdivided as glucocorticoids, mineralocorticoids and sex steroids. These are essential hormones for the body which found their potential in the therapeutics long back. We are still witnessing newer roles of corticosteroids in the endeavour to restrain the diseases. Newer molecules with more desired properties, duration and actions for different disease conditions are now exposed to the world. Topical corticosteroids are primarily glucocorticoids. Now a long list of topical steroids is enlisted in the classification of the World Health Organization [1]. However, the beginning of this journey was not smooth.

1.2 The Early Stages: A 'Planned Serendipity'?

The world was yet to come out of joy of the discovery of serendipity – the penicillin in 1928; the 'Great Depression' of the history started (1929) to spread the shadow of its paw on civilization. The share market was yet to recover from the 'crash' following the 'Great Depression'. People of the USA were stunned with the brutality of 'St. Valentine Day Massacre' by the 'Al Capone' gang in February of 1929 in the city of Chicago [2].

Common people were still trembling with the dysrhythmia in their routine life due to jinx of the 'Great Depression'; the tireless medical scientists had no time to waste for the contemporary developments of the world. Some of them came up with some curious findings which later ushered in a new era. Swingle et al. came up with their finding (1930) that adrenalectomized animals could be treated successfully with the extract of the adrenal gland and the animal could be successfully recovered from coma [3]. This gave rise to the idea that extract of animal adrenocortical tissue could counteract human adrenal failure. That year, scientists from different parts of the world like Tadeus Reichstein in Zurich, Edward Kendall at the Mayo Clinic and Oskar Wintersteiner at Columbia had been able to isolate small amount of active steroid from the adrenal gland. Subsequently, the isolated compounds were found to be different cortical steroids. As chemical analyses of cortical extracts proceeded, mainly in the laboratories, it became evident that it was not a single cortical hormone but a number of steroid compounds are there!. It was the time of World War II, and a rumour was spread in the USA that the German scientists had been able to beat others in discovering the secrets of the adrenal cortex. The developed extract had been able to counter hypoxemia and permitted the pilots of Luftwaffe to fly at the level of 40,000 ft! Incidentally, the rumour was baseless. However, it produced massive gearing up of the research activities in the USA. By 1940 it was understood that there are two categories of compounds: those that cause sodium and fluid retention and those that counteract shock and inflammation. By 1942, sufficient amount of cortisone and cortisol were produced to be sent for testing [4–6]. In 1948, St. Mary Hospital of the Mayo Clinic witnessed the first patient who was treated with cortisone for rheumatoid arthritis. The bedridden lady who was surviving with much pain walked out of the hospital for shopping in a week [7]. This anti-inflammatory effect of corticosteroids was first confirmed by Hench et al. in rheumatoid arthritis [8, 9]. The compounds were named alphabetically as compound A, B, C, D, etc., and the listing was done in 1949. In the same year, the heading of 'cortisone' was made for the first time [10]. In 1950, the efforts of the pioneers like Tadeus Reichstein, Edward Calvin Kendall and Philip Showalter Hench were acknowledged by 'Nobel Prize for Physiology and Medicine' for their work on hormones of the adrenal cortex that eventually culminated in the isolation of cortisone [11]. In 1952, the heading of 'adrenocortical preparation' was made [10].

By 1950–1951, the oral and intra-articular administration of cortisone and hydrocortisone was started. Several lines of research to produce cortisone semi-synthetically showed some success by 1952. Between 1954 and 1958, six synthetic steroids were introduced for systemic anti-inflammatory therapy [5].

1.3 Early Developments: The Commercial Side

Cortisone was first synthesized by Lewis Sarett of Merck & Co., Inc., in the 1930s. The process involved a complicated 36-step process that started with deoxycholic acid, extracted from ox bile. The cost of development was a whooping US $200 per gram, a definitely whooping cost at that time. The high cost was due to the low efficiency of converting deoxycholic acid into cortisone in the process [11].

Cost reduction was possible when Russell Marker, at Syntex, Mexico, utilized wild Mexican yams for a more convenient starting material, diosgenin, which was cheaper also. Conversion of diosgenin into progesterone was a four-step process and now known as 'Marker degradation'. Soon the newly formed company started selling progesterone at US $50 per gram by 1945 and by 1951 at US $2 per gram [12]! Later the company started utilizing the low-cost progesterone which eventually became the preferred precursor in the industrial preparation of cortisone and mass production of all steroidal hormones [11].

Another significant development was in 1952 by D.H. Peterson and H.C. Murray of Upjohn Co. They described a process of microbiological introduction of oxygen using '*Rhizopus* mould' to oxidize progesterone into a compound that was readily converted to cortisone. Research of Percy Julian also aided some interesting progress in the field. The cost reduction was remarkable. Synthesizing large quantities of cortisone from the diosgenin of the Mexican yams resulted in a rapid drop in price to US \$6 per gram and subsequently falling to \$0.46 per gram by 1980 [11, 13].

1.4 The First Topical Use of Corticosteroid: The War-Ravaged World Got a Blessing!

Topical corticosteroid, though first invented in 1951, successful use in human disease was first described in 1952 by Sulzberger and Witten [14]. In their article, Sulzberger and Witten mentioned that topical cortisone acetate ointment is 'without value in the treatment of diseases of the skin'. So they started working with hydrocortisone after procuring crystalline hydrocortisone acetate from the medical division of Merck & Co., Inc., Rahway, New Jersey, whom they acknowledged thankfully in their article. They prepared an ointment with crystalline hydrocortisone acetate 25 mg with lanolin (15%), liquid petrolatum (10%) and white petrolatum to make per gram of ointment and mentioned it as 'compound F' ointment. In their 'innovative' study design, they enrolled patients from their clinical practice and purposefully tried to choose patients with bilateral symmetric dermatological conditions. The purpose of such selection was to use one side for control (ointment base) and compare it to the contralateral site where treatment drug was applied (compound F ointment). The observation period was 4 weeks with follow-up every week. They found 75% (six of the eight cases) of proved or presumptive atopic dermatitis; there was

greater improvement with 'compound F ointment' than the base alone. Similar improvement was also noted by them in a patient with widespread discoid or subacute lupus erythematosus. The study also mentions about a patient, 'Mr. M.S.,' as 'case 3' where improvement was noted even beyond the site of application [15]. To explain this event, Sulzberger mentioned the study of Goldman, Preston and Rockwell of College of Medicine of the University of Cincinnati; they evaluated the result of patch test reactions after intradermal injection of 'compound F' solution and found a zone of inhibition extending beyond the immediate area of intradermal injection. This result was also published in the same year [16]. These two researches opened up the new avenue of topical corticosteroids in human dermatoses.

1.5 Fluorinated Agents: An Endeavour for More Potent and Better Activity

In 1954, Witten, Sulzberger, Zimmerman and Shapiro reported about their research with 9α-fluorohydrocortisone acetate which got published subsequently in 1955. They performed therapeutic assay of topically applied 9α-fluorohydrocortisone acetate in patients with selected dermatoses. Goldfien et al. in 1954 reported that the parenteral preparation when used in Addison's disease showed higher metabolic and therapeutic activity of hydrocortisone, as well as longer duration of action. The assumption was 9α-hydrogen atom, when replaced by a halogen, results in 'many times the glucocorticoid activity' than that of parent cortisone and hydrocortisone. Therefore, Whitten et al. designed their study to find topical activity of 9α-fluorohydrocortisone acetate in comparison to hydrocortisone. They enrolled a total of 62 patients with dermatoses, e.g. atopic dermatitis, allergic eczematous contact dermatitis, nummular eczema, lichen simplex chronicus, etc. which had previously been reported as amenable to topical hydrocortisone acetate and hydrocortisone-free alcohol therapy. Simultaneous paired comparison method of evaluation was possible in 51 of the 62 cases. They reported that fluorohydrocortisone acetate was better than hydrocortisone in 28 out of 51 patients (55%), and in 16 cases (31%), the two compounds were equally effective. They concluded that 9-fluorohydrocortisone acetate was 'slightly more effective' compared to hydrocortisone [17].

The story of topical corticosteroids started progressing with time with development of newer molecules. Alteration of the primary structure of the corticosteroids was successfully utilized to develop newer molecules, many of which showed higher and longer action of the newer compounds than the cortisone or hydrocortisone. However, for the new cortisone-like compounds, the improved effects were mostly reflected by the improved systemic activity. So, a new challenge evolved out to the medicinal chemists that the compounds must be able to penetrate the skin in order to be successful topically. On the other hand, the other challenge was developing compounds which should have minimal systemic effect and primarily exert local activity. So, chemical substitution of the groups in the structure of the steroids was continued to develop new compounds with better functionality and minimizing side effects [4].

Converting $=$O with $-$OH (hydroxylation) of the C11 β of the structure of cortisone resulted in the successful development of hydrocortisone which provided better topical activity. Victor H. Witten of the University of Miami mentioned the discovery of hydrocortisone was not a chance or accidental discovery, rather it was a painstaking effort of the scientists for a long time [10].

In the chronology of development, the next development was addition of a fluorine atom at the 9α position of hydrocortisone. This change increased the potency of the newly developed molecule but produced extensive changes in the fluid and electrolyte balance. The molecule is popularly known as fludrocortisone.

Another fluorine atom was incorporated in the structure at position 6 with further enhancement of potency. But the problem of fluid and electrolyte balance persisted. This molecule was named as flucortolone and is considered as a mid-potency corticosteroid [4].

Later, flumethasone was prepared which contained fluorine atoms at both 6 and 9 positions. However, the problem of fluid and electrolyte balance could not be overcome though the activity was increased.

Further, addition of acetonide group in positions 16 and 17 resulted in the formulation of flurandrenolone acetonide. The preparation though had fluorine in the sixth position; the problem of fluid and electrolyte balance was reduced and had better physico-chemical properties for topical administration [4, 18]. Triamcinolone acetonide was a further improvement with incorporation of a double bond between C 1 and 2 which resulted in higher potency and activity and lowered adverse effects related to fluorine of the ninth position. It was devoid of fluorine at position 6. Fluocinolone acetonide was even better with 'exceptional topical activity' and had explored the advantages of double bond between carbon 1 and 2 (like triamcinolone), fluorine at positions 6 and 9 and acetonide at 16 and 17 positions. It emerged as one of the most potent topical corticosteroids. Fluocinonide was added to the list later which had even more degree of activity, four times more potent to its precursor fluocinolone acetonide and longer duration of action. The drug had excellent anti-inflammatory activity and enhanced lipophilicity and enhanced absorption through the skin which were attributable to esterification at the C-21 position [4]. W.A. Page mentioned in his editorial at the Canadian Medical Association Journal,

"the modern era began in earnest in 1960 with the introduction of the fluorinated corticosteroids triamcinolone, flurandrenolone and flumethasone, each of which was four to six times as potent as hydrocortisone. In 1962 a third generation of topical corticosteroids, betamethasone 17-valerate, fluocinolone and beclomethasone, with 10 to 20 times the potency of hydrocortisone, became available and has subsequently dominated the market-place" [(18)]

1.6   Betamethasone: A Landmark in the Topical Therapy

Betamethasone was a remarkable discovery in the armamentarium of corticosteroids. Initially it was identified and introduced for systemic use by Schering Corporation in 1961. The formulation was oral tablet of 0.6 mg. The topical use formulation came in to picture from 1964. In order to develop more potent corticosteroid, chemical restructuring or modifications continued. Betamethasone valerate was successfully introduced in 1967 as 0.1% cream. This was considered a breakthrough in the topical corticosteroid research because this high-potency compound was having sufficient anti-inflammatory property and was able to treat several difficult dermatoses including psoriasis which were only amenable to systemic corticosteroids earlier [19].

1.7   Further Progress in Topical Therapy: An Effort for Betterment!

Clobetasol, desonide and halcinonide followed the path of betamethasone in the form of good topical activity. In 1965, Canadian physician Norman M. Wrong mentioned in his article that around 50 preparations containing topical steroid alone or in combination were listed in the 'Vademecum International', Canada, in 1965. He also mentioned that these topical steroids are dispensed as ointments, creams, lotions, sprays and foams of different strengths and many of them as combination with other drugs [20].

By the 1970s, the market had the choice of several topical corticosteroids with proven efficacy. The newer agents were more potent. However, the new concern of steroid-related adverse effects raised caution about their use among the physicians. The misuse of corticosteroids was also notified by many [20]. Several drug-induced side effects were noticed in the patients, both systemic and local. Pace (1973) mentioned that "great advances inevitably create new problems. The topical corticosteroids brought many new problems with them, both

local and systemic". He mentioned local reactions like skin atrophy or fungal infection and scabies as a result of reduced local immunity as the points of concern. He also mentioned that the preservatives used in the ointment bases, e.g. parabens (esters of p-hydroxybenzoic acid), may produce allergic sensitization. Systemic absorption from the skin in children was another point he wanted to point out [18].

Another promising molecule, clocortolone pivalate is a relatively new entry in the development path of the topical corticosteroids. This is a mid-potency topical corticosteroid available as a 0.1% emollient cream. It was well understood that the vehicle is also an important factor as well as the parent corticosteroid compound for treatment of dermatological conditions. In this case, the vehicle is formulated for application to a variety of corticosteroid-responsive skin disorders. These include those with inflamed and fissured skin like eczematous dermatoses. The preparation is approved by USFDA, and there is no age restriction in the use of this preparation. This justifies the use of this preparation for seborrhoeic dermatitis and 'diffuse eczematous dermatoses' which are typically common in children. Clocortolone pivalate is unique in chemical structure that provides high lipid solubility to the molecule [21]. The lipophilicity, duration of action and potency of clocortolone were increased due to esterification at C-21 with substitution of a pivalate group. Methylation at C-16 also increases lipophilicity. Therefore the compound exhibits an augmented penetration through the stratum corneum and a higher epidermal concentration. It has been reported that the structural characteristics of this molecule enhance its potency without increasing the potential for topical corticosteroid-related adverse effects. The clinical trials with this preparation reported significantly low incidences of adverse effects and no observed systemic reaction [21–24]. Though a systematic review raised questions about some weaknesses of the clinical trials, overall effectiveness with early onset of action and a good safety profile of this preparation could not be ignored [25].

The list of topical corticosteroids continued increasing (Fig. 1.1). Several new vehicles are

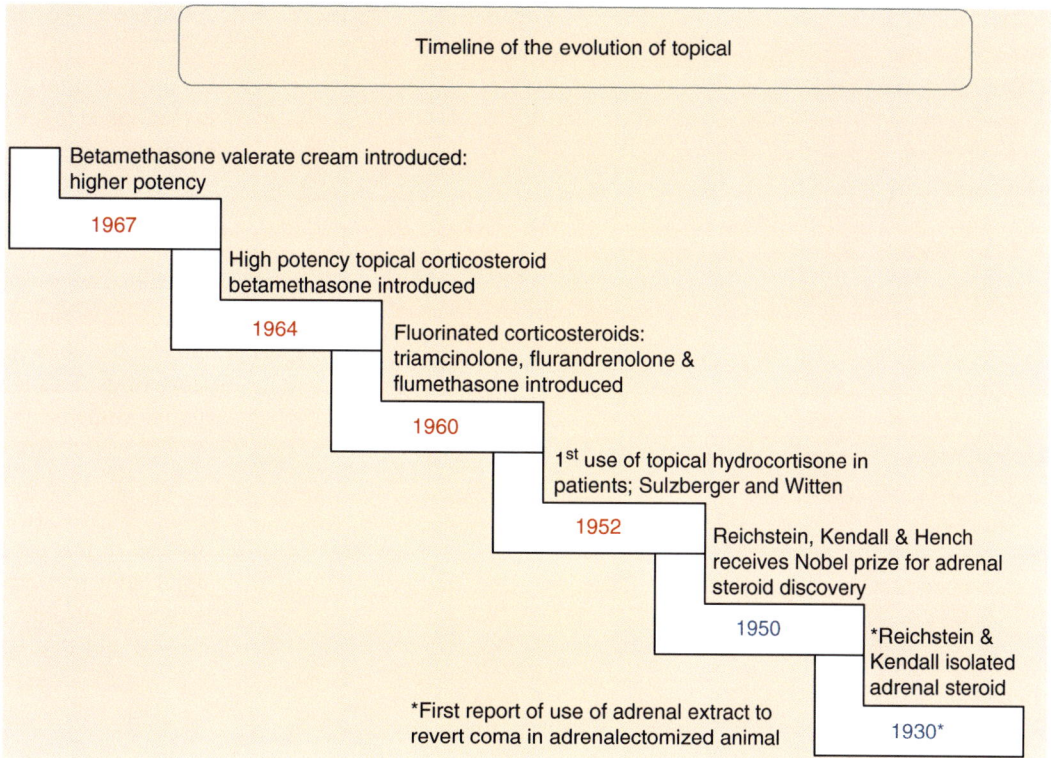

Timeline of the evolution of topical

Betamethasone valerate cream introduced: higher potency
1967

High potency topical corticosteroid betamethasone introduced
1964

Fluorinated corticosteroids: triamcinolone, flurandrenolone & flumethasone introduced
1960

1st use of topical hydrocortisone in patients; Sulzberger and Witten
1952

Reichstein, Kendall & Hench receives Nobel prize for adrenal steroid discovery
1950

*Reichstein & Kendall isolated adrenal steroid

*First report of use of adrenal extract to revert coma in adrenalectomized animal
1930*

Fig. 1.1 Evolution and development of topical corticosteroids

also being utilized for improving topical delivery of the compounds. The agents are different in potency as well as activities. The World Health Organization classified the long list of topical corticosteroids into seven different classes according to their potency [1, 26]. However, newer enlistment will be inevitable as the endeavour for search for more desirable and ideal compound is ongoing.

1.8 Development of the Assay Methods: Scientific Evaluation Was Inevitable

The development of new topical agents inevitably brought the question of comparison of potency and efficacy. Several assay methods were used to compare the potency of the corticosteroid preparations. There was no single specific method to assay the unique therapeutic potentials of corticosteroids. Therefore, a battery of assays

were utilized to screen the compounds for further testing. Fibroblast assay, thymus involution assay, anti-granuloma assay and rat ear assay were some of them. Human vasoconstrictor assay, described by McKenzie and Stoughton in 1962, eventually became one of the most useful assay methods for evaluation of potency of topical corticosteroid [27, 28]. The ability of producing vasoconstriction was found to be related to anti-inflammatory effect in the therapeutic arena [29]. Another significant method of assay which was used to evaluate topical corticosteroids was psoriasis small plaque bioassay [30]. However, the contribution of the vasoconstrictor assay in the evaluation of corticosteroid remained a benchmark for a long time [4].

Conclusion

Topical corticosteroid is a milestone that revolutionized the management of several types of dermatoses. The journey which started in 1930 with the adrenal extracts, finally found its track in the road of topical dermatoses in 1952 with hydrocortisone. The journey always remained challenging. This journey was mostly by manipulation of the steroid molecule to produce compounds with greater lipophilicity, fewer mineralocorticoid properties and high potency. However, addition of new members in the regiment was encouraging, and several new topical agents were designed over the years. In the 1960s, the world witnessed the emergence of the high-potency fluorinated agents like triamcinolone, flurandrenolone, flumethasone or betamethasone. Betamethasone was used topically in for the first time in 1964. It was a discovery which remained as a milestone in the dermatology practice. Unfortunately, adverse drug reactions occur by the same mechanism which resulted in the action of the topical corticosteroids. On the other hand, systemic absorption of the topical agents is another challenge which needs to be addressed. Unless these limitations are overcome, the painstaking journey of development of the topical corticosteroids is yet to be over. Therefore, the world will wait to see the better tomorrows with newer topical agents which will virtually eliminate the risk of systemic absorption and adverse effects one fine morning!

References

1. WHO model prescribing information: drugs used in skin diseases: annex: classification of topical corticosteroids [Internet]. [cited 13 Jan 2017]. Available from: http://apps.who.int/medicinedocs/en/d/Jh2918e/32.html#Jh2918e.32.1.
2. Must Know Events that Occurred in the 1920s [Internet]. About.com Education. [cited 13 Jan 2017]. Available from: http://history1900s.about.com/od/timelines/tp/1920timeline.htm.
3. Swingle WW, Pfiffner JJ. The revival of comatose adrenalectomized cats with an extract of the suprarenal cortex. Science. 1930;72(1855):75–6.
4. Katz M, Gans EH. Topical corticosteroids, structure-activity and the glucocorticoid receptor: discovery and development–a process of "planned serendipity". J Pharm Sci. 2008;97(8):2936–47.
5. Benedek TG. History of the development of corticosteroid therapy. Clin Exp Rheumatol. 2011;29 (5 Suppl 68):S-5–12.
6. Murray JR. The history of corticosteroids. Acta Derm Venereol Suppl (Stockh). 1989;151:4–6; discussion 47–52.
7. Kendall EC. Hormones of the adrenal cortex. Bull N Y Acad Med. 1953;29(2):91–100.
8. Hench PS, Kendall EC. The effect of a hormone of the adrenal cortex (17-hydroxy-11-dehydrocorticosterone; compound E) and of pituitary adrenocorticotropic hormone on rheumatoid arthritis. Proc Staff Meet Mayo Clin. 1949;24(8):181–97.
9. Hench PS, Kendall EC, Slocumb CH, Polley HF. Effects of cortisone acetate and pituitary ACTH on rheumatoid arthritis, rheumatic fever and certain other conditions. Arch Intern Med Chic Ill 1908. 1950;85(4):545–666.
10. Witten VH. History [Internet]. Karger Publishers; 1992 [cited 13 Jan 2017]. Available from: http://www.karger.com/Article/Abstract/419853.
11. Corticosteroid–New World Encyclopedia [Internet]. [cited 12 Jan 2017]. Available from: http://www.newworldencyclopedia.org/entry/Corticosteroid#History.
12. Russell Marker Creation of the Mexican Steroid Hormone Industry–Landmark [Internet]. American Chemical Society [cited 14 Jan 2017]. Available from: https://www.acs.org/content/acs/en/education/whatischemistry/landmarks/progesteronesynthesis.html.
13. Meister PD, Peterson DH, Murray HC, Eppstein SH, Reineke LM, Weintraub A, et al. Microbiological transformations of steroids. II. The preparation of 11 α-Hydroxy- 17 α-progesterone. J Am Chem Soc. 1953;75(1):55–7.
14. Dhar S, Seth J, Parikh D. Systemic side-effects of topical corticosteroids. Indian J Dermatol. 2014;59(5):460–4.
15. Sulzberger MB, Witten VH. The effect of topically applied compound F in selected dermatoses. J Invest Dermatol. 1952;19(2):101–2.
16. Goldman L, Preston R, Rockwell E. The local effect of 17 hydroxycorticosterone-21-acetate (compound F) on the diagnostic patch test reaction. J Invest Dermatol. 1952;18(2):89–90.
17. Witten VH, Sulzberger MB, Zimmerman EH, Shapiro AJ. A therapeutic assay of topically applied 9 alpha-fluorohydrocortisone acetate in selected dermatoses. J Invest Dermatol. 1955;24(1):1–4.
18. Pace WE. Topical corticosteroids. Can Med Assoc J. 1973;108(1):ll-passim.
19. Samson C, Peets E, Winter-Sperry R, Wolkoff H. Betamethasone Valerate—Valisone®—Establishment of a new standard for topical corticosteroid potency [Internet]. Karger Publishers; 1992 [cited 13 Jan 2017]. Available from: http://www.karger.com/Article/Abstract/419877.
20. Wrong NM. The use and abuse of topical steroid therapy. Can Med Assoc J. 1965;92(25):1309–10.
21. Kircik LH. Clocortolone pivalate: a topical corticosteroid with a unique structure. J Drugs Dermatol. 2013;12(2):s3–4.

22. Del Rosso JQ, Kircik L. A comprehensive review of Clocortolone Pivalate 0.1% cream: structural development, formulation characteristics, and studies supporting treatment of corticosteroid-responsive Dermatoses. J Clin Aesthetic Dermatol. 2012;5(7):20–4.
23. Nierman MM. Safety and efficacy of clocortolone pivalate 0.1 percent cream in the treatment of atopic dermatitis, contact dermatitis, and seborrheic dermatitis. Cutis. 1981;27(6):670–1.
24. Rosenthal AL. Clocortolone pivalate: a paired comparison clinical trial of a new topical steroid in eczema/atopic dermatitis. Cutis. 1980;25(1):96–8.
25. Singh S, Mann BK. Clinical utility of clocortolone pivalate for the treatment of corticosteroid-responsive skin disorders: a systematic review. Clin Cosmet Investig Dermatol. 2012;5:61–8.
26. Topical Corticosteroids: World Health Organization Classification of Topical Corticosteroids. 2017 Jan 7 [cited 12 Jan 2017]. Available from: http://emedicine. medscape.com/article/2172256-overview.
27. McKenzie AW, Stoughton RB. Method for comparing percutaneous absorption of steroids. Arch Dermatol. 1962;86(5):608–10.
28. McKenzie AW. Percutaneous absorption of steroids. Arch Dermatol. 1962;86(5):611–4.
29. Place VA, Velazquez JG, Burdick KH. Precise evaluation of topically applied corticosteroid potency. Modification of the Stoughton-McKenzie assay. Arch Dermatol. 1970;101(5):531–7.
30. Dumas KJ, Scholtz JR. The psoriasis bio-assay for topical corticosteroid activity. Acta Derm Venereol. 1972;52(1):43–8.

Topical Corticosteroids: Pharmacology

2

Gagandeep Kwatra and Sandip Mukhopadhyay

Abstract

Topical corticosteroids are widely used for inflammatory and hyperproliferative disorders in dermatology. Numerous topical corticosteroids with high local activity have been developed over the years, with a focus to develop drugs with high efficacy locally and minimum risk for adverse drug reactions. They are available in a number of formulations. Their therapeutic effects are a result of their anti-inflammatory, immunosuppressant, vasoconstrictive and anti-proliferative actions. An appropriate topical corticosteroid is selected on the basis of the dermatological condition to be treated, patient-related factors and the physicochemical properties of the drug. Their use is associated with mainly local adverse drug reactions, but prolonged use and/or use of high-potency topical corticosteroids may cause systemic effects.

Keywords

Topical corticosteroids • Anti-inflammatory • Anti-proliferative • Potency

Learning Points

1. Topical corticosteroids are used extensively by dermatologists for inflammatory and hyperproliferative disorders of the skin.
2. Their anti-inflammatory, anti-proliferative and immunosuppressant actions are responsible for the clinical efficacy.
3. A number of topical corticosteroids, in varying strengths and formulations, are available.
4. Selection of a topical corticosteroid is made on the basis of dermatological condition to be treated, physicochemical properties of the topical corticosteroid and patient-related factors.

G. Kwatra (✉)
Department of Pharmacology, Christian Medical College-Ludhiana, Ludhiana, Punjab, India
e-mail: kwatragagandeep@gmail.com

S. Mukhopadhyay
Department of Pharmacology, Burdwan Medical College, Burdwan, West Bengal, India
e-mail: sandipcmcl@gmail.com

© Springer Nature Singapore Pte Ltd. 2018
K. Lahiri (ed.), *A Treatise on Topical Corticosteroids in Dermatology*,
DOI 10.1007/978-981-10-4609-4_2

5. Local adverse drug reactions are more common than systemic adverse drug reactions (ADRs) with the use of topical corticosteroids.
6. Research in this field is focused on developing molecules with high topical activity and better safety profile.

The successful use of dermatosis patients with hydrocortisone by Sulzberger and Witten in 1952 ushered in a new era in pharmacotherapy of dermatological conditions [1]. Since that time, numerous modifications have been made to develop topical corticosteroid molecules with favourable pharmacokinetic properties, improved efficacy and minimal adverse drug reactions. Topical corticosteroids are now used extensively by dermatologists for myriad conditions.

2.1 Structure-Activity Relationship

Corticosteroids have a C21 structure, consisting of a four-ring cyclophenanthrene nucleus and side chains. There are four rings, named A–D, with three six-membered rings and one five-membered ring. The synthetic corticosteroids used are derived from the natural corticosteroid, cortisol or hydrocortisone [2]. Cortisone was the first corticosteroid tested for dermatological disease but was devoid of topical activity [3]. Hydrocortisone was then developed by reduction of carbonyl group on C11, which was the first topical corticosteroid used and continues to be used in dermatology practice [4]. In the last 4–5 decades, many structural modifications have been made to the molecule in an effort to improve the topical activity of the molecule, while at the same time minimizing the adverse drug reactions.

The presence of double bonds between C4 and C5 and a keto group at C3 provide glucocorticoid and mineralocorticoid property to the corticosteroid molecule. Most of the synthetic molecules also have an –OH group at C21 position on ring D as is also found in the natural corticosteroid molecules. Halogenation, done at 6 α or 9 α position, increases the glucocorticoid and mineralocorticoid activity due to increased binding of the molecule to the glucocorticoid receptor [2]. Addition of a second fluoride or chloride group causes an additional increase in potency. Introduction of a double bond between C1 and C2 improves the glucocorticoid action and decreases the rate of metabolic inactivation, e.g. prednisolone, formed by insertion of double bond C1–2 to hydrocortisone, has a much higher anti-inflammatory activity as compared to hydrocortisone. Triamcinolone and betamethasone are other such examples (Fig. 2.1) [5].

Esterification of the corticosteroid increases its lipophilicity; thus it improves the percutaneous absorption and potency of the corticosteroid, e.g. betamethasone 17-valerate, produced by esterification of betamethasone at C21, has a higher potency than betamethasone and has a higher affinity for the glucocorticoid receptor [5]. Lipophilicity can also be enhanced by masking or removing the 17-dihydroxy acetone side chain or 16-α-hydroxyl group: this results in improved penetration through the stratum corneum [6].

Introduction of an acetonide group between positions C16 and C17 also helps to increase the skin penetration of the topical corticosteroid molecule and subsequent percutaneous absorption. An additional advantage is mitigation of mineralocorticoid effects caused by fluorination at C9 [5].

Undesirable mineralocorticoid activity of the topical corticosteroids can be reduced by adding 16-α-methyl, 16-β methyl or 16-α-hydroxyl group to the halogenated corticosteroid [7].

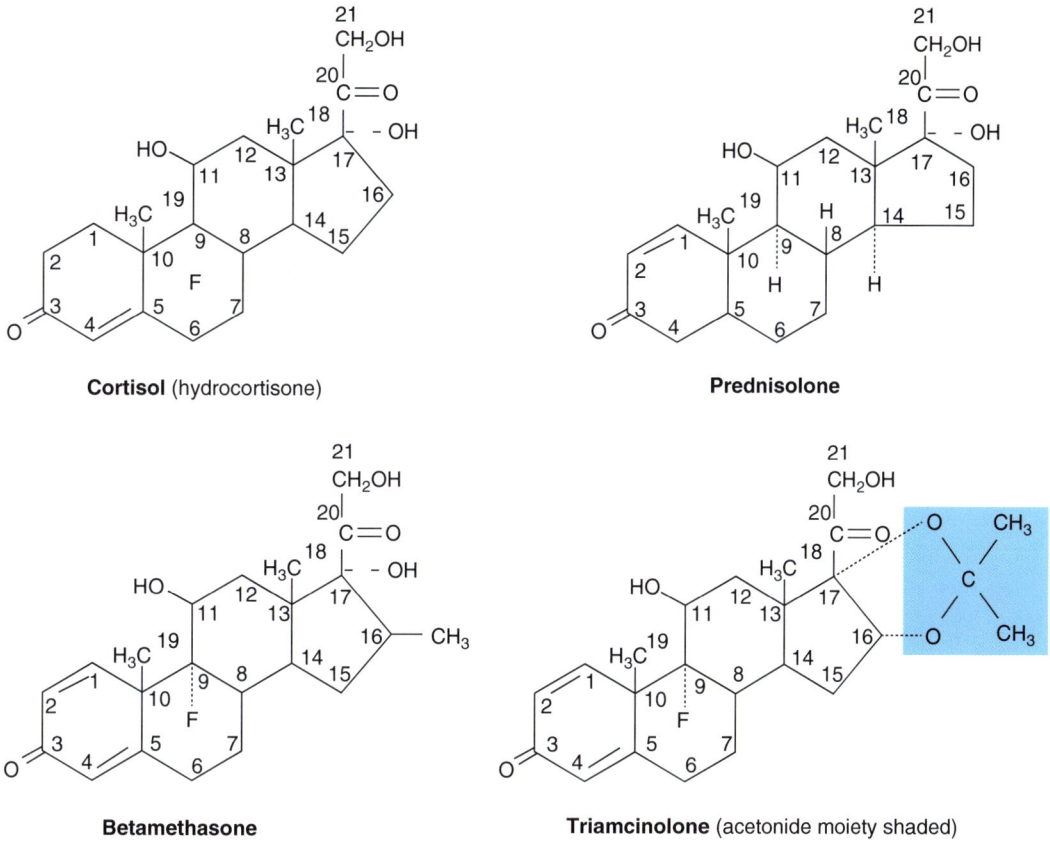

Fig. 2.1 Chemical structure of corticosteroids [9]. Copyright © McGraw-Hill Education. All rights reserved

Medicinal chemists have introduced structural changes to achieve high local glucocorticoid activity, with low potential to cause systemic effects. Analogues which undergo rapid inactivation after absorption are one such example: carbothioate glucocorticoid esters are metabolized to 21-carboxylic acid. Diesters like methylprednisolone aceponate, 17,21-hydrocortisone aceponate, mometasone furoate and carbothiates like fluticasone propionate are glucocorticoids with high topical activity and less propensity to cause skin atrophy and undergo rapid metabolism. They are also termed as 'soft corticosteroids' [8].

Another modification is inactive analogues which get activated at the site of action, e.g. glucocorticoid C21 isobutyryl or propionyl esters that are hydrolyzed to active C21 alcohols by airway-specific esterases [2].

2.2   Potency of Topical Corticosteroids: How to Determine

Many assays using laboratory animals and human volunteers have been used to estimate the clinical efficacy of the topical corticosteroids. Cell cultures, laboratory animals and tests using human volunteers are also used to assess atrophogenic potential of the molecules, as skin atrophy is a common adverse drug reaction reported with the use of topical corticosteroids.

Human vasoconstriction assay, developed by McKenzie and Stoughton, is a commonly used method to estimate the potency of topical corticosteroids. Different dilutions of the drug are applied to the skin and the degree of skin blanching is observed [10]. Some studies have shown a co-relation between the vasoconstriction activity and anti-inflammatory activity in clinical use [11, 12]. Vasoconstriction may not always co-relate with therapeutic assay [13]. A study which compared four ranking systems (vasoconstriction, clinical outcome, therapeutic index and efficacy/safety/cost) found that vasoconstriction assay co-related with clinical efficacy in 62% of agents studied [14]. Currently, however, vasoconstriction property forms the basis for classification of topical corticosteroids.

As the vasoconstriction assay is based on subjective assessment, efforts have been made to make the assessment more objective by laser Doppler velocimetry, capillaroscopy or transepidermal water loss.

Recently, Humbert and Guichard questioned the rationale of using vasoconstrictor effect, which is one of the many possible actions of corticosteroids, as a measure of their anti-inflammatory effect and therapeutic efficacy. They proposed a new classification of topical corticosteroids based on the condition for which it is to be used and measuring the relative effects of the different molecules [15].

The small plaque psoriasis bioassay proposed by Dumas and Scholtz is a modification of the vasoconstrictor assay. In this assay, the corticosteroid formulation is directly tested on psoriatic plaques, rather than on the normal skin, and its anti-inflammatory effect measured [16]. Rat thymus involution assay and antigranuloma assay have also been used to measure the anti-inflammatory effect of topical corticosteroids. Fibroblast assay measures the atrophogenicity property of topical corticosteroids [6].

2.3 Classification of Topical Corticosteroids

The WHO classification divides the topical corticosteroids into seven classes/groups, with group 1 being the most potent and group 7 being the least potent. In this system, potency is based on activity of topical corticosteroid molecule, its concentration and nature of vehicle. The same drug can be placed into different classes with the use of different vehicles [17]. In this classification, the seven classes of corticosteroids are categorized into four groups, wherein class I is considered as ultrahigh-potency, classes II and III as high-potency, classes IV and V as moderate-potency and classes VI and VII as low-potency corticosteroids.

The British National Formulary classification divides the topical corticosteroids into four classes and does not take into consideration the vehicle [18]. Class I is considered to be very potent, while class IV includes drugs with low potency.

The high-potency formulations are recommended for short-term use only and are required for areas like palms and soles and also for chronic or hyperkeratotic lesions. Low- to medium-potency topical corticosteroids are useful for acute inflammatory lesions on the face and intertriginous areas and can be used for a longer term (Table 2.1).

Table 2.1 WHO classification of topical corticosteroids [17]

Potency	Class	Topical corticosteroid	Formulation
Ultrahigh	I	Clobetasol propionate	Cream, 0.05%
		Diflorasone diacetate	Ointment, 0.05%
High	II	Amcinonide	Ointment, 0.1%
		Betamethasone dipropionate	Ointment, 0.05%
		Desoximetasone	Cream or ointment, 0.025%
		Fluocinonide	Cream, ointment or gel, 0.05%
		Halcinonide	Cream, 0.1%
	III	Betamethasone dipropionate	Cream, 0.05%
		Betamethasone valerate	Ointment, 0.1%
		Diflorasone diacetate	Cream, 0.05%
		Triamcinolone acetonide	Ointment, 0.1%
Moderate	IV	Desoximetasone	Cream, 0.05%
		Fluocinolone acetonide	Ointment, 0.025%
		Fludroxycortide	Ointment, 0.05%
		Hydrocortisone valerate	Ointment, 0.2%
		Triamcinolone acetonide	Cream, 0.1%
	V	Betamethasone dipropionate	Lotion, 0.02%
		Betamethasone valerate	Cream, 0.1%
		Fluocinolone acetonide	Cream, 0.025%
		Fludroxycortide	Cream, 0.05%
		Hydrocortisone butyrate	Cream, 0.1%
		Hydrocortisone valerate	Cream, 0.2%
		Triamcinolone acetonide	Lotion, 0.1%
Low	VI	Betamethasone valerate	Lotion, 0.05%
		Desonide	Cream, 0.05%
		Fluocinolone acetonide	Solution, 0.01%
	VII	Dexamethasone sodium phosphate	Cream, 0.1%
		Hydrocortisone acetate	Cream, 1%
		Methylprednisolone acetate	Cream, 0.25%

2.4   Mechanism of Action

Corticosteroids have anti-inflammatory, immunosuppressive, anti-proliferative and vasoconstrictor actions. Many of these actions are mediated by the nuclear glucocorticoid receptor which modulates transcription of proteins. This is considered to be the genomic mechanism and mediates many of the actions produced by the corticosteroids. Additionally, non-genomic mechanisms have been proposed to explain some of the immediate effects which cannot be explained by the classic glucocorticoid-receptor mechanism [19].

The corticosteroid receptor can be present in several isoforms. Corticosteroids produce their effects through the α-isoform, while relatively high levels of β-isoform may cause the resistance to glucocorticoids [2]. The gluco-corticoid receptors are found in most of the cells of the body, which accounts for their widespread systemic effects. In the skin, glucocorticoid receptors have been located in keratinocytes and fibroblasts within the epidermis and dermis [20, 21].

When the receptors are unoccupied by the corticosteroid molecule, they are usually present in the cytoplasm. The inactive receptor is bound to proteins like heat-shock proteins (Hsp) like Hsp90, Hsp70 and immunophilins. The glucocorticoid molecule, being lipophilic, enters the cell by passive diffusion. Within the cell, it binds to the receptor, the heat-shock proteins and immunophilins dissociate from the receptor and the corticosteroid-receptor complex then translocates to the nucleus [2].

Within the nucleus, this receptor-corticosteroid dimer complex then binds to a specific sequence of DNA, known as the glucocorticoid-response element. This interaction induces synthesis of anti-inflammatory proteins and regulator proteins involved in metabolic processes. This process is known as transactivation. The metabolic effects and some of the adverse drug reactions may occur through this process [22].

When the corticosteroid molecule directly/indirectly interacts with regulation of pro-inflammatory genes for transcription factors, such as activator protein 1 (AP1), nuclear factor κ B (NFκB) or interferon regulatory factor-3 (IRF-3), this process is termed as 'transrepression'. This negative regulation brings about anti-inflammatory and immunosuppressive effects [23].

The following non-genomic mechanisms for corticosteroids have been proposed to explain some of their rapid actions:

1. Corticosteroids interact with plasma membrane and mitochondrial membranes to alter their physicochemical properties and activities of membrane-associated proteins [19, 24].
2. Non-genomic glucocorticoid effects could mediate non-genomic effects on immune cells [25].

3. Some of the non-genomic effects could also be brought about by the corticosteroid receptors which are located on the cellular membranes, rather than the cytoplasm [24].

2.5 Pharmacological Actions of Corticosteroids

Corticosteroids are useful in varied dermatological conditions due to their anti-inflammatory, immunosuppressant, vasoconstrictive and anti-proliferative effects (Fig. 2.2).

2.5.1 Anti-Inflammatory and Immuno-Suppressant Effects

Corticosteroids inhibit the functions of most of the cells involved in an inflammatory response: some of these actions are direct, while others are mediated through the receptors. The corticosteroids reduce inflammation actions by the following actions:

1. There is a decrease in the number of polymorphonuclear leucocytes and monocytes at the site of inflammation, and they have a reduced ability to adhere to the vascular endothelium. Their antibacterial and phagocytic activity of the polymorphs is also diminished.
2. There is a reduction of natural killer and antibody-dependent cellular cytotoxicity by lymphocytes.
3. The Langerhans cells are reduced in number and there is diminution of their antigen-presenting function.
4. They inhibit the release of phospholipase A_2 which is involved in the production of prostaglandins, leukotrienes, PAF and other derivatives of arachidonic acid pathway.
5. Decrease in T cell production and increase in T cell apoptosis, partly due to reduced IL-2.
6. There is a decreased expression of ELAM1 (endothelial-leucocyte adhesion molecule-1) and ICAM-1 (intracellular adhesion molecule-1) from the endothelial cells [2].

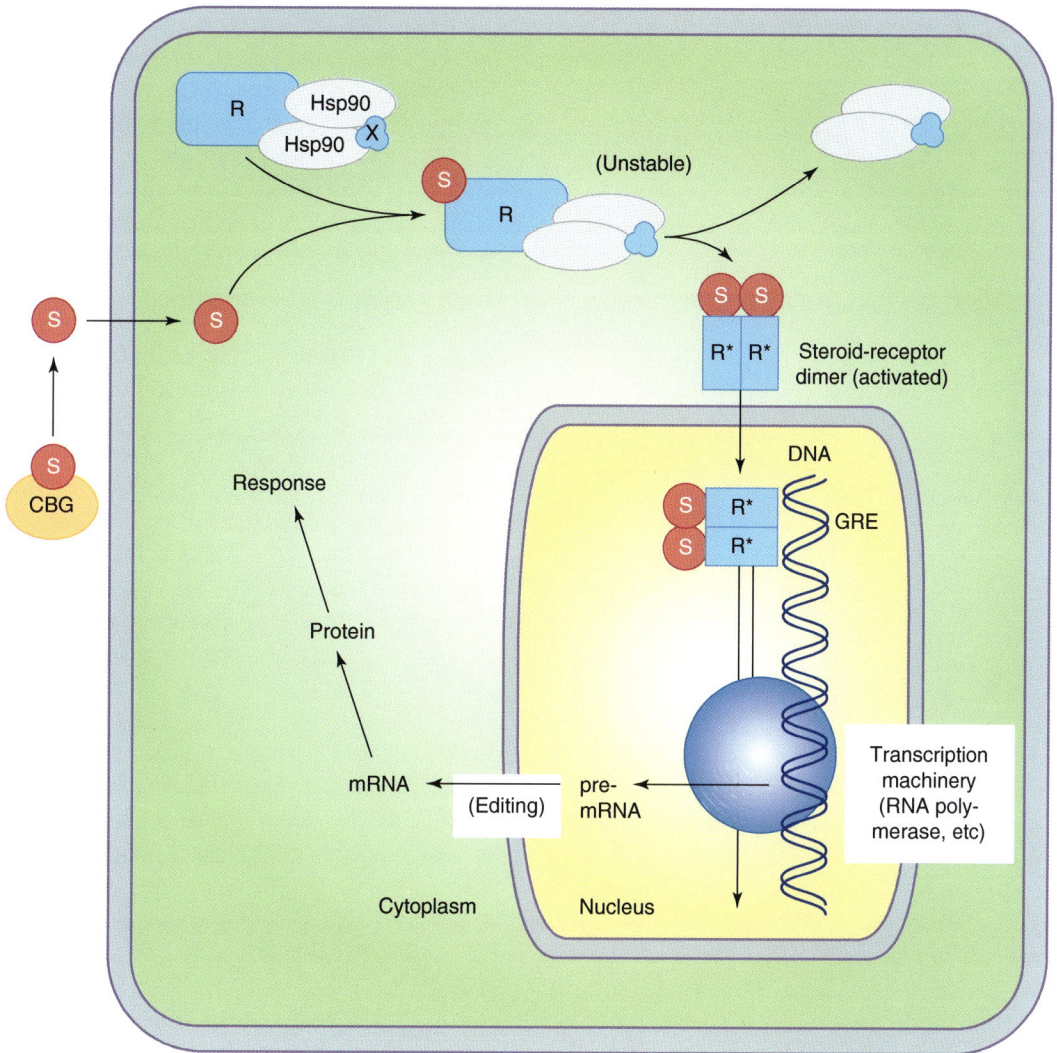

Fig. 2.2 Molecular level mechanism of action of corticosteroids [9]. Copyright © McGraw-Hill Education. All rights reserved

7. They inhibit transcription factors, such as activator protein 1 and nuclear factor κB, which activate pro-inflammatory genes. Lipocortin binds to membrane phospholipids, which is a substrate for phospholipase A_2 and makes it unavailable to form arachidonic acid which generates mediators like prostaglandins and leukotrienes [26, 27].

8. They decrease the release of IL-1α, IL-2, TNF and granulocyte-monocyte stimulating factor.

9. Glucocorticoid-receptor complex inhibits the inducible cyclooxygenase (COX 2) isoform, with minimal inhibition of COX 1. Cyclooxygenase is involved in prostaglandin synthesis [28].

10. They also reduce the levels of inducible nitric oxide (NO) synthetase, which increases NO synthesis. Nitric oxide is a vasodilator and a mediator for inflammation (Table 2.2) [28].

Table 2.2 Important effects of glucocorticoids on primary and secondary immune cells [29]

Monocytes/macrophages
↓ Number of circulating cells (myelopoiesis, release)
↓ Expression of MHC class II molecules and Fc receptors
↓ Synthesis of pro-inflammatory cytokines (e.g. IL-2, IL-6, TNF-a) and prostaglandins
T cells
↓ Number of circulating cells (redistribution effects)
↓ Production and action of IL-2 (most important)
Granulocytes
↓ Number of eosinophile and basophile granulocytes
↓ Number of circulating neutrophils
Endothelial cells
↓ Vessel permeability
↓ Expression of adhesion molecules
↓ Production of IL-1 and prostaglandins
Fibroblasts
↓ Proliferation
↓ Production of fibronectin and prostaglandins

2.5.2 Vasoconstrictor Action

The mechanism of vasoconstrictor action is not clearly understood, but it may be due to blocking of action of vasodilators like histamine and bradykinin [30]. The erythema is reduced due to constriction of capillaries in superficial dermis. The vasoconstrictor action may contribute towards the anti-inflammatory effects. The correlation between vasoconstrictor activity and anti-inflammatory action has been used to grade the potency in the vasoconstrictor assay, mentioned earlier.

2.5.3 Anti-Proliferative Action

Topical corticosteroids are known to reduce mitosis in the epidermis and the basal cell layer becomes less thick. The stratum corneum and granulosum are thinned out. Keratinocyte proliferation and keratinocyte growth factors are also decreased. This is accompanied by a reduced melanocyte production. The dermis also shows signs of atrophy due to inhibition of fibroblast proliferation, migration, chemotaxis and protein synthesis [31]. There is reduced synthesis of collagen and glycosaminoglycans. The dermis

volume shows a reduction due to loss of collagen and glycosaminoglycans and topical corticosteroid-induced vasoconstriction. As these processes continue, the elastin and collagen fibres begin to show abnormal aggregation [7]. These anti-proliferative effects are useful in psoriasis but are also the mechanism for the atrophogenic changes induced by topical corticosteroids.

2.6 Therapeutic Indications

Many inflammatory and hyperproliferative dermatological conditions respond very well to topical corticosteroids. Systemic corticosteroids are used for severe dermatological conditions.

Conditions like atopic dermatitis; stasis dermatitis; psoriasis, especially of genitalia and the face; and nummular eczematous dermatitis are some such examples. Discoid lupus erythematosus, sarcoidosis, pemphigus, vitiligo, etc., respond, but to a lesser extent. Some conditions like keloids and hypertrophic scars may require intra-lesional corticosteroid therapy [32]. Details of indications for the use of topical corticosteroid are presented in the next chapter.

2.7 Formulations

Topical corticosteroids are available in many formulations: creams, ointments, lotions, gel/hydrogel, sprays, shampoo and foam. Some of the newer formulations have a better patient acceptability and help to improve patient compliance.

Vehicles function as carrier for the active topical corticosteroid molecule, hydrate the skin and may help to increase the drug penetration [33]. The absorption and potency of drug depends on the vehicle used, in addition to the chemical structure of the corticosteroid molecule [34]. While selecting the vehicle, due attention needs to be paid to the interactivity of vehicle with the skin and drug molecule; stability, release rate and solubility of the drug in the vehicle; and skin area to be treated [35].

Creams are water-based formulations and have a low occlusive ability. Creams spread easily, without a greasy feel, and are thus preferred by patients. They can be applied to most areas of the body, and preferred in hairy and intertriginous areas, and for wet lesions. The requirement of preservatives is a disadvantage [2, 29].

Ointments are preferred for dry or scaly, lichenified lesions and in areas with thick skin: palms and soles. They increase skin hydration and provide good occlusion. The drug penetration is thus improved. Drug action can be enhanced further by addition of propylene glycol, which increases the solubility of the drug in the vehicle. They are preferred for dry or scaly lesions and for palms and soles but should be avoided in intertriginous areas [2].

Lotions are generally oil-in-water emulsions. They are easy to apply and patient compliance is good. Lotions and foams are used for scalp lesions.

Gels are formulated with a gelling agent and offer ease of application.

Conventionally, ointments have been considered to be more potent than the rest of the formulations, but the use of an optimized vehicle has resulted in equipotent cream, ointment and gel formulations [33].

Besides these conventionally used formulations, there is a lot of interest in developing newer formulations such as nanoparticles, liposomes, microemulsions, ethosomes, etc. [36].

2.8 Selection and Use of Topical Corticosteroids

- Areas with thick stratum corneum, for example, palms and soles, require higher-potency preparations, whereas lower-potency topical corticosteroids are preferred for areas with a thinner stratum corneum, for example, parts of the face, the scrotum and intertriginous areas. There can be an increased penetration of the drug through the skin and, thus, an increased risk of ADRs [38, 39].
- Mild-to-moderate-potency corticosteroids can be used for highly responsive conditions; those which are less responsive need to be treated with higher-potency corticosteroids.
- Another consideration while selecting the topical corticosteroids is the extent of surface area of the skin involved. Systemic adverse drug reactions may occur if extensive skin surface is treated.
- Use of occlusive dressings can increase the permeability up to tenfold. Their use has decreased due to availability of super potent topical corticosteroids.
- The degree of absorption through the skin also varies with disease conditions, e.g. in atopic dermatitis, there is increased absorption of topical corticosteroids through the defective epidermis.
- The use of topical corticosteroids should be avoided on ulcerated or atrophied skin or if there is infectious dermatosis.
- If a systemic adverse drug reaction is suspected, then relevant laboratory investigations should be ordered [2, 37, 38, 39].

2.9 Adverse Drug Reactions (ADRs)

Topical corticosteroids tend to cause local ADRs more commonly, although systemic ADRs have been reported. The ADRs which have been seen commonly are listed in Table 2.3. The use of more potent agents and/or longer duration of therapy increases the chances of developing adverse drug reactions. Surface area of the skin, total amount of drug used, skin integrity and use of occlusive dressing are other risk factors [40].

Table 2.3 Local adverse drug reactions due to topical corticosteroids [13, 42, 43]

- Atrophic changes: striae, telangiectasia, purpura, stellate pseudoscars, ulceration
- Easy bruising
- Steroid acne
- Rosacea
- Aggravation and/or masking of infections
- Allergic contact dermatitis
- Ocular effects: cataract, glaucoma, increased susceptibility to infections, reduced ulcer healing
- Corticosteroid rebound, addiction, tachyphylaxis
- Miscellaneous: hypertrichosis, hypopigmentation

Systemic ADRs are not seen very commonly with the use of topical corticosteroids but may occur when they reach the systemic circulation via percutaneous absorption. High-potency corticosteroid used over large skin surface for prolonged periods increases the chances for developing systemic ADRs. Suppression of the hypothalamic-pituitary axis, growth retardation in children, cataract, glaucoma, avascular necrosis of femur and Cushing's syndrome have been reported; aggravation of diabetes mellitus, hypertension and osteonecrosis have been reported [41].

Children and the elderly have a higher risk of adverse drug reactions due to a higher ratio of total body surface to body weight (about 2.3–3-fold that of adults).

2.10 Contraindications

Topical corticosteroids should not be used when there is known hypersensitivity to the corticosteroid or any component of the vehicle. Ulceration or bacterial, fungal or viral infections being present are relative contra-indications to their use [7].

2.11 Topical Corticosteroids in Special Populations

2.11.1 Pregnancy and Lactation

A Cochrane review conducted in 2015 could not establish a co-relation between the use of topical corticosteroids and congenital abnormalities, preterm delivery or stillbirths, citing reasons of insufficient data. The use of very potent topical corticosteroids during pregnancy may increase the risk of very low-birthweight babies, but there is low evidence for this observation [44].

No adverse effects from the use of topical corticosteroids during lactation are documented, but it is advisable to avoid their use on the nipples before nursing [7].

2.11.2 Geriatric and Paediatric Patients

Low-potency corticosteroids are generally preferred for paediatric patients due to the greater risk of adverse drug reactions due to higher surface area to body weight ratio and fragile skin. In infants, use of diapers may increase drug absorption [39].

Geriatric patients also have a higher propensity to develop adverse drug reactions, more so if there is skin atrophy due to the ageing process [39].

2.12 Recent Advances

Remarkable progress has been made in the development of topical corticosteroids from the time that they were first introduced for treatment of dermatology diseases. Interest in developing new molecules with high topical activity and better safety profile continues. Another area of research is the use of newer formulations like nanosomes, liposomes, etc., for enhanced delivery of drug molecule into the skin [36]. Nitro-glucocorticoids are corticosteroids with an enhanced anti-inflammatory effect. Selective glucocorticoid-receptor agonists (SEGRAs) are drugs which are able to selectively induce transrepression with minimal induction of transactivation and are in various stages of development [45].

References

1. Sulzberger MB, Witten VH. The effect of topically applied compound F in selected dermatoses. J Invest Dermatol. 1952;19(2):101–2.
2. Schimmer BP, Funder WH. ACTH, adrenal steroids, and pharmacology of the adrenal cortex. In: Brunton LL, editor. Pharmacological basis of therapeutics. 13th ed. New York, NY: McGraw-Hill. p. 1209–36.
3. Goldman L, Thomson RG, Trice ER. Cortisone acetate in skin disease: local effect in skin from topical applicants and local injections. AMA Arch Dermatol Syph. 1952;101-2(2):19.
4. Murray JR. The history of corticosteroids. Acta Derm Venereol. 1989;69(Suppl 151):4–6.

5. Katz M, Gans EH. Topical corticosteroids, structure-activity and the glucocorticoid receptor: discovery and development—a process of "planned serendipity". J Pharm Sci. 2008;97:2936–47.

6. Yohn JJ. Weston W.L. Topical glucocorticosteroids. Curr Probl Dermatol. 1990;2:31–63.

7. Warner MR, Camisa C. Topical corticosteroids. In: Wolverton SE, editor. Comprehensive dermatologic drug therapy. 3rd ed. New York, NY: Elsevier Health. p. 487–504.

8. Brazzini B, Pimpinelli N. New and established corticosteroids in dermatology. Am J Clin Dermatol. 2002;3:47–58.

9. Chrousos GP. Adrenocorticosteroids and adrenocortical antagonists. In: Katzung BG, Trevor AJ, editors. Basic and clinical pharmacology. 13th ed. New York, NY: McGraw Hill; 2015. p. 680–95. www.accesspharmacy.com.

10. McKenzie AW, Stoughton RB. Method for comparing percutaneous absorption of steroids. Arch Dermatol. 1962;86:608–10.

11. Cornell RC. Clinical trials of topical corticosteroids in psoriasis: correlations with the vasoconstrictor assay. Int J Dermatol. 1992;31(Suppl 1):38–40.

12. Cornell RC, Stoughton RB. Correlation of the vasoconstriction assay and clinical activity in psoriasis. Arch Dermatol. 1985;121:63–7.

13. Drake L, Dinehart S, Farmer E, et al. Guidelines of care for the use of topical glucocorticosteroids. J Am Acad Dermatol. 1996;35:615–9.

14. Hepburn DJ, Aeling JL, Weston WL. A reappraisal of topical steroid potency. Pediatr Dermatol. 1996;13:239–45.

15. Humbert P, Guichard A. The topical corticosteroid classification called into question: towards a new approach. Exp Dermatol. 2015;24:393–4.

16. Dumas KJ, Scholtz JR. The psoriasis bio-assay for topical corticosteroid activity. Acta Derm Venereol. 1972;52:43–8.

17. WHO model prescribing information: drugs used in skin diseases: Annex: Classification of topical corticosteroids. [Internet] [cited 13 Jan 2017]. Available from: http://apps.who.int/medicinedocs/en/d/Jh2918e/32.html#Jh2918e.32.1.

18. British National Formulary (BNF). 69th ed. London: British Medical Association and Royal Pharmaceutical Society of Great Britain; March 2015.

19. Buttgereit F, Scheffold A. Rapid glucocorticoid effects on immune cells. Steroids. 2002;67(6):529–34.

20. Ponec M, Kempenaar JA, De Kloet ER. Corticoids and cultured human epidermal keratinocytes: specific intracellular binding and clinical efficacy. J Invest Dermatol. 1981;76:211–4.

21. Marks R, Barlow JW, Funder JW. Steroid-induced vasoconstriction:glucocorticoid antagonist studies. J Clin Endocrinol Metab. 1982;54:1075–7.

22. Mc Master A, Ray DW. Drug insight: selective agonists and antagonists of the glucocorticoid receptor. Nat Clin Pract Endocrinol Metab. 2008;4:91–101.

23. Schacke H, Rehwinkel H, Asadullah K, Cato AC. Insight into the molecular mechanisms of glucocorticoid receptor action promotes identification of novel ligands with an improved therapeutic index. Exp Dermatol. 2006;15:565–73.

24. Buttgereit F, Straub RH, Wehling M, Burmester GR. Glucocorticoids in the treatment of rheumatic diseases: an update on the mechanisms of action. Arthritis Rheum. 2004;50:3408–17.

25. Croxtall JD, Choudhury Q, Flower RJ. Glucocorticoids act within minutes to inhibit recruitment of signalling factors to activated EGF receptors through a receptor-dependent, transcription-independent mechanism. Br J Pharmacol. 2000;130:289–98.

26. Burkholder B. Topical corticosteroids: An update. Curr Probl Dermatol. 2000;12:222–5.

27. Mori M, Pimpinelli N, Giannotti B. Topical corticosteroids and unwanted local effects. Improving the benefit/risk ratio. Drug Saf. 1994;10:406–12.

28. Ahluwalia A. Topical glucocorticoids and the skin-mechanisms of action: an update. Mediat Inflamm. 1998;7:183–93.

29. Buttgereit F, Saag KG, Cutolo M, Silva JAP, Bijlsma JWJ. The molecular basis for the effectiveness, toxicity, and resistance to glucocorticoids: focus on the treatment of rheumatoid arthritis. Scand J Rheumatol. 2005;34:14–21.

30. Altura BM. Role of glucocorticoids in local regulation of blood flow. Am J Phys. 1966;211:1393.

31. Hein R, Krieg T. Effects of corticosteroids on human fibroblasts in-vitro. In: Chrostophers E, Schopf E, Kligman AM, et al., editors. Topical corticosteroid therapy: a novel approach to safer drugs. New York, NY: Raven Press; 1988. p. 57–65.

32. Robertson DB, Maibach HI. Dermatologic pharmacology. In: Katzung BG, Trevor AJ, editors. Basic and clinical pharmacology. 13th ed. New Delhi: McGraw Hill; 2015. p. 1033–51.

33. Lee NP, Ariola ER. Topical corticosteroids: back to basics. West J Med. 1999;171:351–3.

34. Ayres PJ, Hooper G. Assessment of the skin penetration properties of different carrier vehicles for topically applied cortisol. Br J Dermatol. 1978;307-17(5):99.

35. Fang JY, Leu YL, Wang YY, Tsai YH. In vitro topical application and in vivo pharmacodynamic evaluation of Nonivamide hydrogels using Wistar rat as an animal model. Eur J Pharm Sci. 2002;15:417–23.

36. Senyigit T, Ozer O. Corticosteroids for skin delivery: challenges and new formulation opportunities. Cited on 30 Jan 2017. Available from http://www.intechopen.com/books/references/glucocorticoids-new-recognition-of-our-familiar-friend/corticosteroids-for-skin-delivery-challenges-and-new-formulation-opportunities.

37. Hill CJH, Rostenberg A. Adverse effects from topical steroids. Cutis. 1978;21:624–8.

38. Lubach D, Bensmann A, Bonemann U. Steroid-induced dermal atrophy: investigations on discontinuous application. Dermatologica. 1989;179:67–72.

39. Valencia IC, Kerdel FA. Topical corticosteroids. In: Fitzpatrick's dermatology in general medicine. 8th ed. New York, NY: McGraw Hill. p. 2659–64.

40. Correale CE, Walker C, Murphy L, Craig TJ. Atopic dermatitis: a review of diagnosis and treatment. Am Fam Physician. 1999;60:1199–210.

41. Mason J, Mason AR, Cork MJ. Topical preparations for the treatment of psoriasis: a systematic review. Br J Dermatol. 2002;146:351–64.

42. Hengge UR, Ruzicka T, Schwartz RA, Cork MJ. Adverse effects of topical glucocorticosteroids. J Am Acad Dermatol. 2006;54:1–15.

43. Coondoo A, Phiske M, Verma S, Lahiri K. Side-effects of topical steroids: a long overdue revisit. Indian Dermatol Online J. 2014;5:416–25.

44. Chi C, Wang S, Wojnarowska F, Kirtschig G, Davies E, Bennett C. Safety of topical corticosteroids in pregnancy. Cochrane Database Syst Rev. 2015;(10):CD007346. doi:10.1002/14651858.CD007346.pub3.

45. Stahn C, Lowenberg M, Hommes DW, Buttgereit F. Molecular mechanisms of glucocorticoid action and selective glucocorticoid receptor agonists. Mol Cell Endocrinol. 2007;275:71–8.

Dermatological Indications and Usage of Topical Corticosteroid

3

Jayakar Thomas and Kumar Parimalam

Abstract

Practice of dermatology has been revolutionised with the introduction of topical corticosteroids (TCS). The ever-expanding search to maximise their effects while minimising their side effects has been complemented by synthesising newer molecules with modified chemical structures. The TCS are a class of primarily synthetic steroids with profound anti-inflammatory and antipruritic action. With this most sought-after therapeutic property, a long list of "steroid responsive dermatoses" has emerged into contemporary dermatologic practice. Success of treatment however depends on the accurate diagnosis and selection of the appropriate steroid molecule with relevant consideration of the delivery vehicle, potency, frequency of application, site of involvement, duration of treatment, and strict vigil on the side effects. One has to remember that no single agent has been proven to have the best benefit-to-risk ratio. This chapter deals concisely with the aforementioned and specially is directed against TCS abuse.

Keywords

Topical corticosteroids • Chemical structure of TCS • Indications of TCS • Methods of usage of TCS

Learning Points
1. Topical corticosteroids (TCS) are a class of primarily synthetic steroids with profound anti-inflammatory and antipruritic action.
2. Most steroid-responsive dermatoses share more than one pathomechanism and are characterised by symptoms that respond to the anti-inflammatory, vasoconstrictive, antimitotic, and immunosuppressive effects of TCS.

J. Thomas (✉)
Professor and Head of Dermatology,
Sree Balaji Medical College & Hospital, Chromepet,
Chennai, India
e-mail: jayakarthomas@gmail.com

K. Parimalam
Professor and Head of Dermatology,
Kilpauk Medical College, Kilpauk, Chennai, India

3. Success of treatment depends on the accurate diagnosis and selection of the appropriate steroid molecule with relevant consideration of the delivery vehicle, potency, frequency of application, duration of treatment, and strict vigil on the side effects.

4. Some indications include all forms of dermatitis, psoriasis, lichen planus, alopecia areata, and vitiligo.

5. TCS are highly effective molecules and very promising in the treatment armamentarium of many dermatological conditions. It is indeed possible to avoid the side effects by judiciously using them.

3.1 Introduction

Topical corticosteroids (TCS) have revolutionised the practice of dermatology ever since they were introduced in the late 1950s. TCS of various potencies and preparations and a wide spectrum of combinations with other products are being synthesised in an effort to maximise the effects while minimising side effects. TCS are a class of primarily synthetic steroids with profound anti-inflammatory and antipruritic action. The major effect of the TCS, namely, the anti-inflammatory effect, was most sought after amongst all other effects of TCS. Chemical structure of TCS was modified in order to reduce the adverse effects. Owing to the arena of properties TCS possess, the list of indications for TCS is lengthening day by day, such that more diseases are being incorporated to the so-called steroid-responsive dermatoses the list of which is given in Table 3.1.

Most of these steroid-responsive dermatoses share more than one pathomechanism and are characterised by symptoms that respond to the anti-inflammatory, vasoconstrictive, antimitotic, and immunosuppressive effects of TCS. Thus TCS has become a cornerstone in the treatment of patients with a variety of skin conditions in all age groups barring young infants up to 2 months of age [1].

Table 3.1 Steroid-responsive skin conditions

Eczema
Atopic dermatitis
Seb. dermatitis
Contact dermatitis
Diaper dermatitis
Photosensitive eczema
Other eczemas
Papulosquamous disorders
Psoriasis
Lichen planus
Autoimmune disorders
Alopecia areata
Vitiligo
Lupus
Blistering disorders
Epidermolysis bullosa
Pemphigus
Bullous pemphigoid
Porphyria
Vascular disorders
Haemangiomas
Inflammatory disease
Intertrigo
Perianal inflammation
Peristomal inflammation
Phimosis
Granulomatous disorders
Others
Urticaria
Urticaria pigmentosa
Lichen scleroses
Burns
Mucocele

Corticosteroid therapy encompasses topical application with or without occlusion and intralesional steroid (ILS) injections. Successful treatment depends on the accurate diagnosis and selection of the appropriate steroid molecule with relevant consideration of the delivery vehicle, potency, frequency of application, duration of treatment, and strict vigil on the side effects.

The usefulness and side effects of topical steroids are a direct result of their anti-inflammatory properties, although no single agent has been proven to have the best benefit-to-risk ratio.

3.1.1 Structure

It is essential to understand the basic structure of a steroid molecule and the modifications responsible for their enhanced potency and diminution of the side effect. Figures 3.1, 3.2, 3.3, and 3.4 are self-explanatory, depicting how the basic structure of hydrocortisone can be modified to improvise the therapeutic effect. This enables physician to choose the molecule to suit the patients' current condition as requirement varies in the same patient with same disease during the course of disease. For example, C16-methyl substitution, interfering with protein binding, and halogenation, seems to reduce the allergenicity of corticosteroid molecules. Hence, when indicated, C16-methylated corticosteroids should be preferentially prescribed.

3.1.2 Strength

Though TCS is available in various strengths, certain dermatoses require higher strength, while others respond well to low-potent steroids. The strength of TCS however should be decided taking into consideration various factors like age of patient, site of involvement and thickness of lesion, vehicle, components of the preparation, and the duration of treatment. The following table gives an idea of different strength required to manage different diseases (Table 3.2). Age-wise choice of TCS in children is given in Table 3.3.

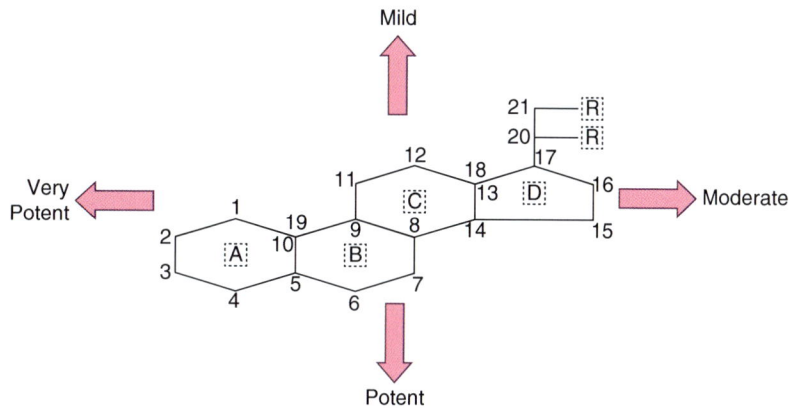

Fig. 3.1 Basic structure of steroid molecule

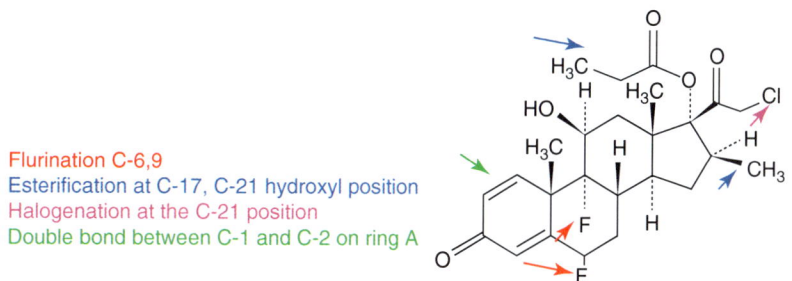

Fig. 3.2 Structural modifications to increase potency

Flurination C-6,9
Esterification at C-17, C-21 hydroxyl position
Halogenation at the C-21 position
Double bond between C-1 and C-2 on ring A

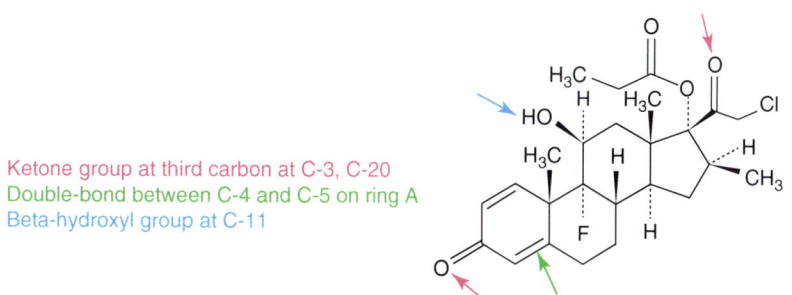

Fig. 3.3 Structural modifications to increase anti-inflammatory action

Ketone group at third carbon at C-3, C-20
Double-bond between C-4 and C-5 on ring A
Beta-hydroxyl group at C-11

Fig. 3.4 Structural modifications to increase safety

Ester at C17
Methyl group at C16

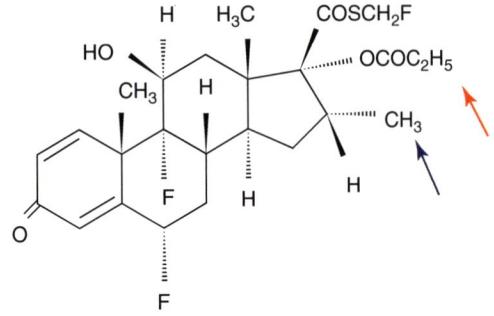

Table 3.2 Conditions treatable with topical steroids in adults

| High-potency steroids (groups I to III) |
| Eczema |
| Atopic dermatitis |
| Acute radiation dermatitis |
| Hyperkeratotic eczema |
| Lichen simplex chronicus |
| Nummular eczema |
| Severe hand eczema |
| Acute contact/irritant dermatitis |
| Psoriasis |
| Lichen planus |
| Lichen sclerosus |
| Alopecia areata |
| Vitiligo |
| Discoid lupus erythematosus |
| Autoimmune blistering disease (pemphigus, pemphigoid) |
| Chronic idiopathic urticaria |
| Urticaria pigmentosa |
| Sarcoidosis |
| **Medium-potency steroids (groups IV and V)** |
| Asteatotic eczema |
| Atopic dermatitis |
| Lichen sclerosus (genital) |
| Nummular eczema |
| Scabies (after treating with scabicide) |
| Seborrhoeic dermatitis |
| Stasis dermatitis |
| Melasma |
| Phimosis |
| Labial adhesion |
| Radiation dermatitis |
| **Low-potency steroids (groups VI and VII)** |
| Diaper dermatitis |
| Eyelid eczema |
| Pityriasis alba |
| Intertrigo |
| Perianal inflammation |
| Peristomal dermatosis |

Table 3.3 Age-wise option for potency of TCS

0–3 months	No TCS
3 months to 1 year	Classes 6, 7
1–2 years	Classes 4, 5
2–12 years	Classes 2, 3
Above 12 years	Class 1

3.1.3 Absorption

One should remember that the absorption is variable in different anatomical sites as seen below. The skin over the eyelids absorbs the most, while that of the sole absorbs the least:

- Eyelids and genitals absorb 30%.
- Face absorbs 7%.
- Armpit absorbs 4%.
- Forearm absorbs 1%.
- Palm absorbs 0.1%.
- Sole absorbs 0.05%.

3.1.4 Safety in Pregnancy and Breastfeeding

Safety of TCS in pregnancy much depends on the placental penetration of the steroid molecule. The enzyme 11-beta-hydroxysteroid dehydrogenase plays a vital role by converting cortisol to cortisone the biologically inactive form. It has been observed that hydrocortisone is relatively safe in pregnancy with only 15% of 3H cortisol crossing the placenta unmetabolised, which is up to 67%

for dexamethasone. In case of methylprednisolone and betamethasone, 45% and 30% of unmetabolised cortisol cross the placental barrier, respectively. Though there is no documented evidence for the development cleft palate/lip or other birth defects, available literature reports placental insufficiency and low birth weight following use of very potent and potent TCS during pregnancy [3–7].

Following are some dos and don'ts worth considering while using TCS in pregnancy:

- Mild/moderate TCS to be preferred to potent/very potent.
- While using potent/very potent, TCS should be advised for as short period as possible and appropriate obstetric follow-up and care should be provided.
- Lipophilic TCS with once a day application are better.
- Until an evidence-based definite safety margin is drawn, TCS should be used with caution during pregnancy.

Mild, moderate, and potent topical corticosteroids are considered safe to use when breastfeeding. Patient should be instructed to wash off any steroid cream applied over breasts before feeding. It is advisable that very potent topical corticosteroids are not recommended to use over the chest while breastfeeding.

3.1.5 Vehicles and Preparation

Steroids may differ in potency based on the vehicle in which they are formulated. Hydration generally promotes steroid penetration. Hence application of TCS after a shower or bath improves effectiveness, which at the same time increases the side effects as well. Cosmetic elegance has also to be born in mind to get better patient adherence and compliance. For example, greasy nature of the ointment may result in poor patient satisfaction. For dermatologic use, topical corticosteroids are available in various dosage forms including creams, dressings (tape), foams,

Table 3.4 Choice of preparation of TCS for different anatomical sites

Choosing the correct preparation of TCS	
Foam, gel	Hairy areas
Lotion, solution	Hairy areas, wider surface
Cream	Face, tender skin
Ointment	Over thick skin and lesion
Emulsion	Hairy areas, wider surface
Shampoo	Hairy areas

gels, lotions, ointments, solutions, and aerosols (suspensions). The choice of a dosage form depends on the location of the lesion, and the condition being treated (Table 3.4) may guide to some extent the choice of formula to be used over different parts of the body.

3.1.6 Combination

Combinations of TCS with other agents like antifungals, antibiotics, keratolytics, and vitamin D are available commercially. Extemporaneous preparation or dilution should not be encouraged. Such a combination of products will result in decreased or variable effectiveness. There are two schools of thoughts about the usefulness of combination of TCS with antibiotics and antifungals, one group in favour and the other against the use of combination products. The authors are of the opinion that judicious use of combinations of TCS with anti-infective agents in carefully selected patients for a limited period will help in faster clinical improvement thereby better patient adherence and complete cure. However, it cannot be overemphasised that prolonged use of combinations should be avoided to reduce the risk of severe, persistent, or recurrent infections especially while dealing with fungal infections more so in children [8].

3.1.7 Frequency of Administration and Duration of Treatment

By and large frequency of application of TCS should not exceed twice a day as more frequent administration does not provide better results. Continuous and prolonged application of TCS can induce tolerance and tachyphylaxis. Ultra-high-potency steroids should not be used for more than 3 weeks continuously. Side effects can be precipitated by mild steroids in prone individuals even in less than a weeks' time [9].

3.1.8 Occlusion

Occlusive dressing therapy is indicated wherever the absorption needs to be increased, whether it is the thick skin or hyperkeratotic lesion. One has to be extremely cautious while using a tape or a plastic film for occlusion. Frequency of occlusive dressing and the duration which is normally 12–24 h determine not only the effect but also the side effects [10].

Intermittent use of occlusive dressings for 12 h daily is recommended to reduce the risk of adverse effects and for greater convenience. If occlusion is indicated over extensive areas, sequential occlusion of only one portion of the body at a time is preferable to whole-body occlusion.

3.1.9 Intralesional Administration

Intralesional steroid (ILS) administration involves injection of a corticosteroid, such as triamcinolone acetonide or betamethasone suspension directly into a lesion on or immediately below the skin. Shorter-acting corticosteroid preparations, such as dexamethasone or betamethasone acetate, are sometimes administered in combination with triamcinolone. ILS injection helps to bypass the barrier of a thickened stratum corneum, thereby reducing the chance of epidermal atrophy and better delivery of steroid in higher concentrations to the site of the pathology.

List of skin conditions that can be effectively treated with is given in Table 3.5.

Table 3.5 Conditions treated with IL steroid injection

Indications for IL steroid injection
Alopecia areata
Keloids
Hypertrophic scars
Nodulocystic acne
Hypertrophic lichen planus
Discoid lupus erythematosus
Lichen simplex chronicus
Resistant plaque psoriasis
Granuloma annulare
Granulomatous cheilitis
Granuloma faciale
Pyoderma gangrenosum
Hidradenitis suppurativa
Necrobiosis lipoidica
Cutaneous sarcoidosis
Infantile haemangiomas
Vitiligo
Mucocele

3.1.10 Side Effect

Side effects induced by TCS should always be born in mind. The use of dermatoscopy should be encouraged which will reveal early signs of atrophy as red lines before they become clinically evident with the naked eye. Early detection of "steroid preatrophy" will help discontinuation of TCS and prevent irreversible damage [11].

3.2 Indications

3.2.1 Atopic Dermatitis

TCS are used in the management of AD in both adults and children and are the mainstay of topical anti-inflammatory therapy. TCS are indicated only in those cases where the conventional emollients have failed to induce desirable clinical effect and in severe cases in order to bring down the inflammation fast. TCS should never be considered as solo therapy in any stage of the disease. Though AD is one of the most common indications for the use of TCS, choice of molecule and formula will vary depending on factors like patient's age, extent and anatomical areas of involvement, severity of xerosis, patient preference, and cost of medication. Twice-daily application of corticosteroids is generally recommended, while according to one school of thought once-daily application is equally good in inducing remission while at the same time reducing the risk of side effects of frequent application. It is also observed that use of TCS as wet wraps is more efficacious than using only moisturizers. Wolkerstorfer et al. have shown that side effects are minimised by diluting the potent TCS to 10% or even 5% of their original strength. However the authors suggest the use of medium-potency TCS instead of dilution [12–21].

TCS are indicated in AD not only for their anti-inflammatory effect but also their antipruritic effect which is the most important aspect in the management of AD. Daily application of TCS is recommended during acute flares, until significant improvement of inflammation is observed clinically, and it is important not to stop TCS abruptly which will lead on to relapse. The success of treatment of AD lies in the effective maintenance of remission which can be achieved by intermittent use of TCS once or twice weekly over areas that commonly help prevent relapses and is found to be more effective than use of emollients alone. With increasing access to literature, and inappropriate knowledge, unnecessary fear in the form of steroid phobia has led to steroid under treatment. It is important therefore to address such factors and counsel both patient and parents to achieve good response.

It is a well-known fact that the skin of an AD patient is commonly colonised with *Staphylococcus aureus* in high densities and AD flares are associated with such an increased colonisation of *S. aureus*. Marked reductions in *Staphylococcus aureus* levels in AD have been observed in those treated with TCS. The use of TCS can reduce the density of *S. aureus* and thereby help in better response in patients with AD as steroid application tends to normalise the cutaneous microbiome on both nonlesional and lesional AD skin. Moreover, there is evidence that TCS not only decreases inflammation but also improves barrier function sufficient enough to reduce bacterial colonisation leading to normalisation of normal flora.

3.2.2 Seborrhoeic Dermatitis (SD)

TCS are considered to be first- or second-line agents for SD, depending upon the severity of disease. The use of TCS for adult SD, regardless of site or severity, is to achieve the most rapid control of signs and symptoms. In many cases, a low- to low-mid-potency TCS is effective in rapidly clearing visible signs and associated symptoms. As SD of the scalp is invariably associated with more severe pruritus when compared to SD of non-hairy areas, there is a need for initial treatment with TCS of higher potency followed lower-potent TCS over the next two weeks. Though low- or mid-potency topical corticosteroids have been successful in reducing itching and inflammation of SD and are as effective as antifungal and other anti-inflammatory agents, it has to be remembered that relapse is more common with use of TCS alone when compared to use of antifungal and other non-steroidal topical therapies. Tapering of frequency and strength may help reduce the risk of relapse. After attaining initial control, mid-potent steroid shampoo can be used as an alternative to or in addition to TCS application used for maintenance. TCS may hasten recurrences and because of rebound effect can lead to dependence; hence, TCS is to be encouraged only for short-term use, while solo therapy with TCS should be discouraged [22–30].

It is preferable to use TCS in combination with other agents like antifungal and keratolytic agents. The choice of potency and formula much depends on the site and severity of SD and age of patient as the same molecule in an ointment is more potent than a cream and lotion. TCS should be used sparingly in SD to avoid adverse effects.

3.2.3   Contact Dermatitis (CD)

TCS are indicated to treat contact dermatitis involving less than 20% body surface area [31–34].

Localised acute allergic CD can be successfully treated with mid- or high-potency TCS such as triamcinolone 0.1% or clobetasol 0.05%. Low-potent TCS such as hydrocortisone are found to be effective in reducing inflammation in children. Potent TCS applied twice daily are useful to treat small areas of moderate-to-severe CD. In the setting of proven allergic CD due to TCS itself, care must be exercised in modifying the molecule to avoid the allergen and to avoid allergy to known cross-reactive agents as well. The usefulness of TCS in the management of irritant CD has not been proven. Levin et al. found TCS to be ineffective in surfactant-induced CD. C16-methyl substitution is likely to reduce the allergenicity of corticosteroid molecules by interfering with protein binding and halogenation. Hence, when indicated, C16-methylated corticosteroids should be preferentially prescribed.

3.2.4   Photosensitive Eczema

TCS are useful in photosensitive eczema, as both anti-inflammatory and immune-modulatory agents. Without the preventive measures like photo protection and use of sunscreens, even TCS will prove ineffective. Depending on the site and severity of disease, the strength and vehicle have to be chosen. Prolonged and continuous use of potent TCS should be avoided for fear of tachyphylaxis and skin atrophy [35].

3.2.5   Lichen Simplex Chronicus (LSC)

TCS are the treatment of choice in LSC as they soften and decrease thickness of the skin in addition to their anti-inflammatory effect. LSC is one condition where occlusive therapy with TCS will be very useful and should be practised wherever possible in order to increase potency and enhance delivery of the agent. Occlusive dressing also helps as physical barrier to the scratching, thereby stopping the itch-scratch cycle. High-potency TCS should not be used over the genital skin and for more than 3 weeks even over the skin on other parts of the body [36–38].

3.2.6   Hand Eczema and Pityriasis Alba

Hand eczema and pityriasis alba are influenced by both exogenous and endogenous factors, making a successful treatment quite challenging. Taking into consideration the severe inflammatory nature of hand eczema and recurrent nature of pityriasis alba, it is better to choose the correct strength and vehicle. TCS are though safe and effective if used judiciously along with emollients, their efficacy nonetheless appears to be limited. It is better to prescribe low-potency TCS of classes 5 and 6 for the treatment of pityriasis alba. Prolonged use of TCS on the face is not recommended, more so in children [39, 40].

3.2.7   Peristomal Dermatoses

Peristomal inflammation is a common problem which needs effective care without affecting the stoma bag adhesion. Lyon et al. have demonstrated that TCS formulated in aqueous/alcohol lotions or carmellose sodium paste are effective in the management of peristomal inflammation without impairing stoma bag adhesion. Before treating with TCS, infections and irritant factors should be identified and corrected. TCS application should be advised for temporary use to control severe disease and for occasional use thereafter. Initial treatment with TCS should not exceed 4 weeks and is applied only at stoma bag changes. TCS formulated in aqueous or alcohol vehicles are preferred to cream or ointment preparations. Strict vigilance for local side effects is mandatory while treating the peristomal skin where the barrier function is already jeopardised [41].

3.2.8 Psoriasis

TCS are the most suitable topical agents for the treatment of psoriasis among all age groups. They have anti-inflammatory, anti-proliferative, immunosuppressive, vasoconstrictive, and antimitotic effects. TCS is the first-line therapy in psoriasis, especially in the event of non-availability of UVB therapy. In appropriate concentration and formula, TCS are still used in treatment of plaques over the face, neck, flexures, and genitalia even in children. Diluted TCS are also used in unstable, erythrodermic, and generalised pustular psoriasis, for a very short period keeping in mind the risk of systemic absorption that cannot be predicted in a breached skin. TCS under occlusion do have a limited place in the management of recalcitrant psoriasis of the scalp, hands, feet, and other areas. Hydrocolloid dressing is found to be superior to plastic film used for occlusive therapy. Low- to mid-potency corticosteroids, classes 5–7, are chosen for facial and intertriginous lesions, while mid-potency, classes 2–4, are chosen for extremities and the scalp. Clobetasol emulsion foam is safe and effective for treatment of psoriasis in patients aged 12 years or older. TCS can be continued till the lesions become flat and inactive [42–45].

Corticosteroid can be given intralesionally in resistant plaques of psoriasis. The concentration is generally 3–10 mg/mL, depending on the size, thickness, and area of the lesion. Triamcinolone hexacetonide (5 mg/mL) or triamcinolone acetonide (10 mg/mL) can be infiltrated intradermally into localised psoriatic lesions by needle injection. Additional injections may be needed every 4–6 weeks. This is of particular value in troublesome, small, resistant lesions where systemic therapy is not required. The remission is prolonged and repetition of the injection may not be required for several months. In psoriasis of fingernails, the nailfold can be injected, with triamcinolone acetonide, but the procedure may be painful and the results are as good as in psoriasis of the skin. Disadvantages of intralesional injections include pain during the injection and potential side effects of local atrophy and systemic absorption.

3.2.9 TCS in Children with Psoriasis

Topical steroids are suitable for the treatment of childhood psoriasis among all age groups. Steroids of classes 5–7 are chosen for facial and intertriginous lesions, while mid-potency classes 2–4 are chosen for extremities and the scalp. TCS treatment should not be discontinued abruptly for fear of developing pustular lesions.

There are different observations as to whether or not TCS used in conjunction can hasten clearance of psoriatic plaques treated with UVB therapy [46–51]. Some studies also indicate that addition of TCS to UVB may lead to more frequent relapse. The authors however feel that addition of TCS to any kind of therapy helps in bringing down the inflammation. Once the inflammation is brought down, instead of discontinuing the therapy, it would be wiser to maintain with non-steroidal topical agents and emollients in order to sustain remission.

TCS are commonly used as polytherapy and combination therapy with other agents which help in the management of psoriasis [52]. Effective combinations with agents like vitamin D3, salicylic acid, and tar help:

- Achieve rapid cure
- Reduce need for prolonged treatment with TCS
- Thereby reduce its side effect of TCS
- Reduce duration and cost of therapy

While treating nail psoriasis, one must keep in mind that psoriasis nail will frequently have superadded fungal infection after treatment of which TCS can be applied to the paronychial skin. Intralesional triamcinolone can also be used in the same region to reduce the subungual inflammation. Severe nail psoriasis can impact significantly on quality of life and is difficult to treat. Dexamethasone iontophoresis may be a useful treatment of this generally recalcitrant condition.

3.2.10 Lichen Planus (LP)

Cutaneous lichen planus is the most itchy papulosquamous disease. TCS particularly class 2 or 3 preparations remain the first-line treatment for cutaneous LP of the skin and mucosa with limited extent. TCS are used to treat painful, erythematous, or erosive oral lesions. Intralesional steroid injections are indicated in hypertrophic oral erosive LP, and that of nail IL injection enhances maximum drug delivery to the affected site. However, care must be taken to avoid side effects like atrophy, depigmentation, and infection [53–55].

While treating oral LP, there is a potential risk of developing oral candidiasis in some patients treated with TCS in orabase. However, the superadded candida growth usually does not affect the healing of LP. Under such circumstances, it is nevertheless important to treat patients with topical or systemic antifungal agents. Use of betamethasone can decrease inflammation by inhibiting polymorphonuclear chemotaxis and reversing the increased capillary permeability. It also inhibits lymphokine production in addition to its inhibitory effect on the Langerhans cells. In selected cases, beclomethasone inhalant as a puff can be used in metered-dose inhaler delivering 50 mcg per puff. Such direct inhaler can deliver the drug to the sites of greatest erythema or erosion. Dental pastes having 0.1% triamcinolone acetonide in 1% carboxy cellulose are also effective in oral LP.

3.2.11 Alopecia Areata (AA)

TCS are widely used in the management of alopecia areata as topical application, as under occlusion, and as intralesional injection. The rate and speed of regrowth are variable, and hence it is advisable that treatment is continued for a min-imum of 3 months before regrowth can be expected and maintain therapy thereafter to prevent recurrence. There are studies indicating the usefulness of TCS in various formulas in the management of AA. Fluocinolone acetonide cream, fluocinolone scalp gel, betamethasone valerate lotion, betamethasone dipropionate cream, clobetasol propionate ointment, dexamethasone in a penetration-enhancing vehicle, and halcinonide cream are some of them showing satisfactory-to-excellent response. It has been documented that remission was maintained well in those patients treated with TCS. However TCS gives best results in small patches, with duration less than 1 year [10, 56–67].

Tosti et al. have shown that TCS used under occlusion gave very good results in their study that was performed in a subgroup of patients whose disease was refractory to other modalities of treatment using. Hair growth was induced in 6 months' time in nearly 30% of the study group and was maintained for 6 months in more than 60% of their patients. However, only less than 20% of their patients showed long-term benefits. According to the authors, regrowth of hair observed only on the treated half of scalp showed that it is the local effect of TCS responsible for the regrowth. Despite the usefulness of TCS in the management of AA, monotherapy with TCS will not be of use in all patients, instead increase the chance of steroid side effects. Folliculitis is the most common adverse effect which can manifest after a few days to weeks. It is important to look for atrophy of the skin which is more difficult to detect on scalp when compared to other body sites. Anaphylaxis though rare, every physician should be prepared to handle the situation when there is an emergency.

IL steroids are found to be superior to TCS and yield best results in adults with limited patchy AA. Typically, 2.5- and 5-mg/mL triamcinolone acetonide concentrations are recommended for the face (beard, eyebrows) and scalp, respectively, not exceeding 20 mg per month/session. Diffusion into the adjacent skin can be minimised with perpendicular placement of the needle with the bevel pointed opposite and 3 mm away from the adjacent border. Studies show no difference in regrowth while using 2.5 mg/mL, 5 mg/mL, or 10 mg/mL, but more cases of reversible skin atrophy were seen in the 10-mg/mL group.

Using the lowest effective concentration minimises local and systemic side effects. By using lower concentration of the drug, it is possible to cover larger area. For example, by using 2.5 mg/mL yields a total of 8 mL volume for a recommended maximum of 20 mg of triamcinolone acetonide per month. This will be useful for treatment of more extensive scalp alopecia areata.

3.2.12 Vitiligo

Treatment of vitiligo with TCS has been shown to be successful in quite a few studies, and it is a simple and safe treatment when used with caution. TCS is better discontinued in patients showing side effects or those who do not show signs of repigmentation in 2 months' time. Results are better in patients with localised involvement having an inflammatory component. The choice of strength of steroid suggested for vitiligo is variable. An easy to follow choice of strength of TCS in vitiligo is as follows:

- Potent TCS for most areas
- Very potent TCS for resistant area
- Moderately potent TCS for the face/eyelids

Intralesional injection of steroid has been recently studied and found to be useful, with repigmentation observed in as early as 3 weeks and very little side effect [68, 69].

3.2.13 Cutaneous Lupus Erythematosus (CLE)

TCS are an essential part of treating all subtypes of CLE. Despite availability of a wide range and potency of TCS and combinations, treatment of CLE is challenging and the resultant scarring is inevitable. Studies have demonstrated high-potency steroid to be more efficacious than low-potency

TCS in CLE. Discoid lupus erythematosus needs to be treated with potent TCS. For the face it is preferable to use desonide 0.05% or triamcinolone 0.1% ointment twice-daily application along with sunscreens. Whereas for other body surface, superpotent TCS such as fluocinonide 0.05% or clobetasol 0.05% ointment twice daily should be advised. Madan et al. have shown combination of TCS with tacrolimus (TCPO) which yield better results than any of the two being used separately. Since cutaneous LE may require prolonged therapy, to minimise side effects of TCS, it is advisable to apply TCS intermittently with steroid-free intervals between weeks of TCS application. To avoid systemic absorption and resultant suppression of HP axis, it is better to keep the use of TCS to less than 45 and 100 gm per week of high- and mid-potent steroid, respectively, without occlusion [70–74].

Deeper lesions including those involving the subcutis will have to be treated with intralesional injection of steroid like triamcinolone acetonide at intervals of at least 3–4 weeks between two injections.

3.2.14 Blistering Disorders

Blistering diseases of mechanobullous, autoimmune, photosensitive, and metabolic aetiology can be treated successfully with TCS. Dumas et al. have successfully treated mild cases of pemphigus vulgaris and pemphigus foliaceus with clobetasol propionate 0.05% cream. Similarly, Abecassis et al. have attained disease clearance in a patient with chronic active hepatitis and epidermolysis bullosa acquisita with clobetasol propionate. New strategies for BP have been proposed by Joly et al. to include topical clobetasol propionate as first-line therapy in the elderly and consider adjuvant therapy only in cases that are resistant to TCS. In autoimmune blistering disorders, TCS should be considered when the disease is mild or when systemic immunosuppressant drugs cannot be used and the patient can't afford other expensive drugs. TCS is also very useful to abate persistent mucosal lesions of pemphigus vulgaris after complete clearance of skin lesions while the patient is on dexamethasone pulse therapy, especially when indirect immunofluorescence is not feasible to assess the antibody levels [75–77].

3.2.15 Haemangiomas

TCS have been used to treat small haemangiomas. Topical steroids are a reasonably good alternative to intralesional steroids for treating superficial haemangioma as IL injections are painful. Clobetasol cream was found to be successful in small superficial haemangiomas at risk of ulceration and lesions over the periocular site. However with the introduction of propranolol and timolol, the need for TCS in the management of IH has come down. Deep haemangiomas can benefit from IL injection of corticosteroids like triamcinolone acetonide [78–82].

3.2.16 Intertrigo and Perianal Inflammation

Medium-potency TCS of groups IV and V may be used in severe intertrigo and perianal inflammation for a short period. Low-potency topical steroids such as fluocinolone 0.01%, hydrocortisone butyrate 0.1%, and hydrocortisone 1% and 2.5% may be effective in dermatitis of the diaper area, eyelids, or face. It is important that appropriate antimycotic treatment is also given to avoid superadded fungal growth. Patients should be monitored for other side effect like atrophy and striae. Authors have noticed striae in obese children with less than a week's use of hydrocortisone [83].

Mild-to-moderate symptoms of perianal inflammation with minimal skin changes can be treated with a weak topical steroid such as 1% hydrocortisone applied morning and night after washing and can be combined with antibacterial or antifungal agents when necessary. Once symp-

toms regress, application should be tapered and replaced with a barrier cream.

3.2.17 Peristomal Inflammation

Calum et al. have documented that TCS formulated in aqueous or alcohol base as a lotion or carmellose sodium paste are very effective in the management of peristomal inflammation without affecting the stoma bag adhesion which is the main concern while treating peristomal area with topical agents. Specific causes like fungal or bacterial infections should be ruled out or treated before advising on a TCS in the peristomal area. There are concerns that long-term use of potent corticosteroids under the occlusion of a stoma bag will result in cutaneous atrophy and systemic absorption. This can be prevented by limiting the duration of initial treatment not exceeding 4 weeks and applying the medicine only at stoma bag changes. In cases of recurring inflammation, TCS application can be suggested every 2–4 weeks to prevent steroid complication [41].

3.2.18 Phimosis/Labial Adhesion

TCS is found to be effective in the management of phimosis in young children and prepubertal boys. Local application of steroid cream to the phimotic foreskin may allow some degree of retraction and avert the need for circumcision. Lund et al. have studied boys with phimosis wherein they had used betamethasone cream and found good results in nearly 75% of boys treated in whom the treatment effect persisted for 18 months. They recommended TCS as the first-line therapy in phimosis which can avoid surgery in up to 85% of cases [84–87].

Betamethasone 0.05% cream appears to be a safe and effective treatment of prepubertal labial adhesions as primary therapy or in patients that have failed previous therapies. Use of TCS may avoid the undesirable side effects of breast budding and hyperpigmentation that can be associated with oestrogen creams.

3.2.19 Lichen Sclerosus

Topical steroids are the treatment of choice for genital LS. Steroid ointments are recommended to reduce inflammation and itching. Strong steroid ointments like clobetasol propionate are the mainstay of treatment for genital LS and are effective in the majority of women. Initial treatment usually requires daily application of the ointment for 1–3 months to resolve the symptoms and reduce inflammation. After the initial course, most women will require maintenance therapy with either less frequent application of the strong steroid ointment or a switch to a less-potent steroid. It is important to use an adequate amount for a sufficient period to bring the disease under control. Steroid injections can be tried if steroid ointments are not effective. Use of potent TCS though improve genital LS, it does not cure the disease in women older than 70 years of age. Even in younger patients who achieve complete remission, according to Vilmer, the result is only temporary. However, treatment of genital LS with TCS plays an important role in the prevention of malignancy as it was found that carcinoma developed in non-treated or irregularly treated lesions of LS, though there are not many statistically significant data documenting the same [88].

3.2.20 Keloid and Hypertrophic Scars

ILS is the maul stay of treatment of keloids. According to Kim et al., the combination therapy (IPL + corticosteroid injection) not only improves the appearance of keloids and hypertrophic scars but also increases the recovery level of skin hydration status in terms of the skin barrier function. Surgical excision with pre- and post-operative ILS injection can be used as the first-line therapy when considering its effect and economic advantage [89, 90].

3.2.21 Melasma

Melasma, a common pigmentary disorder, is one of the indications for using Kligman's formula having TCS as one of the three components. Apart from 0.1% dexamethasone used in the original Kligman's formula, hydrocortisone and fluocinolone acetonide 0.01% are being used in the modified triple combinations. In an Indian study, it has been observed that the best response was seen to the modified Kligman's formula using hydroquinone (2%) + tretinoin (0.025%) + mometasone furoate (0.1%) cream [91, 92].

3.2.22 Burns

It has been suggested that mild TCS like hydrocortisone is an effective treatment and a non-invasive practical option to treat hypergranulation tissue resulting from burn wounds [93].

3.2.23 Chronic Idiopathic Urticaria and Urticaria Pigmentosa

Ellingsen et al. have tried potent TCS under occlusion in cases of chronic idiopathic urticaria and urticarial vasculitis with varying results [94].

3.2.24 TCS as Pretreatment

In patients using testosterone transdermal systems, the incidence and severity of skin irritation at application sites were to be reduced through pretreatment with triamcinolone acetonide 0.1% cream [95].

Shukla et al. have studied 60 patients with carcinoma breast receiving radiotherapy. Radiation-induced wet desquamation of the skin causes pain adding to the agony of these patients. In their study topical beclomethasone dipropionate spray was used as prophylaxis with the purpose of reducing risk of the wet desquamation of the skin in irradiated field. The authors found a statistically significant result in the group pretreated with TCS [96]. According to Schmuth et al., prophylactic and ongoing use of TCS either directly or in an emollient cream can reduce the severity of radiation dermatitis, though it does not prevent the same [97].

3.2.25 Granulomatous Diseases

Many granulomatous diseases of the skin and mucosa respond well to intralesional steroid injections. Diseases like cheilitis granulomatosa, [98] orofacial granulomatosis, [99] and pyoderma gangrenosum [100] respond well to ILS injection. Localised granuloma annulare can be treated with potent TCS with or without occlusion. IL injection can also be tried in adults [101, 102].

Patients with hidradenitis suppurativa (HS) having local, mild disease, or an acute flare may be managed with intralesional corticosteroid injections alone or in combination with antibiotics [103]. Riis et al. have noted significant reductions in physician-assessed erythema, oedema, suppuration, and size of the swelling at follow-up after ILS injection in patients with HS. They conclude that IL steroid injection is beneficial to both physician and patients in the management of flares by reducing pain after 1 day and signs of inflammation in 7 days post-treatment [104].

3.2.26 Sarcoidosis

The role of TCS in the treatment of cutaneous sarcoidosis has long been demonstrated. Clobetasol propionate under hydrocolloid dressing in papular sarcoid and twice-daily application of halobetasol propionate ointment in lupus pernio have shown considerable improvement. ILS injections using triamcinolone acetonide in a concentration of 3–10 mg/mL are more effective than TCS. Some plaques may require a higher concentration up to 20 mg/mL. It should be remembered that increase in concentration also increases the risk of side effects [105–107].

3.2.27 Nodulocystic Acne

Nodulocystic acne is a common yet difficult to treat condition which when untreated leads to severe scarring. IL steroid injection using triamcinolone gives marked and rapid resolution, thereby reducing the duration of systemic agents [108].

3.2.28 Mucocele

According to Baharvand et al., intralesional injection of dexamethasone was an effective, simple, repeatable, cost-effective, and potentially curative method of treatment of mucocele and can be used as a substitute for surgery in the treatment of salivary mucocele. The authors postulate that corticosteroid may promote the shrinkage of dilated salivary ducts or pool like a sclerosing agent, thereby shrinking the mucocele [109].

Conclusion

TCS are highly effective molecules and very promising in the treatment armamentarium of many dermatological conditions. It is indeed possible to avoid the side effects by judiciously using them. With the ongoing research, it will be possible to develop a steroid molecule for topical use with hyper-selective action. With the invent of new steroid molecule that can induce selective transrepression, the choice of TCS will become much easier for the physician to give the best to the patient with minimal if not no side effect.

References

1. Ference JD, Last AR. Choosing topical corticosteroids. Am Fam Physician. 2009;79(2):135–40.
2. Chi CC, Kirtschig G, Aberer W, Gabbud JP, Lipozencić J, Kárpáti S, et al. Guideline on topical corticosteroids in pregnancy. Br J Dermatol. 2011;165(5):943–52.
3. Murphy VE, Fittock RJ, Zarzycki PK, Delahunty MM, Smith R, Clifton VL. Metabolism of synthetic steroids by the human placenta. Placenta. 2007;28:39–46.
4. Mygind H, Thulstrup AM, Pedersen L, Larsen H. Risk of intrauterine growth retardation, malformations and other birth outcomes in children after topical use of corticosteroid in pregnancy. Acta Obstet Gynecol Scand. 2002;81:234–9.
5. Edwards MJ, Agho K, Attia J, Diaz P, Hayes T, Illingworth A, et al. Case–control study of cleft lip or palate after maternal use of topical corticosteroids during pregnancy. Am J Med Genet A. 2003;120:459–63.
6. Chi CC, Mayon-White RT, Wojnarowska FT. Safety of topical corticosteroids in pregnancy: a population-based cohort study. J Invest Dermatol. 2011;131:884–91.
7. Mahé A, Perret JL, Ly F, Fall F, Rault JP, Dumont A. The cosmetic use of skin-lightening products during pregnancy in Dakar, Senegal: a common and potentially hazardous practice. Trans R Soc Trop Med Hyg. 2007;101:183–7.
8. Alston SJ, Cohen BA, Braun M. Persistent and recurrent tinea corporis in children treated with combination antifungal/corticosteroid agents. Pediatrics. 2003;111(1):201–3.
9. Drake LA, Dinehart SM, Farmer ER, Goltz RW, Graham GF, Hordinsky MK, et al. Guidelines of care for the use of topical glucocorticosteroids. J Am Acad Dermatol. 1996;35(4):615–9.
10. Tosti A, Piraccini BM, Pazzaglia M, Vincenzi C. Clobetasol propionate 0.05% under occlusion in the treatment of alopecia totalis/universalis. J Am Acad Dermatol. 2003;49:96–8.
11. Vázquez-López F, Marghoob AA. Dermoscopic assessment of long-term topical therapies with potent steroids in chronic psoriasis. J Am Acad Dermatol. 2004;51:811–3.
12. Wolkerstorfer A, Visser RL, De Waard van der Spek FB, den Hollander JC, Tank B, Oranje AP. Efficacy and safety of wet-wrap dressings in children with severe atopic dermatitis: influence of corticosteroid dilution. Br J Dermatol. 2000;143:999–1004. 38
13. Devillers AC, de Waard-van der Spek FB, Mulder PG, Oranje AP. Treatment of refractory atopic dermatitis using 'wet-wrap' dressings and diluted corticosteroids: results of standardized treatment in both children and adults. Dermatology. 2002;204:50–5.
14. Yentzer BA, Ade RA, Fountain JM, Clark AR, Taylor SL, Borgerding E, et al. Improvement in treatment adherence with a 3-day course of fluocinonide cream 0.1% for atopic dermatitis. Cutis. 2010;86:208–13.
15. Stadler JF, Fleury M, Sourisse M, Rostin M, Pheline F, Litoux P. Local steroid therapy and bacterial skin Flora in atopic dermatitis. Br J Dermatol. 1994;131:536–40.
16. Hung SH, Lin YT, Chu CY, Lee CC, Liang TC, Yang YH, et al. Staphylococcus colonization in atopic dermatitis treated with fluticasone or tacrolimus with or without antibiotics. Ann Allergy Asthma Immunol. 2007;98(1):51–6.
17. Schmitt J, von Kobyletzki L, Svensson A, Apfelbacher C. Efficacy and tolerability of proactive treatment with topical corticosteroids and calcineurin inhibitors for atopic eczema: systematic review and meta-analysis of randomized controlled trials. Br J Dermatol. 2011;164:415–28.
18. Nilsson EJ, Henning CG, Magnusson J. Topical corticosteroids and Staphylococcus Aureus in atopic dermatitis. JAAD. 1992;27(1):29–34.
19. Gonzalez ME, Schaffer JV, Orlow SJ, Orlow SJ, Gao Z, Li H, et al. Cutaneous microbiome effects of fluticasone propionate cream and adjunctive bleach baths in childhood atopic dermatitis. J Am Acad Dermatol. 2016;75:481–93.
20. Glazenburg EJ, Wolkerstorfer A, Gerretsen AL, et al. Efficacy and safety of fluticasone propionate 0.005% ointment in the long-term maintenance treatment of children with atopic dermatitis: differences between boys and girls? Pediatr Allergy Immunol. 2009;20:59–66.
21. Callen J, Chamlin S, Eichenfield LF, Mulder PGH, Oranje AP. A systematic review of the safety of topical therapies for atopic dermatitis. Br J Dermatol. 2007;156:203–21.
22. Del Rosso JQ. Adult Seborrheic dermatitis. A status report on practical topical management. J Clin Aesthet Dermatol. 2011;4(5):32–8.
23. Elewski B. An investigator-blinded, randomized, 4-week, parallel-group, multicenter pilot study to compare the safety and efficacy of a nonsteroidal cream (Promiseb topical cream) and desonide cream 0.05% in the twice-daily treatment of mild to moderate seborrheic dermatitis of the face. Clinics Dermatol. 2009;27:S10–5.
24. Johnson BA, Nunley JR. Treatment of Seborrheic dermatitis. Am Fam Physician. 2000;61(9):2703–10.
25. Clark GW, Pope SM, Jaboori KA. Diagnosis and treatment of Seborrheic dermatitis. Am Fam Physician. 2015;91(3):185–90.
26. Milani M, Di Molfetta SA, Gramazio R, Fiorella C, Frisario C, Fuzio E, et al. Efficacy of betamethasone valerate 0.1% thermophobic foam in seborrhoeic dermatitis of the scalp: an open-label, multicentre, prospective trial on 180 patients. Curr Med Res Opin. 2003;19(4):342–5.

27. Ortonne JP, Nikkels AF, Reich K, Ponce Olivera RM, Lee JH, Kerrouche N, et al. Efficacious and safe management of moderate to severe scalp seborrhoeic dermatitis using clobetasol propionate shampoo 0.05% combined with ketoconazole shampoo 2%: a randomized, controlled study. Br J Dermatol. 2011;165(1):171–6.

28. Rigopoulos D, Ioannides D, Kalogeromitros D, Gregoriou S, Katsambas A. Pimecrolimus cream 1% vs. betamethasone 17-valerate 0.1% cream in the treatment of seborrhoeic dermatitis. A randomized open-label clinical trial. Br J Dermatol. 2004;151(5):1071–5.

29. Firooz A, Solhpour A, Gorouhi F, Daneshpazhooh M, Balighi K, Farsinejad K, et al. Pimecrolimus cream, 1%, vs hydrocortisone acetate cream, 1%, in the treatment of facial seborrheic dermatitis: a randomized, investigator-blind, clinical trial. Arch Dermatol. 2006;142(8):1066–7.

30. Cicek D, Kandi B, Bakar S, Turgut D. Pimecrolimus 1% cream, methylprednisolone aceponate 0.1% cream and metronidazole 0.75% gel in the treatment of seborrhoeic dermatitis: a randomized clinical study. J Dermatolog Treat. 2009;20(6):344–9.

31. Usatine RP, Riojas M. Diagnosis and Management of Contact Dermatitis. Am Fam Physician. 2010; 82(3):249–55.

32. Silverberg NB. Pediatric contact dermatitis treatment and management. Available at http://emedicine.medscape.com/article/911711-treatment#d11. Accessed on 9.1.17.

33. Levin C, Zhai H, Bashir S, Chew AL, Anigbogu A, Stern R, et al. Efficacy of corticosteroids in acute experimental irritant contact dermatitis? Skin Res Technol. 2001;7(4):214–8.

34. Baeck M, Chemelle JA, Rasse C, Terreux R, Goossens A. C16 methyl corticosteroids are far less allergenic than the non-methylated molecules. Contact Dermatitis. 2011;64(6):305–12.

35. Scheinfeld NS. Polymorphous light eruption treatment and management. Drugs & Dis. 2016. Available at http://emedicine.medscape.com/article/1119686-treatment. Accessed 9.1.2017.

36. Brunner N, Yawalkar S. A double-blind, multicenter, parallel-group trial with 0.05% halobetasol propionate ointment versus 0.1% diflucortolone valerate ointment in patients with severe, chronic atopic dermatitis or lichen simplex chronicus. J Am Acad Dermatol. 1991;25(6 Pt 2):1160–3.

37. Datz B, Yawalkar S. A double-blind, multicenter trial of 0.05% halobetasol propionate ointment and 0.05% clobetasol 17-propionate ointment in the treatment of patients with chronic, localized atopic dermatitis or lichen simplex chronicus. J Am Acad Dermatol. 1991;25(6 Pt 2):1157–60.

38. Geraldez MC, Carreon-Gavino M, Hoppe G, Costales A. Diflucortolone valerate ointment with and without occlusion in lichen simplex chronicus. Int J Dermatol. 1989;28(9):603–4.

39. Pinney SS. Pityriasis alba treatment and management. Medscape. Available at http://emedicine.medscape.com/article/910770-treatment.

40. Harper J. Topical corticosteroids for skin disorders in infants and children. Drugs. 1988;36(Suppl 5):34–7.

41. Lyon CC, Smith AJ, Griffiths CEM, Becka MH. Peristomal dermatoses: a novel indication for topical steroid lotions. J Am Acad Dermatol. 2000;43(4):684–7.

42. Thomas J, Parimalam K, Sindhu BR. Childhood psoriasis. Expert Rev Dermatol. 2013;8(5):547–56.

43. Thomas J, Parimalam K. Treating pediatric plaque psoriasis: challenges and solutions. Pediatr Health Med Ther. 2016;7:25–38.

44. Kimball AB, Gold MH, Zib B, Davis MW, Clobetasol Propionate Emulsion Formulation Foam Phase III Clinical Study Group. Clobetasol propionate emulsion formulation foam 0.05%: review of phase II open-label and phase III randomized controlled trials in steroid-responsive dermatoses in adults and adolescents. J Am Acad Dermatol. 2008;59:448–54.

45. Pardasani AG, Feldman SR, Clark AR. Treatment of psoriasis: an algorithm-based approach for primary care physicians. Am Fam Physician. 2000;61(3): 725–33.

46. Menter A, Korman NJ, Elmets CA, Feldman SR, Gelfand JM, Gordon KB, et al. Guidelines of care for the management of psoriasis and psoriatic arthritis. J Am Acad Dermatol. 2009;61(3):451–85.

47. Lidbrink P, Johannesson A, Hammar H. Psoriasis treatment: faster clearance when UVB-dithranol is combined with topical clobetasol propionate. Dermatologica. 1986;172:164–8.

48. Petrozzi JW. Topical steroids and UV radiation in psoriasis. Arch Dermatol. 1983;119:207–10.

49. Larko O, Swanbeck G, Svartholm H. The effect on psoriasis of clobetasol propionate used alone or in combination with UVB. Acta Derm Venereol. 1984;64:151–4.

50. Dover JS, McEvoy MT, Rosen CF, Arndt KA, Stern RS. Are topical corticosteroids useful in phototherapy for psoriasis? J Am Acad Dermatol. 1989;20:748–54.

51. Meola T, Soter NA, Lim HW. Are topical corticosteroids useful adjunctive therapies for the treatment of psoriasis with ultraviolet radiation? A review of the literature. Arch Dermatol. 1991;27:1708–13.

52. van de Kerkhof PC, Kragballe K, Segaert S, Lebwohl M. Factors impacting the combination of topical corticosteroid therapies for psoriasis: perspectives from the international psoriasis council. J Eur Acad Dermatol Venereol. 2011;25(10):1130–9.

53. Sugerman PB. Oral lichen Planus medication. Medscape Updated: Aug 31, 2016. Available at http://emedicine.medscape.com/article/1078327-medication.

54. Chuang T-Y. Lichen planus medication. Updated: Mar 01, 2016. Available at http://emedicine.medscape.com/article/1123213-medication.

55. Sugerman PB. Oral lichen Planus medication. Drugs Dis. 2016. Available at http://emedicine.medscape.com/article/1078327-medication#2. Accessed 9 Jan 2017.

56. Majid I, Keen A. Management of alopecia areata: an update. BJMP. 2012;5(3):a530.

57. Charuwichitratana S, Wattanakrai P, Tanrattanakorn S. Randomized double-blind placebo-controlled trial in the treatment of alopecia areata with 0.25% desoximetasone cream. Arch Dermatol. 2000;136(10):1276–7.

58. Montes LF. Topical halcinonide in alopecia areata and alopecia totalis. J Cutan Pathol. 1997;4:47–50.

59. Tan E, Tay YK, Giam YCH. A clinical study of childhood alopecia areata in Singapore. Pediatr Dermatol. 2002;19:298–301.

60. Ross EK, Shapiro J. Management of hair loss. Dermatol Clin. 2005;23:227–43.

61. Madani S, Shapiro J. Alopecia areata update. J Am Acad Dermatol. 2000;42:549–66.

62. Tosti A, Iorizzo M, Botta GL, Milani M. Efficacy and safety of a new clobetasol propionate 0.05% foam in alopecia areata: a randomized, double-blind placebo-controlled trial. J Eur Acad Dermatol Venereol. 2006;20(10):1243–7.

63. Downs AM, Lear JT, Kennedy CT. Anaphylaxis to intradermal triamcinolone acetonide. Arch Dermatol. 1998;134:1163–4.

64. Devi M, Rashid A, Ghafoor R. Intralesional triamcinolone Acetonide versus topical betamethasone valerate in the management of localized alopecia areata. J Coll Physicians Surg Pak. 2015;25(12):860–2.

65. Chu TW, AlJasser M, Alharbi A, Abahussein O, McElwee K, Shapiro J. Benefit of different concentrations of intralesional triamcinolone acetonide in alopecia areata: an intrasubject pilot study. J Am Acad Dermatol. 2015;73(2):338–40.

66. Chang KH, Rojhirunsakool S, Goldberg LJ. Treatment of severe alopecia areata with intralesional steroid injections. J Drugs Dermatol. 2009;8(10):909–12.

67. Mancuso G, Balducci A, Casadio C, Farina P, Staffa M, Valenti L, et al. Efficacy of betamethasone valerate foam formulation in comparison with betamethasone dipropionate lotion in the treatment of mild-to-moderate alopecia areata: a multicenter, prospective, randomized, controlled, investigator-blinded trial. Int J Dermatol. 2003;42(7):572–5.

68. Lepe V, Moncada B, Castanedo-Cazares JP, Torres-Alvarez MB, Ortiz CA, Torres-Rubalcava AB. A double-blind randomized trial of 0.1% tacrolimus vs. 0.05% clobetasol for the treatment of childhood vitiligo. Arch Dermatol. 2003;139(5):581–5.

69. Wang E, Koo J, Levy E. Intralesional corticosteroid injections for vitiligo: a new therapeutic option. J Am Acad Dermatol. 2014;71(2):391–2.

70. Roenigk HH, Martin JS, Eichorn P, Gilliam JN. Discoid lupus erythematosus. Diagnostic features and evaluation of topical corticosteroid therapy. Cutis. 1980;25:281–5.

71. Tzung TY, Liu YS, Chang HW. Tacrolimus vs. clobetasol propionate in the treatment of facial cutaneous lupus erythematosus: a randomized, double-blind, bilateral comparison study. Br J Dermatol. 2007;156:191–2.

72. Madan V, August PJ, Chalmers RJ. Efficacy of topical tacrolimus 0.3% in clobetasol propionate 0.05% ointment in therapy-resistant cutaneous lupus ery-

thematosus: a cohort study. Clin Exp Dermatol. 2010;35:27–30.

73. Madan V, August PJ, Chalmers RJ, Barikbin B, Givrad S, Yousefi M, et al. Pimecrolimus 1% cream versus betamethasone 17-valerate 0.1% cream in the treatment of facial discoid lupus erythematosus: a double-blind, randomized pilot study. Clin Exp Dermatol. 2009;34:776–80.

74. Eastham ABW. Discoid lupus erythematosus treatment and management. Updated: Feb. http://emedicine.medscape.com/article/1065529-treatment#d10.

75. Joly P, Fontaine J, Roujeau JC. The role of topical corticosteroids in bullous pemphigoid in the elderly. Drugs Aging. 2005;22(7):571–6.

76. Dumas V, Roujeau JC, Wolkenstein P, Revuz J, Cosnes A. The treatment of mild pemphigus vulgaris and pemphigus foliaceus with a topical corticosteroid. Br J Dermatol. 1999;140(6):1127–9.

77. Abecassis S, Joly P, Genereau T, Courville P, André C, Moussalli J, et al. Superpotent topical steroid therapy for epidermolysis bullosa acquisita. Dermatology. 2004;209:164–6.

78. Pandey A, Gangopadhyay AN, Sharma SP, Kumar V, Gupta DK, Gopal SC. Evaluation of topical steroids in the treatment of superficial hemangioma. Skinmed. 2010;8(1):9–11.

79. Metry DW. Management of infantile hemangiomas. Available at http://www.uptodate.com/contents/management-of-infantile-hemangiomas.

80. Garzon MC, Lucky AW, Hawrot A, Frieden IJ. Ultrapotent topical corticosteroid treatment of hemangiomas of infancy. J Am Acad Dermatol. 2005;52:281.

81. Chen MT, Yeong EK, Horng SY. Intralesional corticosteroid therapy in proliferating head and neck hemangiomas: a review of 155 cases. J Pediatr Surg. 2000;35:420.

82. Ceisler EJ, Santos L, Blei F. Periocular hemangiomas: what every physician should know. Pediatr Dermatol. 2004;21(1):1–9.

83. Siddiqi S, Vijay V, Ward M, Mahendran R, Warren S. Pruritus Ani. Ann R Coll Surg Engl. 2008;90(6):457–63.

84. Webster TM, Leonard MP. Topical steroid therapy for phimosis. Can J Urol. 2002;9(2):1492–5.

85. Lund L, Wai KH, Mui LM, Yeung CK. Effect of topical steroid on non-retractile prepubertal foreskin by a prospective, randomized, double-blind study. Scand J Urol Nephrol. 2000;34(4):267–9.

86. Lund L, Wai KH, Mui LM, Yeung CK. An 18-month follow-up study after randomized treatment of phimosis in boys with topical steroid versus placebo. Scand J Urol Nephrol. 2005;39(1):78–81.

87. Myers JB, Sorensen CM, Wisner BP, Furness PD, Passamaneck M, Koyle MA. Betamethasone cream for the treatment of pre-pubertal labial adhesions. J Pediatr Adolesc Gynecol. 2006;19(6):407–11.

88. Renaud-Vilmer C, Cavelier-Balloy B, Porcher R, Dubertret L. Vulvar lichen sclerosus: effect of long-term topical application of a potent steroid on the course of the disease. Arch Dermatol. 2004;40(6):709–12.

89. Kim DY, Park HS, Yoon H-S, Cho S. Efficacy of IPL device combined with intralesional corticosteroid injection for the treatment of keloids and hypertrophic scars with regards to the recovery of skin barrier function: a pilot study. J Dermatol Treat. 2015;26(5):481–4.

90. Jung JY, Roh MR, Kwon YS, Chung KY. Surgery and perioperative intralesional corticosteroid injection for treating earlobe keloids: a Korean experience. Ann Dermatol. 2009;21(3):221–5.

91. Sardesai VR, Kolte JN, Srinivas BN. A clinical study of melasma and a comparison of the therapeutic effect of certain currently available topical modalities for its treatment. Indian J Dermatol. 2013;58:239.

92. Torok HM, Jones T, Rich P, Smith S, Tschen E. Hydroquinone 4%, tretinoin 0.05%, fluocinolone acetonide 0.01%: a safe and efficacious 12 month treatment for melasma. Cutis. 2005;75:57–62.

93. Jaeger M, Harats M, Kornhaber R, Aviv U, Zerach A, Haik J. Treatment of hypergranulation tissue in burn wounds with topical steroid dressings: a case series. Int Med Case Rep J. 2016;9:241–5.

94. Ellingsen AR, Thestrup-Pedersen K. Treatment of chronic idiopathic urticaria with topical steroids. Acta Derm Venereol. 1996;76(1):43–4.

95. Wilson DE, Kaidbey K, Boike SC, Jorkasky DK. Use of topical corticosteroid pretreatment to reduce the incidence and severity of skin reactions associated with testosterone transdermal therapy. Clin Ther. 1998;20(2):299–306.

96. Shukla PN, Gairola M, Mohanti BK, Rath GK. Prophylactic beclomethasone spray to the skin during postoperative radiotherapy of carcinoma breast: a prospective randomized study. Indian J Cancer. 2006;43(4):180–4.

97. Schmuth M, Wimmer MA, Hofer S, Sztankay A, Weinlich G, Linder DM, et al. Topical corticosteroid therapy for acute radiation dermatitis: a prospective, randomized, double-blind study. Br J Dermatol. 2002;146(6):983–91.

98. Sakuntabhai A, MacLeod RI, Lawrence CM. Intralesional steroid injection after nerve block anaesthesia in the treatment of orofacial granulomatosis. Arch Dermatol. 1993;129:477–80.

99. Mignogna MD, Fedele S, Lo Russo L, Adamo D, Satriano A. Effectiveness of small-volume, intralesional, delayed-release triamcinolone injections in orofacial granulomatosis: a pilot study. J Am Acad Dermatol. 2004;51(2):265–8.

100. Chow KP, Ho CV. Treatment of pyoderma gangrenosum. J Am Acad Dermatol. 1996;34:1047–60.

101. Ghadially R. Granuloma annulare treatment and management. Drugs Dis. Updated 2016. Available at http://emedicine.medscape.com/article/1123031-treatment. Accessed 10 Jan 2017.

102. Rallis E, Stavropoulou E, Korfitis C. Granuloma annulare of childhood successfully treated with potent topical corticosteroids previously unresponsive to tacrolimus ointment 0.1%: report of three cases. Clin Exp Dermatol. 2009;34:e475.

103. Maini P. Intralesional corticosteroid injections as a treatment option for acute lesions in patients diagnosed with hidradenitis suppurativa. J Am Acad Dermatol. 2015;72(5):AB51.

104. Riis PT, Boer J, Prens EP, Saunte DM, Deckers IE, Emtestam L, et al. Intralesional triamcinolone for flares of hidradenitis suppurativa (HS): a case series. J Am Acad Dermatol. 2016;75(6):1151–5.

105. Volden G. Successful treatment of chronic skin diseases with clobetasol propionate and a hydrocolloid occlusive dressing. Acta Derm Venereol. 1992;72:69.

106. Khatri KA, Chotzen VA, Burrall BA. Lupus pernio: successful treatment with a potent topical corticosteroid. Arch Dermatol. 1995;131:617.

107. Prystowsky S, Sanchez M. Management of cutaneous sarcoidosis. Uptodate 2011. Available at http://cursoenarm.net/UPTODATE/contents/mobipreview.htm?21/17/21777/abstract/15.

108. Lee SJ, Hyun MY, Park KY, Kim BJ. A tip for performing intralesional triamcinolone acetonide injections in acne patients. J Am Acad Dermatol. 2014;71(4):e127–e12.

109. Baharvand M, Sabounchi S, Mortazavi H. Treatment of labial mucocele by intralesional injection of dexamethasone: case series. JDMT. 2014;3(3):128–33.

An Evidence Based Approach of Use of Topical Corticosteroids in Dermatology

4

Anupam Das and Saumya Panda

Abstract

Topical corticosteroids form the backbone of treating numerous dermatological conditions. If used judiciously and appropriately, these drugs can be referred to as the "magic molecules". On extensive literature search, we have found substantial evidences in favour of using topical corticosteroids in atopic eczema, localized vitiligo, psoriasis (both scalp and non-scalp), chronic hand eczema and localized bullous pemphigoid. However, contrary to conventional wisdom, we did not find any high-level scientific evidence supporting the prescription of these agents in cutaneous lichen planus, sarcoidosis and seborrhoeic dermatitis. In addition, evidence suggests recommended judicious use of mild to moderate steroids (if required) in pregnancy and lactation and there is no risk of any foetal abnormality.

Keywords

Topical corticosteroids • Randomized controlled trials • Meta-analysis • Systematic reviews

Learning Points

1. Application of twice-weekly potent TC (topical corticosteroids) to stable eczema can reduce the number of flare-ups in both, adults and children.
2. Skin thinning and suppression of the pituitary–adrenal axis are not seen if TCs are correctly used.
3. Class 3 TCs are highly effective in treating generalized or localized vitiligo. However, atrophy, telangiectasia, hypertrichosis and acneiform papules are the commonly reported adverse effects with long-term use of TCs documented in this condition.
4. Both class III and class IV TCs are effective in inducing remission in non-scalp psoriasis but frequency and duration of application must be tapered down during maintenance phase to avoid cutaneous and systemic adverse

A. Das • S. Panda (✉)
Department of Dermatology, KPC Medical College and Hospital, Jadavpur, Kolkata, India
e-mail: saumyapan@gmail.com

© Springer Nature Singapore Pte Ltd. 2018
K. Lahiri (ed.), *A Treatise on Topical Corticosteroids in Dermatology*,
DOI 10.1007/978-981-10-4609-4_4

effects. Scalp psoriasis responds exceptionally well to TCs.

5. TCs are widely used as first-line therapy in cutaneous lichen planus, but high-level scientific evidence is absent. There is not a single RCT supporting the use of TCs in cutaneous lichen planus. However, there are evidences in favour of prescribing TCs in oral lichen planus.

6. Class I TCs are effective in patch and plaque stages of MF (early-stage IA/IB MF), but evidence in the favour of using them is lacking.

7. TCs have emerged as the first-line treatment for both localized and mild bullous pemphigoid, however, the results cannot be extrapolated to extensive disease.

8. In chronic hand eczema, TCs have been found to be beneficial but the choice between short bursts of potent TCs versus continuous application of mild TCs is difficult, on account of scarcity of evidence.

9. Evidence in favour of using TCs in cutaneous sarcoidosis, infantile hemangiomas, seborrhoeic dermatitis is lacking.

10. In pregnancy and lactation, mild to moderate topical corticosteroids can be safely prescribed, without the fear of associated risk of foetal growth restriction. However, this is not applicable to potent steroids and areas with high absorption rates.

4.1   Introduction

Since the introduction in early 1950s, topical corticosteroids (TC) have become the most commonly prescribed drugs by dermatologists in an out-patient setting. These agents form the mainstay of treatment for many skin conditions. If used appropriately, they are safe and effective, and side effects are generally uncommon. Not only dermatologists, steroids have been rampantly prescribed by general physicians, paediatricians, gynaecologists and specialists of numerous disciplines.

Unfortunately, TCs are increasingly being abused by doctors and patients. Topical steroid addiction (TSA) and red burning skin syndrome (RBSS) are legitimate clinical entities which are well recognized these days [1]. As a result, the problem of steroid phobia is being increasingly recognized by physicians worldwide which, sometimes, is associated with simple fear, due to patient ignorance. Besides, current advice to patients to apply topical corticosteroids contributes to steroid phobia to some extent, further aggravating the probability of poor compliance, clinical response and therapeutic failure. However, it must be noted that legible prescriptions by qualified dermatologists contain topical corticosteroids of mild potency in majority of the cases, and these are unlikely to cause any harm. But the patients do not understand these subtle facts. This leads to propagation of a wrong message that topical corticosteroids of any potency, irrespective of the amount and duration of application, lead to irreversible side effects [2].

In this chapter, we have reviewed the various indications of topical corticosteroids in dermatology with an overview of the evidences available in the support of using these drugs in various dermatoses. Wherever possible, we have tried our best to collate the evidences, and analyse them in such a manner that both the opposing concerns may be addressed, and we may come up with a balanced view on TC use in clinical dermatology. As a disclaimer, we must inform the readers that this chapter is not meant to be a comprehensive review of evidence of TC usage in dermatology, given the limitations of space. We have tried, instead, to place on record the evidence of these agents in the clinical indications in which these are most commonly used.

4.2 Discussion and Evidences

4.2.1 Eczema

Eczema is a non-infective, chronic, inflammatory dermatosis clinically characterized by inflamed, pruritic, erythematous and/or dry skin [3]. Various therapeutic modalities are available to control eczema and amongst them, TCs are the most widely used. The majority of patients with eczema respond well to emollients as and when required. [4, 5] According to the traditional approach, it is prudent to prescribe TCs during acute flares and withdraw the same once the symptoms are controlled. However, recent authors are of the opinion that pro-active approach is better than the more commonly followed reactive approach. [6] According to the latest evidence, it is favourable to go for high dose corticosteroids during the exacerbation of the disease and continuing with low dose corticosteroids when the acute episode is under control.

Besides, step-up and step-down approach can be followed which refers to increasing the potency of the steroid in acute flares and lowering the potency in periods of remission. [7] Overall, a systematic review of the best strategies for using topical corticosteroids in the treatment of established eczema is, therefore, required [8].

Here is a brief overview of some of the major randomized controlled trials comparing the use of different TCs in eczema.

Name of study	Type of study	Intervention	Outcome measures	Result
Almeyda et al. [9]	Randomized, double-blind, paired-comparison trial	10% urea and 1% hydrocortisone vs cream 0.1% betamethasone 17-valerate cream applied twice daily for 3 weeks	Lesion response: excellent, good, none, deterioration	1% hydrocortisone controls atopic eczema without the hazards of potent fluorinated corticosteroids and it is as effective as 0.1% betamethasone 17-valerate
Andersen et al. [10]	Randomized, double-blind, left–right multicentre study	Mildison lipocream 1% hydrocortisone ointment twice daily vs Uniderm cream 1% hydrocortisone ointment twice daily	Global severity of symptoms, global improvement of skin lesions, investigator and patient preference	Little efficacy difference between treatments, yet patients preferred the Mildison lipocream 1% hydrocortisone ointment
Bagatell et al. [11]	Double-blind, randomized and balanced-parallel-group trial	Alclometasone dipropionate cream 0.05% vs hydrocortisone cream 1.0% thrice daily for 3 weeks	Erythema, induration, pruritus Investigator global evaluation	71% alclometasone patients showed marked improvement compared to 69% hydrocortisone patients
Beattie et al. [12]	Randomized, single-observer trial	Hydrocortisone 1% once daily vs Hydrocortisone 1% twice daily. Both groups were instructed to apply emollient as and when required	Six Area, Six Sign Atopic Dermatitis (SASSAD) severity score, Infants Dermatology Quality of Life Index (IDQOL), Dermatitis Family Impact (DFI) and Side effects	conventional therapy with hydrocortisone and emollients alone is as effective as wet-wrap therapy for infants with moderately severe, widespread AD
Binder et al. [13]	Randomized, double-blind, paired-comparison trial	Fluocinonide 0.05% cream twice daily vs Betamethasone valerate 0.01% cream twice daily for 2 weeks	Lesion improvement	Fluocinolone was superior to betamethasone in 70% of patients but difficult to interpret magnitude of effect

(continued)

(continued)

Name of study	Type of study	Intervention	Outcome measures	Result
Bleehen et al. [14]	Randomized, double-blind, parallel-group controlled trial	Fluticasone propionate 0.05% cream OD vs Fluticasone propionate 0.05% cream BD for 4 weeks	Patient diary cards for itch, rash and sleep disturbance and physician assessed six signs and global assessment	Improvement within first week in 80% patients in o.d. vs 85% in b.d. groups but method and concealment of randomization was unclear
Bleeker et al. [15]	Randomized, double-blind trial	halcinonide 0.1% cream twice daily vs clobetasol propionate 0.05% cream twice daily for 2 weeks	Decrease in erythema, oedema, transudation, lichenification, scaling, pruritus and pain	92% 'excellent' or 'good' clinical response for both groups
Duke et al. [16]	Randomized, parallel-group design, blind evaluator study	Alclometasone dipropionate 0.05% ointment bd vs clobetasone butyrate 0.05% ointment bd for 3 weeks	Clinical score erythema, induration, pruritus, and physician global assessment	75% improvement in alclometasone group compared with 68% improvement in clobetasone group
Fisher et al. [17]	Randomized, double-blind, left-right comparison trial	Fluocinonide 0.05% cream tds vs Betamethasone valerate 0.1% cream tds for 3 weeks	Clinical response relative to status of lesion	Mean clinical response better in fluocinonide than betamethasone on a scale of 1–5
Foelster-Holst et al. [18]	Randomized controlled trial	Topical corticosteroid prednicarbate with vs without partial wet-wrap dressing	Local SCORAD	Wet-wrap therapy with a topical corticosteroid is an effective treatment option in patients with exacerbated AD
Glazenburg et al. [19]	Randomized, double-blind, controlled trial	Placebo ointment bd vs fluticasone propionate 0.005% ointment bd for 16 weeks	SCORAD	Addition of twice-weekly FP to standard maintenance therapy significantly reduces the risk of relapse in children with moderate severe AD
Grimalt et al.a [5]	Open randomized controlled study	Micronized desonide 0.1% cream Locatop and/or desonide 0.1% cream Locapred with vs without emollient (Exomega)	Scoring Atopic Dermatitis Index (SCORAD), and infants' and parents' quality of life by Infant's Dermatitis Quality of Life Index and Dermatitis Family Impact scores	Emollients significantly reduced the high-potency topical corticosteroid consumption in infants with AD
Haneke et al. [20]	Randomized, double-blind, left–right comparison trial	0.1% methylprednisolone aceponate ointment o.d vs 0.1% betamethasone valerate b.d. for 4 weeks	Patient and doctor global assessments	Actual data not found and method and concealment of randomization not clear
Hanifin et al. [21]	Randomized, investigator-blind, left–right comparison trial	desonide 0.05% lotion bd vs desonide 0.05% lotion bd plus a moisturizing cream tds for 4 weeks	erythema, dryness or scaling, pruritus, excoriations, lichenification, oozing or crusting, and induration or papules	Addition of a moisturizer to a low-potency corticosteroid lotion was effective in treating mild-to-moderate atopic dermatitis
Hanifin et al. [22]	Randomized, double-blind parallel trial	Intermittent fluticasone propionate or vehicle, once daily 4 days per week for 4 weeks followed by once daily 2 days per week for 16 weeks	Global assessment score	Once stabilized with fluticasone treatment, the risk of relapse significantly reduced by extended intermittent dosing with fluticasone cream in addition to regular emollient therapy

Haribhakti et al. [23]	Randomized, double-blind, controlled trial	Clobetasone butyrate cream bd vs Hydrocortisone cream bd for 2–3 weeks	erythema, dryness or scaling, pruritus, excoriations, lichenification, oozing or crusting	Reductions in pre-treatment total scores have been greater for Clobetasone as compared to hydrocortisone, the difference becoming significant at the end of 3 weeks of treatment
Hebert et al. [24]	Multicentre, randomized, blinded, vehicle-controlled studies	desonide hydrogel 0.05% bd vs hydrogel vehicle bd for 4 weeks	SCORAD	Desonide hydrogel 0.05% was extremely well tolerated and provided statistically significant improvements in all primary ($P < 0.001$) and secondary ($P < 0.006$) efficacy endpoints in both studies
Hoybye et al. [25]	Randomized, single-blind, parallel-group and multicentre trial	Mometasone furoate cream o.d. vs hydrocortisone 17-butyrate cream b.d. for 6 weeks	Patient VAS for severity of eczema, 0–3 score for doctor-assessed erythema, infiltration and pruritus, global evaluation scores of 1–6	No difference in efficacy between the two treatments
Jorizzo et al. [26]	Randomized, investigator-masked, parallel-group design trial	Desonide 0.05% ointment vs hydrocortisone 1% ointment b.d. for 5 weeks	Physician global improvement, erythema, lichenification excoriations, oozing and crusting, induration and papules Pruritus assessed subjectively	68% desonide group and 40% hydrocortisone group had marked improvement at 5 weeks
Kirkup et al. [27]	Multicentre, randomized, double-blind, parallel-group trial	One study compared FP with hydrocortisone (HC) 1% cream (FP 70, HC 67) and the other with hydrocortisone butyrate (HCB) 0.1% cream (FP 67, HCB 62). Treatments were applied twice daily, for 2–4 weeks until the AD was stabilized, and thereafter intermittently ('as required') for up to 12 weeks	Pruritus, erythema, scaling, lichenification, oozing, excoriation, overall global impression	FP demonstrated a high level of efficacy and maintenance of disease control with a tolerability similar to HC 1%
Koopmans et al. [28]	Randomized, double-blind, controlled trial	0.1% hydrocortisone 17-butyrate cream b.d. vs o.d. plus vehicle o.d. for 4 weeks	Patient and doctor assessed overall severity Clinical features assessed were erythema, induration, pruritus and excoriation	78% o.d. vs 93% b.d. noticed considerable improvement

(continued)

(continued)

Name of study	Type of study	Intervention	Outcome measures	Result
Korting et al. [29]	Randomized, double-blind, left–right comparison trial	0.039% liposomal betamethasone dipropionate vs 0.054% commercial propylene glycol gel for 2 weeks	Investigator assessed ten signs and symptoms of eczema and proportion of patients with major improvement or healed and global effect on a 0–5 scale	80% patients had major improvement in liposome group compared with 60% patients in reference group
Lassus et al. [30]	Randomized double-blind, parallel-group trial	Alclometasone dipropionate cream 0.05% b.d. vs hydrocortisone butyrate cream 0.1% b.d. for 2 weeks	Erythema, induration, pruritus Physician global evaluation of improvement	76–100% marked improvement in 40% of alclometasone patients and 35% of hydrocortisone patients
Lebwohl et al. [31]	Randomized, evaluator-blind, parallel-group trial	0.1% mometasone furoate cream o.d. vs 0.2% hydrocortisone valerate cream b.d. for 3 weeks	Investigator assessed seven signs and symptoms on a 0–3 scale (0 = none, 3 = severe) and global assessment % improved	Mean improvement in severity score (no baselines given) at day 21 (% of patients with 100% clearance), 87.4% for mometasone and 79.7% for hydrocortisone valerate at Day 21
Lucky et al. [32]	Single-centre, randomized, parallel, open-label study	Desonide 0.05% ointment vs hydrocortisone 2.5% ointment b.d. for 4 weeks	Hypothalamic pituitary–adrenal (HPA) axis (cortisol levels)	−1.6 and −1.3% change in cortisol levels over baseline at 4 weeks for desonide and hydrocortisone groups, respectively
Marchesi et al. [33]	Randomized, third-party blind evaluator, parallel-group controlled trial	Mometasone furoate ointment 0.1% o.d. vs betamethasone dipropionate ointment 0.05% b.d. for 3 weeks	Investigator assessed erythema, induration and pruritus on a 0–3 scale, global evaluation % improvement	100% patients in both groups had experienced good improvement by week 3
Morley et al. [34]	Randomized, double-blind controlled trial	0.05% clobetasone butyrate cream or ointment b.d. vs 0.et al.% flurandrenolone cream or ointment b.d. for 1 week	Clinician-assessed lesions as healed, improved, static or worse plus clinician/ patient preference for right/left side	Data to assess effect of treatment absent
Msika et al. [35]	Randomized controlled trial	Corticosteroids with or without a new emollient cream	SCORAD and quality of life index	Twice-daily application of a new natural emollient proved to be a major steroid sparing alternative, improved the lichenification and excoriation and also, it improved the quality of life in children and their parents
Olholm Larsen et al. [36]	Randomized controlled trial	Mildison lipocream (1% hydrocortisone in 65/35% oil-in-water emulsion) bd vs Uniderm cream (1% hydrocortisone cream) b.d. for 4 weeks	SCORAD	Significant improvement in both groups

Oliveira et al. [37]	Randomized, double-blind, comparative trial	Mometasone furate 0.1% cream bd vs Desonide 0.5% cream o.d.	SCORAD and quality of life index	Significantly better outcome in mometasone group
Pei et al. [38]	Randomized, single-blind, controlled trial	wet-wrap dressings with 0.1% mometasone furoate and 0.005% fluticasone propionate ointments	SCORAD and global assessment score	Both were effective in the treatment of atopic dermatitis, and that wet wraps are useful in further improving refractory disease in children
Peserico et al. [39]	Double-blind, placebo-controlled, randomized, parallel-group study	Emollient with or without methylprednisolone aceponate (MPA) 0.1% cream twice weekly	Time to relapse, relapse rate and disease status, the patient's assessment of intensity of itch, the Eczema Area and Severity Index, the IGA score, affected body surface area, Dermatology Life Quality Index (DLQI) and children's DLQI (CDLQI), patient's and investigator's global assessment of response and patient's assessment of quality of sleep	MPA twice weekly plus an emollient provides an effective maintenance treatment regimen to control AD
Rafanelli et al. [40]	Randomized, third-party blind parallel-group trial	0.1% Mometasone furoate cream od vs 0.05% Clobetasone cream bd for 3 weeks	Pruritus, erythema and DLQI	Mometasone cream was very effective
Rajka et al. [41]	Randomized, double-blind, left–right comparison trial	Hydrocortisone 17-butyrate (Locid®) 0.1% fatty cream bd vs Desonide (Apolar®) 0.1% ointment bd for 4 weeks	Investigator assessed global severity and severity grades of erythema, induration and scaling	Mean global severity score over baseline of 2.8 reduced to 1.3 for hydrocortisone and 1.7 for desonide
Rampini et al. [42]	Randomized, double-blind trial	Methylprednisolone aceponate 0.1% cream b.d. vs prednicarbate 0.25% cream b.d.	Objective and subjective symptoms of erythema, exudation, scaling, hyperkeratosis, itching, burning Global therapeutic response	100% prednicarbate patients showed complete clearing compared to 97.3% of other group
Rampini et al. [42]	Randomized, double-blind trial	Methylprednisolone aceponate 0.1% o.d. ointment vs prednicarbate 0.25% cream b.d.	Objective and subjective symptoms of erythema, exudation, scaling, hyperkeratosis, itching, burning Global therapeutic response	98.1% prednicarbate patients showed complete clearing compared to 96.3% of other group
Reidhav et al. [43]	Randomized, double-blind controlled trial	Betamethasone valerate 0.1% cream od vs mometasone furoate 0.1% cream od for 4 weeks	Patient assessed pruritus and smarting pain on 0–3 scale, evaluator assessed erythema, scaling, lichenification, excoriation, papules, and vesicles	Both showed good improvement without any significant difference

(continued)

(continued)

Name of study	Type of study	Intervention	Outcome measures	Result
Richelli et al. [44]	Randomized parallel trial	Clobetasone 17-butyrate lotion b.d. (8 am and 3 pm) vs b.d. (3 pm and 8 pm) or o.d. (9 pm) for 3 weeks	Itching, burning, pain, erythema, oedema, exudation, blisters, bullae, scabs, scaling, lichenification, pooled into a mean score Serum cortisol and ACTH tests	No obvious differences between three groups
Rubio et al. [45]	Randomized controlled, double-blind trial	fluticasone propionate cream 0.05% bd vs vehicle cream bd for 16 weeks	Pruritus, erythema, scaling, excoriation, lichenification	Excellent improvement with fluticasone
Ruzicka et al. [46]	Randomized, double-blind controlled trial	mometasone furoate with a water content of 33% (Monovo® Cream) and with a smooth consistency versus the commercially available fatty cream of mometasone furoate (Ecural® Fettcreme)	efficacy, cosmetic properties, and patients' acceptance	new formulation was preferred by the patients
Savin et al. [47]	Randomized, double-blind controlled trial	Betamethasone dipropionate ointment 0.05% vs hydrocortisone ointment 1% b.d. for 3 weeks	Clinical effectiveness: excellent(>75%), good (50–75%), fair (25–50%), poor (<25%)	50% betamethasone 'excellent' or 'good' response compared with 22% hydrocortisone
Thomas et al. [48]	Randomized, double-blind, parallel clinical trial	1% hydrocortisone ointment bd vs 0.1% betamethasone valerate ointment bd for 3 days followed by white soft paraffin for four days	Scratch-free days, number of relapses, median duration of relapses, number of undisturbed nights, disease severity (six area, six sign atopic dermatitis severity scale), scores on two quality of life measures (children's life quality index and dermatitis family impact questionnaire), and number of patients in whom treatment failed in each arm	short burst of a potent topical corticosteroid is just as effective as prolonged use of a milder preparation
Torok et al. [49]	Investigator-blinded, parallel, randomized study	clocortolone pivalate cream 0.1% (Cloderm® Cream 0.1%) and tacrolimus ointment 0.1% (Protopic Ointment 0.1%) bd vs clocortolone pivalate cream 0.1% bd vs tacrolimus ointment 0.1% bd	Global response	Concomitant therapy minimized the adverse effects of both treatments taken alone and potentially improved overall response

Traulsen et al. [50]	Randomized, double-blind, left–right comparison trial	Hydrocortisone buteprate cream 0.1% o.d. vs betamethasone valerate 0.1% cream o.d. for 2 weeks	Erythema, infiltration, lichenification, scaling, vesiculation, papules, excoriations and pruritus on a 0–4 scale Patient-assessed efficacy and investigator global assessment	There were no significant differences between the two treatments
Trookman et al. [51]	Single-centre, randomized, evaluator-blinded, parallel-comparison, non-inferiority study	Desonide gel 0.05% bd vs desonide ointment 0.05% bd for 4 weeks	Disease severity, body surface area involvement, subjective assessments of symptoms, corneometry, transepidermal water loss, and the patient's preference for vehicle attributes	Desonide hydrogel was preferred by patients
Ulrich et al. [52]	Randomized, double-blind study	0.05% Halometasone cream b.d. vs 0.25% Prednicarbate cream b.d. (both topical steroids) for 2 weeks	Clinical effectiveness (doctor-assessed, fivepoint scale), onset of clinical effectiveness (doctor-assessed), adverse effects and cosmetic acceptability (patient-assessed fivepoint scale)	Clinical effectiveness: no significant difference between groups; onset: no difference at Day 1 or 4 between groups; adverse effects: none reported and cosmetic acceptability: 51% vs 46% rated it 'excellent'
Veien et al. [53]	Randomized, double-blind, left–right comparison trial	Hydrocortisone 17-butyrate (Locoid) cream 0.1% vs hydrocortisone (Uniderm) 1% cream for 4 weeks	Global severity of all lesions	Complete clearance of skin symptoms was found in 60% hydrocortisone 17-butyrate-treated patients compared with 30% hydrocortisone 1% treated patients
Vernon et al. [54]	Randomized, double-blind parallel-group trial	Mometasone furoate 0.1% cream vs hydrocortisone 1.0% cream o.d. for 6 weeks	Doctor-assessed erythema, lichenification, skin surface disruption (crusting, scaling), excoriation, and pruritus on a 0–3 scale, % body surface area and global evaluation	Mean percentage improvement in total sign/symptom score was 95% for mometasone vs 75% for hydrocortisone
Wolkerstorfer et al. [55]	Randomized, double/single-blind/open/cluster, controlled trial	Fluticasone propionate 0.05% cream o.d. vs clobetasone butyrate 0.05% cream b.d. for 4 weeks	SCORAD composite scale of extent and intensity of eight signs	At week 4, three fluticasone patients and one clobetasone patient clinically healed
Yasuda et al. [56]	Randomized, double-blind study	Hydrocortisone 17-butyrate 0.1% loemeid ointment vs triamcinolone acetonide 0.1% ointment or hydrocortisone acetate 1% ointment for 1 week	Decrease in erythema, scaling, oedema, subjective symptoms such as pruritus and burning sensation and improvement of lesions	Hydrocortisone 17-B superior to triamcinolone and comparable to hydrocortisone

(continued)

The aforementioned trials showed remarkable improvement in 13–100% of patients, following treatment with TCs for 1–12 weeks. Nineteen studies showed significantly better response to topical corticosteroids, when compared with placebo. To be precise, the older trials (in terms of the year they were published) showed more favourable response to TCs. On the other hand, three studies could not demonstrate a significant difference between the groups receiving topical corticosteroids and placebo. Five RCTs have clearly demonstrated that the number of acute episodes of flare can be significantly reduced by intermittent treatment with a potent topical corticosteroid. Three RCTs and two small within-patient comparison studies have investigated the role of wet-wrap bandages on the top of TCs. To summarize, we cannot recommend the 'best' TC, because there is not a single RCT, which has compared the effectiveness, safety and tolerability of all the available preparations of similar potency. Besides, there is no high-level scientific evidence supporting the application of twice-daily over once-daily TCs. However, it can be definitely concluded that application of twice-weekly potent TC to cases of stable eczema can significantly reduce the number of acute episodes in adults and children. However, the long-term safety profile of such intermittent therapy is yet to be found [57].

In a systematic review of treatments for atopic eczema, short term randomized controlled trials evaluated the effects of topical corticosteroids on pituitary–adrenal axis. It must be noted that these studies could not demonstrate any harm on the axis [58]. There is no high-level scientific evidence that correct use of topical steroids (proper potency, duration and amount) can lead to thinning of skin.

4.2.2 Vitiligo

Vitiligo is an acquired cutaneous disorder of pigmentation, characterized by destruction of melanocytes. Available therapeutic modalities include topical and systemic corticosteroids, topical immunomodulators, photo(chemo)therapy, surgery and depigmentation of normally pigmented skin. Immunosuppressive therapy with highly potent topical corticosteroids (clobetasol) gives excellent results in cases of localized stable vitiligo [59–61].

In this section, we have tabulated the evidences available in favour of using topical corticosteroids in vitiligo.

Name of study	Type of study	Intervention	Outcome measures	Result
Koopmans-van Dorp et al. [62]	Randomized controlled trial	Betamethasone 17-valerate in a dimethyl sulfoxide cream base vs placebo	Repigmentation in the vitiliginous areas	42% patients receiving steroids showed excellent repigmentation
Bleehen et al. [63]	Randomized controlled trial	0.1% betamethasone valerate (BV) or with 0.05% clobetasol propionate (CP) creams vs placebo for 3 months	Repigmentation in the vitiliginous areas	Excellent results with topical steroids
Clayton et al. [64]	Randomized double-blind controlled trial	0.05% clobetasol propionate in a cream base vs cream base alone	Repigmentation in the vitiliginous areas	Active product was significantly superior to the cream base alone
Kandil et al. [65]	Randomized controlled trial	0.1% betamethasone valerate in 50% isopropyl alcohol vs alcohol base	Repigmentation in the vitiliginous areas	Higher percentage of lesions had complete repigmentation with active product in comparison to placebo

Lepe et al. [66]	Randomized double-blind trial	0.1% tacrolimus vs 0.05% clobetasol	Characteristics of pigment, time of response, symptoms, telangiectasias, and atrophy	Tacrolimus and clobetasol propionate, both were equally effective
Sanclemente et al. [67]	Randomized, matched-paired, double-blind trial	0.05% betamethasone vs. topical catalase/dismutase superoxide (C/DSO) for 10 months	Skin repigmentation by digital morphometry	Topical C/DSO and 0.05% betamethasone, both showed good results
Kumaran et al. [68]	Randomized trial	Betamethasone dipropionate (0.05%) cream bd vs calcipotriol ointment (0.005%) bd vs betamethasone dipropionate (0.05%) in the morning and calcipotriol (0.005%) in the evening	Skin repigmentation by digital morphometry	Combined therapy showed faster and stable repigmentation and with lesser side effects
Xing et al. [69]	Open, uncontrolled trial	topical calcipotriol 0.005%vs betamethasone dipropionate 0.05% ointment bd for 12 weeks	Skin repigmentation by digital morphometry	Calcipotriene 0.005% and betamethasone dipropionate 0.05% ointment is effective
Agarwal et al. [70]	Randomized, placebo-controlled, double-blind, parallel study	oral levamisole (150 mg for adults and 100 mg for children) on 2 consecutive days in a week plus mometasone furoate cream (0.1%) once a day vs oral placebo plus mometasone furoate cream once a day for 6 months	Cessation of spread of vitiligo. DLQI, CDLQI, World Health Organization Quality of Life Brief Questionnaire	Levamisole was not much effective in arresting disease progression. Cessation of spread of disease was similar in both groups (both received mometasone)
Akdeniz et al. [71]	Randomized parallel-group study	Topical calcipotriol, NB-UVB, and betamethasone (1) vs NB-UVB and topical calcipotriol (2) vs NBUVB alone (3) for 6 months	Percentage improvement in repigmentation, DLQI and VAS	Statistically significant difference between groups 1 and 3
Kathuria et al. [72]	Randomized parallel-group study	0.1% tacrolimus ointment twice daily vs 0.05% fluticasone propionate cream once daily for 6 months	Percentage of repigmentation	Both tacrolimus and fluticasone propionate produced variable results in segmental vitiligo
Khalid et al. [73]	Randomized parallel-group study	Topical PUVAsol vs clobetasol propionate (0.05%) cream bd for 6 months. Each group received treatment for 6 weeks followed by a gap of 2 weeks	Repigmentation	Clobetasol showed favourable response
Köse et al. [74]	Randomized parallel-group study	0.1% mometasone furoate cream (M-Furo) once daily vs 1% pimecrolimus cream (Elidel) twice daily for 12 weeks	Degree of repigmentation	Mometasone cream was found to be effective in vitiligo on any part of the body but Pimecrolimus was effective on the face only, in childhood localized vitiligo

(continued)

(continued)

Name of study	Type of study	Intervention	Outcome measures	Result
Lim-Ong et al. [75]	Randomized, double-blind, placebo-controlled, within-participants, left/right comparison study	Clobetasol propionate ointment and NBUVB vs placebo and NBUVB for 6 months	Repigmentation and Cessation of spread	Group receiving clobetasol showed better response
Sassi et al. [76]	Randomized parallel-group study	308 nm laser phototherapy twice weekly in combination with hydrocortisone 17-butyrate cream twice daily vs 308 nm laser phototherapy twice weekly alone	Percentage repigmentation and Patient-rated quality of life: Skindex-29	Recalcitrant vitiligo of face and neck showed good results with combination of excimer laser phototherapy with topical hydrocortisone 17-butyrate cream
Wazir et al. [77]	Randomized parallel-group study	Topical mometasone furoate 0.01% ointment vs Topical tacrolimus 0.03% ointment and mometasone furoate 0.01% for 6 months	Repigmentation measured by comparing the treated areas with pretreatment photographs with responses graded on a scale from 0–5	Mometasone when combined with tacrolimus showed good results
Westerhof et al. [78]	Randomized, parallel-group, left/right comparison study	Fluticasone propionate 0.5% (FP) alone on one side of the body and FP + UVA on the other vs UVA alone on one side, and FP + UVA on the other for 9 months	Repigmentation	Combination treatment with FP and UV-A is much more effective in reaching complete repigmentation than are FP and UV-A used alone
Yaghoobi et al. [79]	Randomized parallel-group study	0.05% clobetasol propionate cream in isopropyl alcohol 65° preparation (in equal proportion) for the body and 0.1% triamcinolone acetonide cream for the face and flexures, used twice daily vs 0.05% clobetasol propionate cream in isopropyl alcohol 65° preparation (in equal proportion) for the body and 0.1% triamcinolone acetonide cream for the face and flexures with oral zinc sulphate capsules for 4 months	Percentage of repigmentation, assessed at 1, 3, 4 months after beginning of treatment	Clobetasol, triamcinolone and zinc showed excellent results in vitiligo

A meta-analysis, an additional systematic review, and several RCTs showed that class 3 TCs are effective in comparison with placebo, either alone or more so in combination with NB-UVB, or psoralen plus UVA light (using sunlight or artificial light sources), in treating generalized and localized vitiligo. There is some RCT evidence that topical clobetasol propionate is of equivalent effectiveness with tacrolimus in treating this condition. All studies examining the effect of TCs reported adverse effects, with the more frequent being atrophy, telangiectasia, hypertrichosis and acneiform papules [80].

4.2.3   Psoriasis

Topical steroids are used since ages to treat mild-to-moderate plaque psoriasis. These are available in different potencies and formulations but their use relies mostly on the basis of individual experience. Here is a brief summary of evidences in favour of using topical steroids in psoriasis [81, 82].

Name of study	Type of study	Intervention	Outcome measures	Result
Shupack et al. [83]	Randomized double-blind, parallel clinical trial	Diflorasone diacetate ointment 0.05% versus betamethasone dipropionate ointment 0.05%	Erythema, scaling, induration or the investigator's global evaluation	Both showed good results but no statistically significant difference between the two groups with respect to erythema, scaling, induration or the investigator's global evaluation
Sears et al. [84]	Double-blind, randomized, placebo-controlled	Hydrocortisone buteprate 0.1% cream vs placebo	Erythema, scaling, induration or the investigator's global evaluation	Hydrocortisone group showed good results
Peharda et al. [85]	Randomized double-blind, parallel clinical trial	Mometasone furoate 0.1% ointment and betamethasone dipropionate 0.05% ointment	Erythema, scaling, induration or the investigator's global evaluation	Both showed good results but betamethasone group was better
Lebwohl et al. [86]	Randomized, double-blind, placebo-controlled study	Clobetasol propionate 0.05% foam bd vs placebo	Investigator's and subject's global assessment of the response and severity of erythema, scaling, and plaque thickness	Clobetasol propionate foam is more effective than placebo in the treatment of non-scalp psoriasis
Koo et al. [87]	Randomized, controlled, double-masked, parallel-group, multicentre	Mometasone furoate 0.1%-salicylic acid 5% ointment versus mometasone furoate 0.1%ointment	Severity of erythema, induration, and scaling	Mometasone furoate-salicylic acid ointment provides more effective treatment of moderate-to-severe psoriasis than does mometasone furoate ointment alone and is safe and well tolerated
Medansky et al. [88]	Single-centre, randomized, double-masked, intraindividual, bilateral-paired comparative trial	Mometasone furoate 0.1%-salicylic acid 5% ointment twice daily versus fluocinonide 0.05%ointment twice daily for 21 days	Signs of psoriasis (i.e., erythema, induration, and scaling) and overall clinical response	Mometasone furoate 0.1%-salicylic acid 5% ointment was more efficacious than and equally as safe as fluocinonide 0.05% ointment

(continued)

(continued)

Name of study	Type of study	Intervention	Outcome measures	Result
Tiplica et al. [89]	Randomized, parallel multicentre trial	Mometasone furoate 0.1% and salicylic acid 5% for 7 days followed by mometasone furoate 0.1% for 14 days vs mometasone furoate 0.1% for 21 days	Psoriasis Area Severity Index (PASI) score and Dermatology Life Quality Index (DLQI)	The sequential treatment mometasone furoate 0.1% and salicylic acid 5% followed by mometasone furoate 0.1% proves to be efficient, safe and an excellent option and better than the other group
Guenther et al. [90]	Multicentre, investigator-blinded, parallel-group study	Tazarotene 0.1% gel once daily plus mometasone furoate 0.1% cream once daily versus calcipotriene 0.005% ointment twice daily for 8 weeks	Global improvement, plaque elevation, scaling, erythema, and percentage of body surface area involvement, efficacy of study treatment compared with previous therapies, comfort of treated skin, outlook for long-term control of psoriasis, and overall impression of treatment	Both groups showed excellent response, but the one receiving both tazarotene and mometasone was better
Green et al. [91]	Multicentre, investigator-masked, randomized, parallel-group	Tazarotene 0.1% gel alone vs tazarotene plus a high-potency topical corticosteroid (fluocinonide 0.05% ointment, mometasone furoate 0.1% ointment, or diflorasone diacetate 0.05% ointment), vs tazarotene plus a mid-high-potency topical corticosteroid (betamethasone dipropionate 0.05% cream, fluticasone propionate 0.005% ointment, or diflorasone diacetate 0.05% cream) all applied once daily for 12 weeks	Global improvement, plaque elevation, scaling, erythema, and pruritus. Patients also rated their treatment in terms of efficacy, tolerability and satisfaction	Betamethasone dipropionate 0.05% cream (a mid-high-potency steroid) was the best option followed by mometasone furoate 0.1% ointment (a high-potency steroid) and diflorasone diacetate 0.05% ointment (a high-potency steroid)
Katz et al. [92]	Randomized, prospective double-blind bilateral comparative clinical trial	Fluocinonide 0.05% cream (Lidex) vs fluocinonide 0.05% cream (Vasoderm)	Reduction in erythema, induration, scale and overall severity	Lidex' cream demonstrated significantly greater reduction in erythema, induration, scale and overall severity in psoriatic activity

Koo et al. [93]	Randomized, multicentre sequential study	Clobetasol foam plus calcipotriene ointment or either agent as monotherapy for 2 weeks	Reduction in erythema, induration, scale and overall severity	combination of clobetasol foam and calcipotriene ointment is significantly more effective than monotherapy for short-term treatment
Ellis et al. [94]	Multicentre, evaluator-blind, parallel-group study	New formulation of betamethasone dipropionate 0.05% cream, augmented formulation (AF), od vs fluocinonide 0.05% cream bd	Erythema, induration, and scaling, as well as the physicians' and patients' global evaluations of response	Results significantly favoured betamethasone dipropionate AF over fluocinonide
Greenspan et al. [95]	Double-blind, randomized, parallel study	0.05% desonide lotion vs 0.05% desonide cream tds for 3 weeks	Reduction in erythema, induration, scale and overall severity	New lotion formulation of desonide was equivalent in both efficacy and safety to a 0.05% cream formulation
Frost et al. [96]	Double-blind, randomized, parallel-group	Alclometasone dipropionate vs desonide ointments (0.05%) bd for 3 weeks	Erythema, induration and scaling	Both showed excellent results but differences between the groups were not statistically significant, but trends consistently favoured alclometasone
Cornell et al. [97]	Randomized, parallel-group, double-blind study	Amcinonide ointment 0.1 percent twice daily and fluocinonide ointment 0.05 percent three times daily for 2 weeks	Erythema, induration and scaling	Amcinonide ointment 0.1 percent applied twice a day was found to be as effective and acceptable to patients as was fluocinonide ointment 0.05 percent applied three times a day in the treatment of psoriasis
Angelo et al. [98]	Double-blind, randomized, right-left comparison study	Once-daily tazarotene 0.1% cream with that of once-daily clobetasol propionate 0.05% cream for 12 weeks	Erythema, induration and scaling	Topical tazarotene 0.1% cream was less effective than topical clobetasol propionate 0.05% cream in the treatment of plaque psoriasis

(continued)

(continued)

Name of study	Type of study	Intervention	Outcome measures	Result
Senter et al. [99]	Double-masked, randomized, concurrently controlled clinical trial	Once-daily fluocinonide (Lidex), combined with three-times-a-day application of its vehicle vs four-times-a-day Lidex for 4 weeks	Erythema, induration and scaling	Once-a-day application of fluocinonide was equally effective as four-times-a-day application
Bernhard et al. [100]	Randomized, double-blind, and vehicle-controlled	0.05% halobetasol ointment over vehicle bd for 2 weeks	Plaque elevation, erythema and scaling	0.05% halobetasol ointment was much favourable than the vehicle
Fleming et al. [101]	Randomized, parallel-group, double-blind, exploratory study	Calcipotriol plus betamethasone dipropionate gel compared with its active components in the same vehicle and the vehicle alone	Erythema, induration and scaling	Two-compound gel was safe and more efficacious than its individual ingredients
Gottlieb et al. [102]	Multicentre, randomized, double-blinded, placebo-controlled study	Clobetasol propionate foam 0.05% bd vs placebo for 2 weeks	Erythema, induration and scaling, Patient's Global Assessment score	Clobetasol propionate foam 0.05% is safe and effective for the treatment of plaque-type psoriasis
Jarratt et al. [103]	Multicentre, randomized, double-blinded, vehicle-controlled, parallel-group, comparative study	Clobetasol propionate spray 0.05% vs vehicle for 4 weeks	Scaling, erythema, plaque elevation, pruritus and overall disease severity	Clobetasol propionate spray 0.05% administered twice daily for 4 weeks was effective and safe
Kaufmann et al. [104]	Randomized double-blind study	Combination ointment with betamethasone dipropionate ointment, calcipotriol ointment and ointment vehicle	Scaling, erythema, plaque elevation, pruritus and overall disease severity	Calcipotriol/ betamethasone dipropionate combination ointment used once daily is well tolerated and more effective than either active constituent used alone
Mraz et al. [105]	Randomized parallel clinical study	Clobetasol propionate (CP) 0.05% (Clobex Spray; Galderma Laboratories, L.P., Fort Worth, TX, USA vs Olux Foam; Stiefel/ Connetics Corp., Coral Gables, FL, USA)	Scaling, erythema, plaque elevation, pruritus and overall disease severity, DLQI	Spray was better than foam
Singh et al. [106]	Randomized, observer-blind clinical trial	Augmented betamethasone dipropionate 0.05% cream once daily in the first and third weeks and calcipotriene 0.005% ointment twice daily in the second and fourth weeks. Vs augmented betamethasone once daily for 4 weeks	Scaling, erythema, plaque elevation, pruritus and overall disease severity, DLQI, PASI	Use of augmented betamethasone and calcipotriene on alternate weeks was more effective than daily corticosteroid

Stein et al. [107]	Randomized, double-blind, placebo-controlled, paired-comparison, split-body study	*Betamethasone Valerate Foam* Vs placebo bd for 12 weeks	Scaling, erythema, plaque elevation, pruritus and overall disease severity	*Betamethasone Valerate Foam* Was highly effective
Aggerwal et al. [108]	Randomized parallel-group design, evaluator-blind clinical study	Alclometasone cream 0.05% and clobetasone butyrate cream 0.5% bd for 3 weeks	Erythema, induration and scaling, physician's global assessment	alclometasone and clobetasone had comparable efficacy and safety
Blum et al. [109]	Double-blind, parallel-group, multicentre comparative trial	0.05% halobetasol propionate ointment and 0.1% betamethasone valerate ointment	Erythema, induration and scaling	0.05% halobetasol propionate ointment proved significantly superior
Choonhakarn et al. [110]	Randomized, comparative, double-blind trial	Topical aloevera (AV) cream vs 0.1% triamcinolone cetonide (TA) cream	Psoriasis Area Severity Index (PASI) and the Dermatology Life Quality Index (DLQI)	AV cream may be more effective than 0.1% TA cream
Decroix et al. [111]	Randomized, controlled comparative, double-blind trial	Clobetasol propionate lotion vs vehicle bd for 4 weeks	Erythema, induration and scaling, Dermatology Life Quality Index (DLQI)	Clobetasol propionate lotion was efficient, safe, and well tolerated
Fredriksson et al. [112]	Randomized, comparative, double-blind, left–right trial	Budesonide vs and betamethasone-17,21-dipropionate	Itching, scaling, erythema and induration were recorded on a 5-point scale	Statistically significant results favouring the budesonide ointment were obtained
Goldberg et al. [113]	Randomized double-blind, parallel-group, multicentre trial	0.05% halobetasol propionate ointment vs 0.05% clobetasol propionate ointment for 2 weeks	Itching, scaling, erythema and induration	Halobetasol was superior to clobetasol
Jacobson et al. [114]	Randomized double-blind, parallel-group, comparative trial	Clobetasol propionate 0.05 percent ointment vs betamethasone dipropionate 0.05 percent ointment	Itching, scaling, erythema and induration	Clobetasol was better
Jegasothy et al. [115]	Randomized double-blind, parallel comparison study	0.05% clobetasol propionate cream and 0.05% fluocinonide cream for 2 weeks	Investigators' overall judgement of clinical response, degree of severity of specific signs and symptoms, and patients' evaluation of improvement	Clobetasol was statistically significantly superior to fluocinonide
Krueger et al. [116]	Investigator-blinded, randomized, bilateral paired-comparison study	flurandrenolide (4 microg/cm2) tape versus 0.05% diflorasone diacetate ointment	Erythema, scaling, induration and treatment success	The efficacy of flurandrenolide tape in the treatment of psoriatic plaques surpasses that of diflorasone diacetate ointment.

(continued)

(continued)

Name of study	Type of study	Intervention	Outcome measures	Result
Kuokkanen et al. [117]	Randomized double-blind comparative trial	0.25% desoximetasone ointment with 0.05% fluocinonide ointment bd for 2 weeks	Erythema, scaling and induration	Desoximetasone-treated side showed a significantly better improvement than on the fluocinonide-treated side
Leibsohn et al. [118]	Randomized double-blind comparative trial	Diflorasone diacetate ointment 0.05% or betamethasone dipropionate ointment 0.05% twice a day for 3 weeks	Erythema, oedema, lichenification, induration, scaliness, excoriations, pruritus and soreness	Both medications were effective and statistically significant differences existed between treatment groups
Lowe et al. [119]	Multicentre, investigator-blind, randomized, active- and vehicle-controlled, parallel-group study	clobetasol propionate lotion compared vs clobetasol pro'ionate emollient cream vs vehicle for 4 weeks	Erythema, scaling and induration, DLQI	Clobetasol propionate lotion was significantly more effective than vehicle lotion and was comparable in efficacy to the emollient cream
Mensing et al. [120]	Double-blind, parallel-group, multicentre comparative trial	0.05% halobetasol propionate ointment and 0.05% betamethasone dipropionate ointment bd for 4 weeks	Erythema, scaling and induration	Halobetasol was superior
Molin et al. [121]	Randomized multicentre double-blind, parallel-group study	Calcipotriol, 50 micrograms/g, in a cream formulation vs betamethasone 17-valerate cream for 8 weeks	Erythema, scaling and induration, PASI, DLQI	Both were effective but there was no statistically significant difference
Olsen et al. [122]	Multicentre, double-blind, randomized, vehicle-controlled parallel-group trial	Fluticasone propionate 0.005% ointment vs placebo bd for 4 weeks	Erythema, scaling and induration	Fluticasone ointment was clearly shown to be superior
Roberts et al. [123]	Randomized, double-blind, parallel-group, multicentre study	Fluticasone propionate ointment, 0.005%, and betamethasone-17,21-dipropionate ointment, 0.05% for 12 weeks	Erythema, scaling and induration	Fluticasone ointment, 0.005%, was not significantly different from betamethasone ointment, 0.05%
Bruce et al. [124]	Randomized, double-blind, parallel-group, active-controlled trial	Calcipotriene ointment 0.005% versus fluocinonide ointment 0.05% bd for 6 weeks	Scaling, erythema, plaque elevation, and for overall disease severity, physician's global assessment	Calcipotriene was superior to fluocinonide
Fabry et al. [125]	Multicentre, between-patient, comparative trial	0.05 halometasone ointment vs ointment, containing 0.25% fluocortolone +0.25% fluocortolone caproate	Scaling, erythema, plaque elevation, and for overall disease severity, physician's global assessment	Halometasone ointment yielded a higher success rate
Huntley et al. [126]	Randomized, double-blind study	Amcinonide vs betamethasone dipropionate ointments, bd for two weeks	Scaling, erythema, plaque elevation	Both groups showed good response

To summarize, both class III and class IV TCs are very effective in inducing remission, but class IV appears superior. It remains unclear whether once- or twice-daily dosing is to be recommended, but frequency as well as duration should be tapered down in a maintenance phase because of concerns with cutaneous and systemic adverse effects. Of the cutaneous complications, skin atrophy is the commonest, but it is less of an issue in psoriatics than with, say, atopics. However, the continuous use of very potent or ultrapotent TCs may cause irreversible skin atrophy and striae, may cause psoriasis to become unstable, and may have systemic effects when used over a large surface area [127]. The ointment formulations appear to be the most effective, but there are many alternative galenicals to increase feasibility and treatment adherence without losing too much effectiveness [128].

Scalp psoriasis, though responds to a wide array of topical therapies but topical corticosteroids form the first line of management and the response is excellent [81, 82]. The evidences in favour of steroids are tabulated below:

Name of study	Type of study	Intervention	Outcome measures	Result
Olsen et al. [128]	Double-blind vehicle-controlled parallel-group study	Clobetasol propionate 0.05% vs placebo bd for 2 weeks	Scaling, erythema, plaque elevation, morning plasma cortisol	Clobetasol propionate 0.05% scalp application appears to be a safe and an effective treatment for scalp psoriasis
Ellis et al. [129]	Double-blind vehicle-controlled parallel-group study	Amcinonide lotion 0.1% vs placebo bd	Scaling, erythema, plaque elevation	Amcinonide lotion 0.1% is effective treatment
Franz et al. [130]	Randomized, multicentre, double-blind, active-and placebo-controlled trial	Betamethasone valerate foam 0.12% vs placebo bd for 4 weeks	Scaling, erythema, plaque elevation, suppression of the hypothalamic–pituitary–adrenal (HPA) axis	The novel foam formulation with enhanced betamethasone valerate bioavailability had greater efficacy in the treatment of scalp psoriasis without an increased toxicity
Katz et al. [131]	Randomized, multicentre, investigator-blinded, parallel-group study	Twice-daily augmented betamethasone dipropionate 0.05% lotion vs clobetasol propionate 0.05% solution for 2 weeks	Erythema, pruritus, induration, scaling, global clinical response	Both were equally effective, but betamethasone dipropionate lotion provided a faster onset of relief for scaling and induration
Van De Kerkhof et al. [132]	Randomized, multicentre, double-blind, parallel-group study	Calcipotriol plus betamethasone dipropionate vs calcipotriol vs betamethasone dipropionate bd for 8 weeks	Erythema, pruritus, induration, scaling, global clinical response	Two-compound scalp formulation was well tolerated and more effective
Willis et al. [133]	Randomized, double-blind, multicentre study	Desoximetasone gel 0.05% vs fluocinonide gel 0.05% bd	Erythema, pruritus, induration, scaling	Both were equally effective but desoximetasone was slightly better tolerated
Rey gagne et al. [134]	Multicentre, randomized, investigator-masked, parallel-group study	Clobetasol propionate shampoo 0.05% vs calcipotriol solution 0.005%	Erythema, pruritus, induration, scaling, global clinical response	Clobetasol propionate demonstrated significantly superior efficacy to calcipotriol solution

(continued)

(continued)

Name of study	Type of study	Intervention	Outcome measures	Result
Pauporte et al. [135]	Randomized, double-blind, vehicle-controlled multicentre study	Fluocinolone acetonide 0.01% in oil vs placebo for 3 weeks	Erythema, pruritus, induration, scaling, global clinical response	Fluocinolone group had significantly better response
Klaber et al. [136]	Multicentre, prospective, randomized, double-blind, parallel-group study	Calcipotriol Solution (50 Micrograms/Ml) and Betamethasone 17-Valerate Solution (1 Mg/Ml) bd for 4 weeks	Erythema, pruritus, induration, scaling, global clinical response	Betamethasone group was significantly better
Jemec et al. [137]	Multicentre, randomized, double-blind study	*Calcipotriene plus betamethasone vs calcipotriene vs betamethasone vs placebo bd for 8 weeks*	Erythema, pruritus, induration, scaling, global clinical response	Calcipotriene plus betamethasone dipropionate scalp formulation was more effective than either of the individual components or the vehicle alone
Jarratt et al. [138]	Multicentre, randomized, vehicle-controlled, double-masked and parallel-group study	Clobetasol propionate shampoo 0.05% vs placebo for 4 weeks	Erythema, pruritus, induration, scaling, global clinical response	The novel short contact shampoo formulation of clobetasol propionate was efficacious, safe and well tolerated
Feldman et al. [139]	Randomized, single-blind, open-label study	Betamethasone valerate in foam vehicle od vs bd for 4 weeks	Erythema, pruritus, induration, scaling	BMV foam was effective with both once-a-day and twice-a-day use
Duweb et al. [140]	Randomized, double-blind clinical study	Topical calcipotriol 50 micrograms/g/ml solution vs. betamethasone valerate 1% lotion bd for 6 weeks	Thickness, redness, scaliness of plaque	Both drugs were effective and well tolerated
Buckley et al. [141]	Randomized, double-blind clinical study	Calcipotriol plus Betamethasone Dipropionate Scalp Formulation Vs betamethasone od for 8 weeks	Thickness, redness, scaliness of plaque	Calcipotriol plus betamethasone dipropionate scalp formulation was superior to betamethasone dipropionate alone
Andreassi et al. [142]	Open, investigator-blinded, multicentre, randomized, crossover study	Betamethasone valerate mousse (BVM) vs standard therapies (steroid or calcipotriol)	Erythema, pruritus, induration, scaling,	BVM is more effective than lotion-based standard therapy

The results in scalp psoriasis are similar to that seen in chronic plaque psoriasis elsewhere in the body.

4.2.4 Lichen Planus

Lichen planus (LP) is a common chronic inflammatory dermatosis associated with cell-mediated immunological dysfunction. Cutaneous lesions are often intensely pruritic and require rigorous intervention. Besides, symptomatic oral LP is painful and complete healing is rare, which necessitates active intervention. Topical corticosteroids are conventionally used as first-line therapy in cutaneous lichen planus, but high-level scientific evidence is absent. However, topical corticosteroids show good results in oral lichen planus and the evidences have been summarized below [143–146].

Name of study	Type of study	Intervention	Outcome measures	Result
Voute et al. [147]	Randomized, placebo-controlled, parallel clinical trial	Fluocinonide in adhesive cream (0.025%) vs placebo 6 times a day for 9 weeks	Pain and clinical score	Fluocinonide group showed excellent results
Conrotto et al. [148]	Double-blind, randomized controlled trial	Topical clobetasol propionate 0.025% in hydroxy ethyl cellulose bd vs topical ciclosporin 1.5% in hydroxy ethyl cellulose bd for 2 months	Pain and clinical score, adverse effects	Clobetasol was more effective than ciclosporin in inducing clinical improvement but it was associated with higher incidence of side effects
Yoke et al. [149]	Double-blind, randomized controlled trial	Topical ciclosporin solution 0.1% tds vs triamcinolone acetonide 0.1% in Orabase tds for 8 weeks	Pain and clinical score	Triamcinolone group showed better results
Gorouhi et al. [150]	Investigator-blinded parallel-group randomized clinical trial	Pimecrolimus 1% cream qid vs: triamcinolone acetonide 0.1% paste qid for 2 months	Pain, clinical score and quality of life	Both topical pimecrolimus and triamcinolone acetonide therapy showed excellent results
Corrocher et al. [151]	Randomized, double-blind, clinical trial	Topical tacrolimus 0.1% ointment 2 mL qid vs topical clobetasol 0.05% ointment 2 mL qid for 4 weeks	Pain severity, burning sensation, and mucosal lesion extension	Tacrolimus 0.1% ointment was more effective than clobetasol propionate 0.05% ointment
Laeijendecker et al. [152]	Randomized, double-blind, clinical trial	Tacrolimus 0.1% ointment qid vs triamcinolone acetonide 0.1% in hypromellose 20% ointment qid for 6 weeks	Clinical score, adverse effects	Topical tacrolimus 0.1% ointment induced a better initial therapeutic response than triamcinolone acetonide 0.1% ointment but it was associated with frequent relapses
Hegarty et al. [153]	Randomized, crossover study	Sequence fluticasone (FP) and betamethasone (BSP) vs sequence betamethasone and fluticasone (Fluticasone spray (50 lg), 2 puffs applied to lesions 4 times daily, for 6 weeks and betamethasone sodium phosphate 500 lg (0.5 mg in 10 mL water), 3 min mouth rinse 4 times daily, for 6 weeks)	Pain, clinical score, quality of life, adverse effects	FP and BSP were both effective but FP was more acceptable
Rodstrom et al. [154]	Randomized double-blind clinical trial	Clobetasol propionate 0.05% in Orabase (50/50) twice a day for the first 3 weeks, once a day for the second 3 weeks, once every other day for the third 3 weeks vs triamcinolone acetonide 0Æ1% ointment twice a day for the first 3 weeks, once a day for the second 3 weeks, once every other day for the third 3 weeks (total 9 weeks)	Pain, clinical score, quality of life, adverse effects	Clobetasol propionate was found to be more effective than triamcinolone acetonide with respect to clinical improvement at the end of 3 weeks but at the end of 6 weeks, no significant difference was found

(continued)

(continued)

Name of study	Type of study	Intervention	Outcome measures	Result
Campisi et al. [155]	Randomized controlled single-blind phase IV clinical trial	Topical clobetasol propionate in microspheres 0.025%, two applications daily for the first month and one application daily for the second month vs topical clobetasol propionate 0.025% in a dispersion of a lipophilic ointment in a hydrophilic phase, two applications daily for the first month and one application daily for the second month	Pain and clinical score	New topical drug delivery system increased symptom remission, compliance and effectiveness of clobetasol propionate
Carbone et al. [156]	Randomized, double-blind, placebo-controlled trial	Topical clobetasol 0.025% in hydroxy ethyl cellulose bd vs topical clobetasol 0.05% in hydroxy ethyl cellulose bd for 2 months	Pain, clinical score, relapses, adverse effects	Both showed excellent results, without any statistically significant difference
Malhotra et al. [157]	Randomized comparative study	Betamethasone 5 mg as a single daily dose orally on 2 consecutive days every week (3 months), then 4 mg (1 month), then 3 mg (1 month), then 2 mg (1 month) vs topical triamcinolone acetonide (0.1%) paste	Pain, clinical score, adverse effects	Betamethasone OMP showed faster response
Ghabanchi et al. [158]	Randomized comparative study	Mucoadhesive prednisolone tablet (5 mg) bd vs triamcinolone acetonide paste (0.1%) tds for 2 weeks	Clinical score	Both were equally effective

There is no evidence for the efficacy of TCs in cutaneous LP, although it is usually recommended as the first-line treatment [159]. This an indicator of the fact that, like several other more uncommon inflammatory dermatoses, in LP too, the use of TCs is fairly undocumented, but not necessarily unwarranted, as the advent of TC as a group of agents happened in the age of empiricism when the use of medicines was dictated by hypothetical reasoning rather than being guided by evidence generated from RCTs.

Only limited evidence exists for the efficacy of TCs in oral LP. Also there is no evidence that topical calcineurin inhibitors are more effective than TCs in oral LP [160].

4.2.5 Mycosis Fungoides

The commonest form of cutaneous T-cell lymphoma (CTCL) is mycosis fungoides (MF), which accounts for approximately 60% of cases. Several reviews and guidelines on the management of mycosis fungoides have been published. Topical corticosteroids (lotions, creams or ointments) have been successfully used in the treatment of mild, patch-stage MF [161] but evidence in the favour of using them is lacking [162].

The lack of controlled studies and a short median follow-up of 9 months weaken the impact of the results. No evidence of impact on disease-specific survival or overall survival was reported. Current evidence based recommendation is: TCs, especially class I (potent) compounds, are effective at temporarily clearing patches and plaques in some patients with early-stage IA/IB MF.

4.2.6 Bullous Pemphigoid

Bullous pemphigoid (BP) is an acquired common autoimmune blistering dermatosis characterized by the development of autoantibodies against the components of the basement membrane zone of the skin. Numerous therapeutic modalities are available to manage this condition. However, superpotent topical steroids have emerged as a first-line therapy for limited disease [163]. Two randomized clinical trials have been published in favour of topical steroids and the summary has been tabulated as under:

Name of study	Type of study	Intervention	Outcome measures	Result
Joly et al. [164]	Randomized non-blind comparative trial	Clobetasol propionate vs prednisone, 0.5 mg/kg (moderate disease) and 1 mg/kg (severe disease)	Cessation of appearance of new lesions and rate of healing of old lesions	100% disease control in both groups with moderate disease, but patients with extensive disease had better control with clobetasol. Besides, adverse effects were significantly less in clobetasol group
Joly et al. [165]	Randomized non-blind comparative trial	Clobetasol propionate: mild dose (10–30 g/d depending on the severity of disease and weight) vs standard dose (40 g/d)	Cessation of appearance of new lesions and rate of healing of old lesions	The disease control was excellent in both the groups, along with 70% reduction in the cumulative doses of cream used in mild regimen. Also, mortality was less in patients with moderate disease treated with the mild regimen

The two RCTs suggest the use of TCs as first-line for the treatment for both localized and mild disease. Relatively few and mild side effects are associated with TC use in BP; however, their use in extensive disease may be limited by more side effects and practical factors.

4.2.7 Cutaneous Sarcoidosis

Sarcoidosis is a granulomatous disease with multisystem involvement. Topical high-potency fluorinated corticosteroids (with or without occlusive dressing) have been successfully used in localized cutaneous sarcoidosis, but high-level scientific evidence is lacking [166, 167].

4.2.8 Hand Eczema

Chronic hand eczema is an extremely common and notorious entity encountered by general physicians and dermatologists. Currently, evidence based guidelines for the management of this condition are lacking. However, there are a few randomized clinical trials favouring the use of topical corticosteroids.

Name of study	Type of study	Intervention	Outcome measures	Result
Gola et al. [168]	Randomized double-blind comparative trial	Fluticasone propionate 0.05% cream and clobetasol ointment 0.05%	Redness; scaling; lichenification	Clobetasol group showed better response
Faghihi et al. [169]	Randomized, double-blind, right to left, prospective, clinical trial	0.05% Clobetasol +2.5% zinc sulphate' cream versus '0.05% Clobetasol alone' cream	Redness; scaling; lichenification and pruritus	0.05% Clobetasol +2.5% zinc sulphate' cream was more effective than '0.05% Clobetasol alone' cream
Agarwal et al. [170]	Observer blinded randomized comparative trial	Clobetasol propionate 0.05% cream bd vs oral azathioprine 50 mg daily plus clobetasol propionate 0.05% cream bd	Redness; scaling; lichenification and pruritus, HECSI score (hand eczema severity index)	Both the groups showed good results but low dose oral azathioprine therapy was found to be an effective adjunctive treatment modality
Granlund et al. [171]	Randomized, double-blind study	Oral cyclosporine at 3 mg/kg/day with topical 0.05% betamethasone-17,21-dipropionate (BDP) cream	Redness; scaling; lichenification and pruritus, Eczema Disability Index (EDI)	Both groups showed good clinical response. However, low-dose cyclosporine proved to be a successful alternative treatment in non-responsive conditions. Total EDI score decreased significantly and to the same degree in both groups

There is insufficient evidence on which to base a choice between short bursts of potent TCs compared with continuous application of mild TCs. There is little evidence of steroid sparing effect of emollients, although these are widely prescribed. There is an insufficient evidence of an additive effect of topical antibacterial agents. There is an insufficient evidence of the superiority of topical calcineurin inhibitors to TCs [172].

4.2.9 Infantile Hemangiomas

Superficial infantile cutaneous hemangiomas are difficult to treat. Two small case series using ultrapotent topical corticosteroids for periocular hemangiomas have been reported. However, evidence in favour of using this therapy for other sites is lacking. Garzon et al. assessed the cessation of growth, shrinkage or flattening of the lesion and lightening of the surface colour. 74% of the cases demonstrated either good or partial response to ultrapotent topical corticosteroids [173]. In another study by Pandey et al., mometasone furoate was applied twice daily and compared with intralesional triamcinolone acetonide injections at monthly intervals at 1–2 mg/kg. Topical steroids were found to be a good alternative to intralesional steroids for treating superficial hemangiomas [174]. For the small but significant complicated His that require intervention, steroids were considered first-line therapy. It has now been superseded by oral propranolol.

4.3   Miscellaneous Conditions

Alopecia Areata One RCT demonstrated that potent TCs are marginally more effective than placebo when used continuously for a minimum of 3 months. In observational case series, children between the ages of 3 and 10 years appear most likely to respond [175].

Anogenital Pruritus In idiopathic cases, TCs may be helpful, but they may mask malignancy and other underlying disease [176].

Cutaneous Lupus Erythematosus All the controlled trials of TC were of short duration, but the evidence supports the use of potent TCs in DLE. Although TC use may be associated with skin atrophy, it is probably not important in DLE, which produces severe scarring and atrophy in itself [177].

Melasma There has been one systematic review [178] and one trial of 17 participants followed for 3 months [179]. Although the study reports that betamethasone was effective as a depigmenting agent ($P < 0.05$), the numbers were very small and seven of 16 women in the study found no therapeutic difference between treatment and placebo. There is controversy over the balance between benefits and harms of using TCs in the treatment of melasma, especially since long-term use on face can cause skin thinning and telangiectasia.

Perioral Dermatitis There is insufficient evidence (level of evidence: D) on the effects of non-fluorinated steroids in patients with perioral dermatitis. A split-face RCT of hydrocortisone butyrate versus 1% hydrocortisone alcohol cream is available [180]. Two patients with perioral dermatitis showed a moderate rebound of the eruption after withdrawal of topical treatment, in each case on the hydroxybutyrate-treated side of the face. In view of the study design and the small number of patients, it is difficult to draw conclusions.

Seborrheic Dermatitis Surprisingly, few RCTs have examined the efficacy of TCs.

4.4   Pregnancy and Lactation

Women with skin conditions often need topical corticosteroids during pregnancy. However, the knowledge about the effects of topical corticosteroids on the foetus is scarce. The current best evidence supports the use of mild to moderate topical corticosteroids in comparison to potent/superpotent alternatives in pregnancy, because of the associated risk of foetal growth restriction with the latter. There is no significantly increased risk of orofacial clefts, preterm delivery, growth retardation and foetal death when mild to moderate topical corticosteroids are used in pregnancy. Depending on the severity of the dermatoses, women should use topical corticosteroids of the least potency required and the duration and amount of application of the drug must be monitored judiciously. The risk of adverse events is increased when areas with high absorption (genitals, eyelids and flexures) are treated with topical steroids [181].

References

1. Fukaya M, Sato K, Sato M, et al. Topical steroid addiction in atopic dermatitis. Drug Healthcare Patient Safety. 2014;6:131–8.
2. Bewley A, Dermatology Working Group. Expert consensus: time for a change in the way we advise our patients to use topical corticosteroids. Br J Dermatol. 2008;158:917–20.
3. Dirven-Meijer PC, Glazenburg EJ, Mulder PGH, Oranje AP. Prevalence of atopic dermatitis in children younger than 4 years in a demarcated area in central Netherlands: the West Veluwe Study Group. Br J Dermatol. 2008;158:846–7.
4. Oranje AP, de Waard-van der Spek FB, Ordonez C, De Raeve L, Spierings M, van der Wouden JC. Emollients for eczema (Protocol). Cochrane Database Syst Rev. 2010;(1):CD008304.
5. Grimalt R, Mengeaud V, Cambazard F, et al. The steroid-sparing effect of an emollient therapy in infants with atopic dermatitis: a randomized controlled study. Dermatology. 2007;214:61–7.

6. Bieber T. Atopic dermatitis. Ann Dermatol. 2010;22:125–37.

7. Atopic eczema in under 12s: diagnosis and management. https://www.nice.org.uk/guidance/cg57. Last accessed on 20 Feb 2017.

8. Moed H, Yang Q, Oranje AP, Panda S, van der Wouden JC. Different strategies for using topical corticosteroids for established eczema. Cochrane Database Syst Rev. 2012;(10):CD010080.

9. Almeyda J, Burt BW. Double blind controlled study of treatment of atopic eczema with a preparation of hydrocortisone in a new drug delivery system versus betamethasone 17-valerate. Br J Dermatol. 1974;91:579–83.

10. Andersen BL, Andersen KE, Nielsen R, Stahl D, Niordson A, Roders GA. Treatment of dry atopic dermatitis in children. A double-blind comparison between mildison Lipocream™ (1% hydrocortisone) and Uniderm™ (1% hydrocortisone) ointment. Clin Trials J. 1988;25:278–84.

11. Bagatell FK, Barkoff JR, Cohen HJ, Lasser AE, McCormick GE, Rex IH, et al. A multi-center comparison of alclometasone dipropionate cream 0.05% and hydrocortisone cream 1.0% in the treatment of atopic dermatitis. Curr Ther Res Clin Exp. 1983;33:46–52.

12. Beattie PE, Lewis-Jones MS. A pilot study on the use of wet wraps in infants with moderate atopic eczema. Clin Exp Dermatol. 2004;29:348–53.

13. Binder R, McCleary J. Comparison of fluocinonide in a double-blind study with betamethasone valerate. Curr Ther Res Clin Exp. 1972;14:35–8.

14. Bleehen SS, Chu AC, Hamann I, Holden C, Hunter JA, Marks R. Fluticasone propionate 0.05% cream in the treatment of atopic eczema: a multicentre study comparing once-daily treatment and once-daily vehicle cream application versus twice-daily treatment. Br J Dermatol. 1995;133:592–7.

15. Bleeker J. Double-blind comparison between two new topical corticosteroids, halcinonide 0.1% and clobetasol propionate cream 0.05%. Curr Med Res Opin. 1975;3:225–8.

16. Duke EE, Maddin S, Aggerwal A. Alclometasone dipropionate in atopic dermatitis: a clinical study. Curr Ther Res Clin Exp. 1983;33:769–74.

17. Fisher M, Kelly AP. Multicenter trial of fluocinonide in an emollient cream base. Int J Dermatol. 1979;18:660–4.

18. Foelster-Holst R, Nagel F, Zoellner P, Spaeth D. Efficacy of crisis intervention treatment with topical corticosteroid prednicarbat with and without partial wet-wrap dressing in atopic dermatitis. Dermatology. 2006;212:66–9.

19. Glazenburg EJ, Wolkerstorfer A, Gerretsen AL, Mulder PG, Oranje AP. Efficacy and safety of fluticasone propionate 0.005% ointment in the long-term maintenance treatment of children with atopic dermatitis: differences between boys and girls? Pediatr Allergy Immunol. 2009;20:59–66.

20. Haneke E. The treatment of atopic dermatitis with methylprednisolone aceponate (mpa), a new topical corticosteroid. J Dermatol Treat. 1992;3(Suppl 2):13–5.

21. Hanifin JM, Hebert AA, Mays SR, Paller AS, Sherertz EF, Wagner AM, et al. Effects of a lowpotency corticosteroid lotion plus a moisturizing regimen in the treatment of atopic dermatitis. Curr Ther Res Clin Exp. 1998;59(4):227–33.

22. Hanifin J, Gupta AK, Rajagopalan R. Intermittent dosing of fluticasone propionate cream for reducing the risk of relapse in atopic dermatitis patients. Br J Dermatol. 2002;147:528–37.

23. Haribhakti PB. Comparative Study of Clobetasone Butyrate Cream (eumovate) and Hydrocortisone Cream in Children with Eczema. Indian J Dermatol Venereol Leprol. 1982;48:344–7.

24. Hebert AA, Cook-Bolden FE, Basu S, Calvarese B, Trancik RJ, Desonide Hydrogel Study Group. Safety and efficacy of desonide hydrogel 0.05% in pediatric subjects with atopic dermatitis. J Drugs Dermatol. 2007;6:175–81.

25. Hoybye S, Balk Moller S, De Cunha BF, Ottevanger V, Veien NK. Continuous and intermittent treatment of atopic dermatitis in adults with momethasone furoate vs. hydrocortisone 17-butyrate. Curr Ther Res Clin Exp. 1991;50:67–72.

26. Jorizzo J, Levy M, Lucky A, Shavin J, Goldberg G, Dunlap F, et al. Multicenter trial for long-term safety and efficacy comparison of 0.05% desonide and 1% hydrocortisone ointments in the treatment of atopic dermatitis in pediatric patients. J Am Acad Dermatol. 1995;33:74–7.

27. Kirkup ME, Birchall NM, Weinberg EG, et al. Acute and maintenance treatment of atopic dermatitis in children – two comparative studies with fluticasone propionate (0.05%) cream. J Dermatol Treat. 2003;14:141–8.

28. Koopmans B, Lasthein Andersen B, Mork NJ, Austad J, Suhonen RE. Multicentre randomized double-blind study of locoid lipocream fatty cream twice daily versus locoid lipocream once daily and locobase once daily. J Dermatol Treat. 1995;6:103–6.

29. Korting HC, Zienicke H, Schafer-Korting M, BraunFalco O. Liposome encapsulation improves efficacy of betamethasone dipropionate in atopic eczema but not in psoriasis vulgaris. Eur J Clin Pharmacol. 1990;39:349–51.

30. Lassus A. Clinical comparison of alclometasone dipropionate cream 0.05% with hydrocortisone butyrate cream 0.1% in the treatment of atopic dermatitis in children. J Int Med Res. 1983;11:315–9.

31. Lebwohl M, Lane A, Savin R, Drake L, Berman B, Lucky A, et al. A comparison of once-daily application of mometasone furoate 0.1% cream compared with twice-daily hydrocortisone valerate 0.2% cream in pediatric atopic dermatitis patients who failed to respond to hydrocortisone. Int J Dermatol. 1999;38:604–6.

32. Lucky AW, Grote GD, Williams JL, Tuley MR, Czernielewski JM, Dolak TM, et al. Effect of desonide ointment, 0.05%, on the hypothalamic pituitary-adrenal axis of children with atopic dermatitis. Cutis. 1997;59:151–3.

33. Marchesi E, Rozzoni M, Pini P, Cainelli T. Comparative study of mometasone furoate and betamethasone dipropionate in the treatment of atopic dermatitis. G Ital Dermatol Venereol. 1994;129:IX–XII.

34. Morley N, Fry L, Walker S. Clinical evaluation of clobetasone butyrate in the treatment of children with atopic eczema, and its effect on plasma corticosteroid levels. Curr Med Res Opin. 1976;4:223–8.

35. Msika P, De Belilovsky C, Piccardi N, et al. New emollient with topical corticosteroid-sparing effect in treatment of childhood atopic dermatitis: SCORAD and quality of life improvement. Pediatr Dermatol. 2008;25:606–12.

36. Olholm Larsen P, Brandrup F, Roders GA. Report on a double-blind, left-right study comparing the clinical efficacy of mildison (hydrocortisone 1%) Lipocream™ with Uniderm™ (hydrocortisone 1%) cream in the treatment of children with atopic dermatitis. Curr Ther Res Clin Exp. 1988;44:421–5.

37. Prado de Oliveira ZN, Cuce LC, Arnone M. Comparative evaluation of efficacy, tolerability and safety of 0.1% topical momethasone furoate and 0.05% desonide in the treatment of childhood atopic dermatitis. An Bras Dermatol. 2002;77:25–33.

38. Pei AYS, Chan HHL, Ho KM. The effectiveness of wet wrap dressings using 0.1% mometasone furoate and 0.005% fluticasone proprionate ointments in the treatment of moderate to severe atopic dermatitis in children. Pediatr Dermatol. 2001;18:343–8.

39. Peserico A, Stadtler G, Sebastian M, et al. Reduction of relapses of atopic dermatitis with methylprednisolone aceponate cream twice weekly in addition to maintenance treatment with emollient: a multicentre, randomized, double-blind, controlled study. Br J Dermatol. 2008;158:801–7.

40. Rafanelli A, Rafanelli S, Stanganelli I, Marchesi E. Mometasone furoate in the treatment of atopic dermatitis in children. J Eur Acad Dermatol Venereol. 1993;2:225–30.

41. Rajka G, Verjans HL. Hydrocortisone 17-butyrate (locoid) 0.1% fatty cream versus desonide (apolar) 0.1% ointment in the treatment of patients suffering from atopic dermatitis. J Int Med Res. 1986;14:85–90.

42. Rampini E. Methylprenisolone aceponate (mpa) – use and clinical experience in children. J Dermatol Treat. 1992;3(Suppl 2):27–9.

43. Reidhav I, Svensson A. Betamethasone valerate versus mometasone furoate cream once daily in atopic dermatitis. J Dermatol Treat. 1996;7:87–8.

44. Richelli C, Piacentini GL, Sette L, Bonizzato MC, Andreoli A, Boner AL. Clinical efficacy and tolerability of clobetasone 17-butyrate 0.5% lotion in children with atopic dermatitis. Curr Ther Res Clin Exp. 1990;47:413–7.

45. Rubio E, et al. Allergic diseases of the skin and drug allergies – 2015. Randomized controlled, double blind trial of topical twice weekly fluticasone propionate maintenance treatment to reduce risk of relapse in mild or moderate atopic dermatitis in children. World Allergy Org J. 2013;6(Suppl 1):P102.

46. Ruzicka T, Willers C, Wigger-Alberti W. Efficacy and patient-reported outcomes of a new mometasone cream treating atopic eczema. Skin Pharmacol Physiol. 2012;25(6):305–12.

47. Savin RC. Betamethasone dipropionate in psoriasis and atopic dermatitis. Conn Med. 1976;40:5–7.

48. Thomas KS, Armstrong S, Avery A, et al. Randomised controlled trial of short bursts of a potent topical corticosteroid versus prolonged use of a mild preparation for children with mild or moderate atopic eczema. BMJ. 2002;324:768.

49. Torok HM, Maas-Irslinger R, Slayton RM. Clocortolone pivalate cream 0.1% used concomitantly with tacrolimus ointment 0.1% in atopic dermatitis. Cutis. 2003;72:161–6.

50. Traulsen J. Hydrocortisone buteprate versus betamethasone valerate for once-daily treatment of atopic dermatitis. J Dermatol Treat. 1997;8:109–14.

51. Trookman NS, Rizer RL. Randomized controlled trial of desonlde hydrogel 0.05% versus desonide ointment 0.05% in the treatment of mild-to-moderate atopic dermatitis. J Clin Aesth Dermatol. 2011;4:34–8.

52. Ulrich R, Andresen I. Double-blind comparative trial involving 0.5% halomethasone (Sicorten™) cream versus 0.25% prednicarbate cream in patients with acute episodes of atopic dermatiti. Fortschr Med. 1991;109:49–50. 53–54

53. Veien NK, Hattel T, Justesen O, Norholm A, Verjans HL. Hydrocortisone 17-butyrate (Locoid) 0.1% cream versus hydrocortisone (Uniderm) 1% cream in the treatment of children suffering from atopic dermatitis. J Int Med Res. 1984;12:310–3.

54. Vernon HJ, Lane AT, Weston W. Comparison of mometasone furoate 0.1% cream and hydrocortisone 1.0% cream in the treatment of childhood atopic dermatitis. J Am Acad Dermatol. 1991;24:603–7.

55. Wolkerstorfer A, Strobos MA, Glazenburg EJ, Mulder PGH, Oranje AP. Fluticasone propionate 0.05% cream once daily versus clobetasone butyrate 0.05% cream twice daily in children with atopic dermatitis. J Am Acad Dermatol. 1998;39:226–31.

56. Yasuda T. Clinical experiences with hydrocortisone 17-butyrate. Dermatologica. 1976;152(Suppl 1):221–9.

57. Thomas K, Charman C, Nankervis H, Ravenscroft J, Williams HC. Atopic eczema. In: Williams HC, Bigby M, Herxheimer A, Naldi L, Rzany B, Dellavalle RP, et al., editors. Evidence-based dermatology. 3rd ed. Chichester: Wiley Blackwell; 2014. p. 13–8.

58. Hoare C, Li Wan Po A, Williams H. Systematic review of treatments for atopic eczema. Health Technol Assess. 2000;4:1–191.

59. Forschner T, Buchholtz S, Stockfleth E. Current state of vitiligo therapy–evidence-based analysis of the literature. J Dtsch Dermatol Ges. 2007;5:467–75.

60. Whitton ME, Pinart M, Batchelor J, Leonardi-Bee J, González U, Jiyad Z, Eleftheriadou V, Ezzedine K. Interventions for vitiligo. Cochrane Database Syst Rev. 2015;(2):CD003263.

61. Njoo MD, Spuls PI, Bos JD, Westerhof W, et al. Nonsurgical repigmentation therapies in vitiligo. Meta Anal Liter Arch Dermatol. 1998;134:1532–40.

62. Koopmans-van Dorp B, Goedhart-van Dijjk B, Neering H, van Dijk E. Treatment of vitiligo by local application of betamethasone 17-valerate in a dimethyl sulfoxide cream base. Dermatologica. 1973;146:310–4.

63. Bleehen SS. The treatment of vitiligo with topical corticosteroids. Light and electronmicroscopic studies. Br J Dermatol. 1976;94(Suppl 12):43–50.

64. Clayton R. A double-blind trial of 0-05% clobetasol proprionate in the treatment of vitiligo. Br J Dermatol. 1977;96:71–3.

65. Kandil E. Treatment of vitiligo with 0-1 per cent betamethasone 17-valerate in isopropyl alcohol–a double-blind trial. Br J Dermatol. 1974;91:457–60.

66. Lepe V, Moncada B, Castanedo-Cazares JP, Torres-Alvarez MB, Ortiz CA, Torres-Rubalcava AB. A double-blind randomised trial of 0.1% tacrolimus vs 0.05% clobetasol for the treatment of childhood vitiligo. Arch Dermatol. 2003;139:581–5.

67. Sanclemente G, Garcia JJ, Zuleta JJ, Diehl C, Correa C, Falabella R. A double-blind randomized trial of 0.05% betamethasone vs. topical catalase/dismutase superoxide in vitiligo. J Eur Acad Dermatol Venereol. 2008;22:1359–64.

68. Kumaran MS, Kaur I, Kumar B. Effect of topical calcipotriol, betamethasone dipropionate and their contribution in the treatment of localized vitiligo. J Eur Acad Dermatol Venereol. 2006;20:269–73.

69. Xing C, Xu A. The effect of combined calcipotriol and betamethasone dipropionate ointment in the treatment of vitiligo: an open, uncontrolled trial. J Drugs Dermatol. 2012;11:e52–4.

70. Agarwal S, Ramam M, Sharma VK, Khandpur S, Pal H, Pandey RM. A randomised placebo-controlled double-blind study of levamisole in the treatment of limited and slowly spreading vitiligo. Br J Dermatol. 2005;153:163–6.

71. Akdeniz N, Yavuz IH, Gunes Bilgili S, et al. Comparison of efficacy of narrow band UVB therapies with UVB alone, in combination with calcipotriol, and with betamethasone and calcipotriol in vitiligo. J Dermatolog Treat. 2014;25:196–9.

72. Kathuria S, Khaitan BK, Ramam M, Sharma VK. Segmental vitiligo: a randomized controlled trial to evaluate efficacy and safety of 0.1% tacrolimus ointment vs 0.05% fluticasone propionate cream. Indian J Dermatol Venereol Leprol. 2012;78:68–73.

73. Khalid M, Mujtaba G, Haroon TS. Comparison of 0.05% clobetasol propionate cream and topical PUVAsol in childhood vitiligo. Int J Dermatol. 1995;34:203–5.

74. Köse O, Arca E, Kurumlu Z. Mometasone cream versus pimecrolimus cream for the treatment of childhood localized vitiligo. J Dermatol Treat. 2010;21:133–9.

75. Lim-Ong M, Leveriza RMS, Ong BET, Frez MLF. Comparison between narrow-band UVB with topical corticosteroid and narrow-band UVB with placebo in the treatment of vitiligo: a randomized controlled trial. J Phillipine Dermatol Soc. 2005;14:17–25.

76. Sassi F, Cazzaniga S, Tessari G, Chatenoud L, Reseghetti A, Marchesi L, et al. Randomized controlled trial comparing the effectiveness of 308-nm excimer laser alone or in combination with topical hydrocortisone 17-butyrate cream in the treatment of vitiligo of the face and neck. Br J Dermatol. 2008;159:1186–91.

77. Wazir SM, Paracha MM, Khan SU. Efficacy and safety of topical mometasone furoate 0.01% vs. tacrolimus 0.03% and mometasone furoate 0.01% in vitiligo. J Pak Assoc Dermatol. 2010;20:89–92.

78. Westerhof W, Nieuweboer-Krobotova L, Mulder PG, Glazenburg EJ. Left-right comparison study of the combination of fluticasone propionate and UVA vs either fluticasone propionate or UVA alone for the long-term treatment of vitiligo. Arch Dermatol. 1999;135:1061–6.

79. Yaghoobi R, Omidian M, Bagherani N. Comparison of therapeutic efficacy of topical corticosteroid and oral zinc sulfate-topical corticosteroid combination in the treatment of vitiligo patients: a clinical trial. BMC Dermatol. 2011;11:7.

80. Manriquez JJ, Niklitschek SM. Vitiligo. In: Williams HC, et al., editors. Evidence-based dermatology. 3rd ed. Chichester: Wiley; 2014. p. 44–9.

81. Castela E, Archier E, Devaux S, et al. Topical corticosteroids in plaque psoriasis: a systematic review of efficacy and treatment modalities. J Eur Acad Dermatol Venereol. 2012;26(Suppl 3):36–46.

82. Samarasekera EJ, Sawyer L, Wonderling D, Tucker R, Smith CH. Topical therapies for the treatment of plaque psoriasis: systematic review and network meta-analyses. Br J Dermatol. 2013;168:954–67.

83. Shupack JL, Jondreau L, Kenny C, et al. Diflorasone diacetate ointment 0.05% versus betamethasone dipropionate ointment 0.05% in moderate-severe plaque-type psoriasis. Dermatology. 1993;186:129–32.

84. Sears HW. A double-blind, randomized, placebo-controlled evaluation of the efficacy and safety of hydrocortisone buteprate 0.1% cream in the treatment of psoriasis. Adv Ther. 1997;14:140–9.

85. Peharda V, Gruber F, Prpic L, Kastelan M, Brajac I. Comparison of mometasone furoate 0.1% ointment and betamethasone dipropionate 0.05% ointment in the treatment of psoriasis vulgaris. Acta Dermatovenerol Croat. 2000;8:223–6.

86. Lebwohl M, Sherer D, Washenik K, et al. A randomized, double-blind, placebo-controlled study of clobetasol propionate 0.05% foam in the treatment of nonscalp psoriasis. Int J Dermatol. 2002;41:269–74.

87. Koo J, Cuffie CA, Tanner DJ, et al. Mometasone furoate 0.1%-salicylic acid 5% ointment versus mometasone furoate 0.1% ointment in the treatment of moderate-to-severe psoriasis: a multicenter study. Clin Ther. 1998;20:283–91.

88. Medansky RS, et al. Mometasone furoate 0.1%-salicylic acid 5% ointment twice daily versus fluocinonide 0.05% ointment twice daily in the management of patients with psoriasis. Clin Ther. 1997;19:701–9.

89. Tiplica GS, Salavastru CM. Mometasone furoate 0.1% and salicylic acid 5% vs. mometasone furoate 0.1% as sequential local therapy in psoriasis vulgaris. J Eur Acad Dermatol Venereol. 2009;23:905–12.

90. Guenther LC, Poulin YP, Pariser DM. A comparison of tazarotene 0.1% gel once daily plus mometasone furoate 0.1% cream once daily versus calcipotriene 0.005% ointment twice daily in the treatment of plaque psoriasis. Clin Ther. 2000;22:1225–38.

91. Green L, Sadoff W. A clinical evaluation of tazarotene 0.1% gel, with and without a high- or mid-high-potency corticosteroid, in patients with stable plaque psoriasis. J Cutan Med Surg. 2002;6:95–102.

92. Katz HI, Gross E, Buxman M, et al. A double-blind, vehicle-controlled paired comparison of halobetasol propionate cream on patients with plaque psoriasis. J Am Acad Dermatol. 1991;25:1175–8.

93. Koo J, Blum RR, Lebwohl M. A randomized, multicenter study of calcipotriene ointment and clobetasol propionate foam in the sequential treatment of localized plaque-type psoriasis: short- and long-term outcomes. J Am Acad Dermatol. 2006;55:637–41.

94. Ellis CN, Katz HI, Rex IHJ, et al. A controlled clinical trial of a new formulation of betamethasone dipropionate cream in once-daily treatment of psoriasis. Clin Ther. 1989;11:768–74.

95. Greenspan A, Herndon JH Jr, Baker MD, Cheney T. Controlled evaluation of 0.05% desonide lotion and desonide cream in psoriasis. Curr Therapeu Res Clin Exp. 1993;53:614–20.

96. Frost P, Horwitz SN. Clinical comparison of alclometasone dipropionate and desonide ointments (0.05%) in the management of psoriasis. J Int Med Res. 1982;10:375–8.

97. Cornell RC. Comparison of amcinonide ointment 0.1 percent twice daily and fluocinonide ointment 0.05 percent three times daily in the treatment of psoriasis. Cutis. 1983;31:566–9.

98. Angelo JS, Kar BR, Thomas J. Comparison of clinical efficacy of topical tazarotene 0.1% cream with topical clobetasol propionate 0.05% cream in chronic plaque psoriasis: a double-blind, randomized, right-left comparison study. Indian J Dermatol Venereol Leprol. 2007;73:65.

99. Senter TP, Stimson DH, Charles G, et al. Comparison of two therapeutic regimens using the same topical corticoid for stable psoriasis. West J Med. 1983;139:657–62.

100. Bernhard J, Whitmore C, Guzzo C, et al. Evaluation of halobetasol propionate ointment in the treatment of plaque psoriasis: report on two double-blind, vehicle-controlled studies. J Am Acad Dermatol. 1991;25:1170–4.

101. Fleming C, Ganslandt C, Guenther L, et al. Calcipotriol plus betamethasone dipropionate gel compared with its active components in the same vehicle and the vehicle alone in the treatment of psoriasis vulgaris: a randomised, parallel group, double-blind, exploratory study. Eur J Dermatol. 2010;20:465–71.

102. Gottlieb AB, Ford RO, Spellman MC. The efficacy and tolerability of clobetasol propionate foam 0.05% in the treatment of mild to moderate plaque-type psoriasis of nonscalp regions. J Cutan Med Surg. 2003;7:185–92.

103. Jarratt MT, Clark SD, Savin RC, et al. Evaluation of the efficacy and safety of clobetasol propionate spray in the treatment of plaque-type psoriasis. Cutis. 2006;78:348–54.

104. Kaufmann R, Bibby AJ, Bissonnette R, et al. A new calcipotriol/betamethasone dipropionate formulation (Daivobet) is an effective once-daily treatment for psoriasis vulgaris. Dermatology. 2002;205:389–93.

105. Mraz S, Leonardi C, LE C'n, et al. Different treatment outcomes with different formulations of clobetasol propionate 0.05% for the treatment of plaque psoriasis. J Dermatolog Treat. 2008;19:354–9.

106. Singh S, Reddy DC, Pandey SS. Topical therapy for psoriasis with the use of augmented betamethasone and calcipotriene on alternate weeks. J Am Acad Dermatol. 2000;43:61–5.

107. Stein LF, Sherr A, Solodkina G, et al. Betamethasone valerate foam for treatment of nonscalp psoriasis. J Cutan Med Surg. 2001;5:303–7.

108. Aggerwal A, Maddin S. Alclometasone dipropionate in psoriasis: a clinical study. J Int Med Res. 1982;10:414–8.

109. Blum G, Yawalkar S. A comparative, multicenter, double blind trial of 0.05% halobetasol propionate ointment and 0.1% betamethasone valerate ointment in the treatment of patients with chronic, localized plaque psoriasis. J Am Acad Dermatol. 1991;25:1153–6.

110. Choonhakarn C, Busaracome P, Sripanidkulchai B, et al. A prospective, randomized clinical trial comparing topical Aloe vera with 0.1% triamcinolone acetonide in mild to moderate plaque psoriasis. J Eur Acad Dermatol Venereol. 2010;24:168–72.

111. Decroix J, Pres H, Tsankov N, et al. Clobetasol propionate lotion in the treatment of moderate to severe plaque-type psoriasis. Cutis. 2004;74:201–6.

112. Fredriksson T, Salde L. A double-blind trial of budesonide and betamethasone- 17,21-dipropionate in psoriasis. Curr Med Res Opin. 1982;8:171–7.

113. Goldberg B, Hartdegen R, Presbury D, et al. A double-blind, multicenter comparison of 0.05% halobetasol propionate ointment and 0.05%

clobetasol propionate ointment in patients with chronic, localized plaque psoriasis. J Am Acad Dermatol. 1991;25:1145–8.

114. Jacobson C, Cornell RC, Savin RCA. comparison of clobetasol propionate 0.05 percent ointment and an optimized betamethasone dipropionate 0.05 percent ointment in the treatment of psoriasis. Cutis. 1986;216:218–20.

115. Jegasothy B, Jacobson C, Levine N, et al. Clobetasol propionate versus fluocinonide creams in psoriasis and eczema. Int J Dermatol. 1985;24:461–5.

116. Krueger GG, O'Reilly MA, Weidner M, et al. Comparative efficacy of once-daily flurandrenolide tape versus twice-daily diflorasone diacetate ointment in the treatment of psoriasis. J Am Acad Dermatol. 1998;38:186–90.

117. Kuokkanen K. Comparison of 0.25% desoxymethasone ointment with 0.05% fluocinonide ointment in psoriasis. Curr Med Res Opin. 1976;4:703–5.

118. Leibsohn E. Comparison of diflorasone diacetate and betamethasone dipropionate ointment in the treatment of psoriasis. J Int Med Res. 1982;10: 22–7.

119. Lowe N, Feldman SR, Sherer D, et al. Clobetasol propionate lotion, an efficient and safe alternative to clobetasol propionate emollient cream in subjects with moderate to severe plaque-type psoriasis. J Dermatolog Treat. 2005;16:158–64.

120. Mensing H, Korsukewitz G, Yawalkar S. A double-blind, multicenter comparison between 0.05% halobetasol propionate ointment and 0.05% betamethasone dipropionate ointment in chronic plaque psoriasis. J Am Acad Dermatol. 1991;25:1149–52.

121. Molin L, Cutler TP, Helander I, et al. Comparative efficacy of calcipotriol (MC903) cream and betamethasone 17-valerate cream in the treatment of chronic plaque psoriasis. A randomized, double-blind, parallel group multicentre study. Calcipotriol Study Group. Br J Dermatol. 1997;136:89–93.

122. Olsen EA. Efficacy and safety of fluticasone propionate 0.005% ointment in the treatment of psoriasis. Cutis. 1996;57:57–61.

123. Roberts DT. Comparison of fluticasone propionate ointment, 0.005%, and betamethasone-17,21-dipropionate ointment, 0.05%, in the treatment of psoriasis. Cutis. 1996;57:27–31.

124. Bruce S, Epinette WW, Funicella T, et al. Comparative study of calcipotriene (MC 903) ointment and fluocinonide ointment in the treatment of psoriasis. J Am Acad Dermatol. 1994;31:755–9.

125. Fabry H, Yawalkar SJ. A comparative multicentre trial of halometasone ointment and fluocortolone plus fluocortolone caproate ointment in the treatment of psoriasis. J Int Med Res. 1983;11:26–30.

126. Huntley AC, Isseroff R. Amcinonide vs. betamethasone dipropionate ointments in the treatment of psoriasis. Cutis. 1985;35:489–92.

127. Nast A, Spuls P, Nijsten T. Treatment of psoriasis. In: Williams HC, et al., editors. Evidence-based dermatology. 3rd ed. Chichester: Wiley Blackwell. p. 175–99.

128. Olsen EA, Cram DL, Ellis CN, et al. A double-blind, vehicle-controlled study of clobetasol propionate 0.05% (Temovate) scalp application in the treatment of moderate to severe scalp psoriasis. J Am Acad Dermatol. 1991;24:443–7.

129. Ellis CN, Horwitz SN, Menter A. Amcinonide lotion 0.1% in the treatment of patients with psoriasis of the scalp. Curr Therapeu Res Clin Exp. 1988;44:315–24.

130. Franz TJ, Parsell DA, Halualani RM, et al. Betamethasone valerate foam 0.12%: a novel vehicle with enhanced delivery and efficacy. Int J Dermatol. 1999;38:628–32.

131. Katz HI, Lindholm JS, Weiss JS, et al. Efficacy and safety of twice-daily augmented betamethasone dipropionate lotion versus clobetasol propionate solution in patients with moderate-to-severe scalp psoriasis. Clin Ther. 1995;17:390–401.

132. Van de Kerkhof PCM, Hoffmann V, Anstey A, et al. A new scalp formulation of calcipotriol plus betamethasone dipropionate compared with each of its active ingredients in the same vehicle for the treatment of scalp psoriasis: a randomized, double-blind, controlled trial. Br J Dermatol. 2009;160:170–6.

133. Willis I, Cornell RC, Penneys NS, et al. Multicenter study comparing 0.05% gel formulations of desoximetasone and fluocinonide in patients with scalp psoriasis. Clin Ther. 1986;8:275–82.

134. Reygagne P, Mrowietz U, Decroix J, et al. Clobetasol propionate shampoo 0.05% and calcipotriol solution 0.005%: a randomized comparison of efficacy and safety in subjects with scalp psoriasis. J Dermatolog Treat. 2005;16:31–6.

135. Pauporte M, Maibach H, Lowe N, et al. Fluocinolone acetonide topical oil for scalp psoriasis. J Dermatolog Treat. 2004;15:360–4.

136. Klaber MR, Hutchinson PE, Pedvis-Leftick A, et al. Comparative effects of calcipotriol solution (50 micrograms / ml) and betamethasone 17-valerate solution (1 mg/ml) in the treatment of scalp psoriasis. Br J Dermatol. 1994;131:678–83.

137. Jemec GBE, Ganslandt C, Ortonne J, et al. A new scalp formulation of calcipotriene plus betamethasone compared with its active ingredients and the vehicle in the treatment of scalp psoriasis: a randomized, double-blind, controlled trial. J Am Acad Dermatol. 2008;59:455–63.

138. Jarratt M, Breneman D, Gottlieb AB, et al. Clobetasol propionate shampoo 0.05%: a new option to treat patients with moderate to severe scalp psoriasis. J Drugs Dermatol. 2004;3:367–73.

139. Feldman SR, Ravis SM, Fleischer ABJ, et al. Betamethasone valerate in foam vehicle is effective with both daily and twice a day dosing: a single-blind, open-label study in the treatment of scalp psoriasis. J Cutan Med Surg. 2001;5:386–9.

140. Duweb GA, Abuzariba O, Rahim M, et al. Scalp psoriasis: topical calcipotriol 50 micrograms/g/ml solution vs. betamethasone valerate 1% lotion. Int J Clin Pharmacol Res. 2000;20:65–8.

141. Buckley C, Hoffmann V, Shapiro J, et al. Calcipotriol plus betamethasone dipropionate scalp formulation is effective and well tolerated in the treatment of scalp psoriasis: a phase II study. Dermatology. 2008;217:107–13.

142. Andreassi L, Giannetti A, Milani M. Efficacy of betamethasone valerate mousse in comparison with standard therapies on scalp psoriasis: an open, multicentre, randomized, controlled, cross-over study on 241 patients. Br J Dermatol. 2003;148:134–8.

143. Bernard C, Camille F, Olivier C. Treatment of lichen planusan evidence-based medicine analysis of efficacy. Arch Dermatol. 1998;134:1521–30.

144. Cheng S, Kirtschig G, Cooper S, Thornhill M, Leonardi-Bee J, Murphy R. Interventions for erosive lichen planus affecting mucosal sites. Cochrane Database Syst Rev. 2012;(2):CD008092.

145. Lodi G, Carrozzo M, Furness S, Thongprasom K. Interventions for treating oral lichen planus: a systematic review. Br J Dermatol. 2012;166:938–47.

146. Zakrzewska JM, Chan ES, Thornhill MH. A systematic review of placebo-controlled randomized clinical trials of treatments used in oral lichen planus. Br J Dermatol. 2005;153:336–41.

147. Voute ABE, Schulten EAJM, Langendijk PNJ, et al. Fluocinonide in an adhesive base for treatment of oral lichen planus. Oral Surg Oral Med Oral Pathol. 1993;75:181–5.

148. Conrotto D, Carbone M, Carrozzo M, et al. Ciclosporin vs. clobetasol in the topical management of atrophic and erosive oral lichen planus: a double-blind, randomized controlled trial. Br J Dermatol. 2006;154:139–45.

149. Yoke PC, Tin GB, Kim MJ, et al. A randomized controlled trial to compare steroid with cyclosporine for the topical treatment of oral lichen planus. Oral Surg Oral Med Oral Pathol Oral Radiol Endod. 2006;102:47–55.

150. Gorouhi F, Solhpour A, Beitollahi JM, et al. Randomized trial of pimecrolimus cream versus triamcinolone acetonide paste in the treatment of oral lichen planus. J Am Acad Dermatol. 2007;57:806–13.

151. Corrocher G, Di Lorenzo G, Martinelli N, et al. Comparative effect of tacrolimus 0.1% ointment and clobetasol 0.05% ointment in patients with oral lichen planus. J Clin Periodontol. 2008;35:244–9.

152. Laeijendecker R, Tank B, Dekker SK, et al. A comparison of treatment of oral lichen planus with topical tacrolimus and triamcinolone acetonide ointment. Acta Derm Venereol. 2006;86:227–9.

153. Hegarty AM, Hodgson TA, Lewsey JD, et al. Fluticasone propionate spray and betamethasone sodium phosphate mouthrinse: a randomized cross-over study for the treatment of symptomatic oral lichen planus. J Am Acad Dermatol. 2002;47:271–9.

154. Rodstrom PO, Hakeberg M, Jontell M, et al. Erosive oral lichen planus treated with clobetasol propionate and triamcinolone acetonide in Orabase: a double-blind clinical trial. J Dermatolog Treat. 1994;5:7–10.

155. Campisi G, Giandalia G, De Caro V, et al. A new delivery system of clobetasol-17-propionate (lipid-loaded microspheres 0Æ025%) compared with a conventional formulation (lipophilic ointment in a hydrophilic phase 0Æ025%) in topical treatment of atrophic/erosive oral lichen planus. A Phase IV, randomized, observer-blinded, parallel group clinical trial. Br J Dermatol. 2004;150:984–90.

156. Carbone M, Arduino PG, Carrozzo M, et al. Topical clobetasol in the treatment of atrophic-erosive oral lichen planus: a randomized controlled trial to compare two preparations with different concentrations. J Oral Pathol Med. 2009;38:227–33.

157. Malhotra AK, Khaitan BK, Sethuraman G, et al. Betamethasone oral mini-pulse therapy compared with topical triamcinolone acetonide (0Æ1%) paste in oral lichen planus: a randomized comparative study. J Am Acad Dermatol. 2008;58:596–602.

158. Ghabanchi J, Bahri Najafi R, Haghnegahdar S. Treatment of oral inflammatory diseases with a new mucoadhesive prednisolone table versus triamcinolone acetonide paste. IRCMJ. 2009;11:155–9.

159. Fazel N. Cutaneous lichen planus: a systematic review of treatments. J Dermatolog Treat. 2015;26:280–3.

160. Le Cleach L, Chosidow O. Lichen planus. In: Williams HC, et al., editors. Evidence-based dermatology. 3rd ed. Chichester: Wiley Blackwell; 2014. p. 200–5.

161. Kim EJ, Hess S, Richardson SK, et al. Immunopathogenesis and therapy of cutaneous T cell lymphoma. J Clin Invest. 2005;115:798–812.

162. Trautinger F, Knobler R, Willemze R, et al. EORTC consensus recommendations for the treatment of mycosis fungoides/Sézary syndrome. Eur J Cancer. 2006;42:1014–30.

163. Teresa García-Romero M, Werth VP. Randomized controlled trials needed for bullous pemphigoid interventions. Arch Dermatol. 2012;148(2):243–6.

164. Joly P, Roujeau JC, Benichou J, et al. A comparison of oral and topical corticosteroids in patients with bullous pemphigoid. N Engl J Med. 2002;346:321–7.

165. Joly P, Roujeau JC, Benichou J, et al. A comparison of two regimens of topical corticosteroids in the treatment of patients with bullous pemphigoid: a multicenter randomized study. J Invest Dermatol. 2009;129:1681–7.

166. Volden G. Successful treatment of chronic skin diseases with clobetasol propionate and a hydrocolloid occlusive dressing. Acta Derm Venereol. 1992;72:69–71.

167. Baughman RP, Lower EE. Evidence-based therapy for cutaneous sarcoidosis. Clin Dermatol. 2007;25:334–40.

168. Gola M, D'Erme AM, Milanesi N. Clinical efficacy of two topical corticosteroids in the management of chronic hand eczema. G Ital Dermatol Venereol. 2015;150:293–6.

169. Faghihi G, Iraji F, Shahingohar A, Saidat AH. The efficacy of '0.05% Clobetasol + 2.5% zinc sulphate'

cream vs. '0.05% Clobetasol alone' cream in the treatment of the chronic hand eczema: a double-blind study. J Eur Acad Dermatol Venereol. 2008;22:531–6.

170. Agarwal US, Besarwal RK. Topical clobetasol propionate 0.05% cream alone and in combination with azathioprine in patients with chronic hand eczema: an observer blinded randomized comparative trial. Indian J Dermatol Venereol Leprol. 2013;79:101–3.

171. Granlund H, Erkko P, Eriksson E, Reitamo S. Comparison of the influence of cyclosporine and topical betamethasone-17,21-dipropionate treatment of severe chronic hand eczema. Acta Dermatol Venereol. 1996;76:371–6.

172. Christoffers WA, Schuttelaar M-LA, Coenraads P-J. Hand eczema. In: Williams HC, et al., editors. Evidence-based dermatology. Chichester: Wiley Blackwell. p. 117–26.

173. Garzon MC, Lucky AW, Hawrot A, Frieden IJ. Ultrapotent topical corticosteroid treatment of hemangiomas of infancy. J Am Acad Dermatol. 2005;52:281–6.

174. Pandey A, Gangopadhyay AN, Sharma SP, Kumar V, Gupta DK, Gopal SC. Evaluation of topical ste-

roids in the treatment of superficial hemangioma. Skinmed. 2010;8:9–11.

175. Olsen E, Hordinsky M, McDonald-Hull S, et al. Alopecia areata investigational assessment guidelines. National Alopecia Areata Foundation. J Am Acad Dermatol. 1999;40:242–6.

176. Oztas MO, Oztas P, Onder M. Idiopathic perianal pruritus: washing compared with topical corticosteroids. Postgrad Med J. 2004;80:295–7.

177. Jessop S, Whitelaw D. Cutaneous lupus erythematosus. In: HC Williams et al (eds.) Evidence-based dermatology, 3rd edn, pp. 523-30Wiley Blackwell, Chichester

178. Rajaratnam R, Halpern J, Salim A, et al. Interventions for melasma. Cochrane Database Syst Rev. 2010;(7):CD003583.

179. Neering H. Treatment of melasma (chloasma) by local application of steroid cream. Dermatologica. 1975;151:349–53.

180. Sneddon I. A trial of hydrocortisone butyrate in the treatment of rosacea and perioral dermatitis. Br J Dermatol. 1973;89:505–8.

181. Chi CC, Kirtschig G, Aberer W, et al. Evidence-based (S3) guideline on topical corticosteroids in pregnancy. Br J Dermatol. 2011;165:943–52.

Ethical Use of Topical Corticosteroids

5

Abir Saraswat

Abstract

Topical corticosteroids are very useful drugs in the treatment of various inflammatory and pigmentary dermatoses. However, they are susceptible to overuse and misuse by virtue of their anti-inflammatory and pigment-lightening properties. It is therefore important for all clinicians to keep in mind the ethical underpinnings of the basic tenets of topical corticosteroid use. Basic aspects of medical ethics like truth telling, patient autonomy, and non-malfeasance are discussed in the context of topical corticosteroid use, so that prescribers can be aware of the potential pitfalls that lie in their way. The broad clinical prerequisites of ethical topical corticosteroid use are also dealt with briefly.

Keywords

Topical corticosteroids • Adverse effets • Medical ethics

Learning Points

1. A working clinical diagnosis and a thorough knowledge of clinical pharmacology of corticosteroid being prescribed are the two essentials of ethical use of TC.
2. Full explanation of the pros and cons of TC therapy should be done to the patient and all efforts should be made to ensure correct use. However, the patient's wishes should be respected if he/she doesn't want to use them.
3. "First do no harm" should be the guiding principle, especially if the disease in question is not a classical corticosteroid-responsive dermatosis or the use is for esthetic benefit.

A. Saraswat
Indushree Skin Clinic, Indiranagar, Lucknow, India
e-mail: abirsaraswat@yahoo.com

© Springer Nature Singapore Pte Ltd. 2018
K. Lahiri (ed.), *A Treatise on Topical Corticosteroids in Dermatology*,
DOI 10.1007/978-981-10-4609-4_5

5.1 Introduction

Topical corticosteroids (TCs) are some of the most extensively used therapeutic agents in the treatment of skin diseases. They are very widely prescribed not only by dermatologists but also general practitioners, pediatricians, gynecologists, and other specialists. They have antipruritic, anti-inflammatory, anti-proliferative, and pigment-lightening activity on the skin [1]. This wide-ranging activity profile leads to their frequent use in dermatology prescriptions. A recent prescription audit from an Indian dermatology clinic revealed that close to 30% of all prescriptions contained a TC [2]. A study from primary-care physicians in Bahrain reported that 13% of the prescriptions to infants contained one or more TC and almost half of them were moderately potent or potent [3]. In addition to prescription use, mild topical corticosteroids have over-the-counter status in most countries and are considered generally safe for unsupervised use. In India, although topical corticosteroids are Schedule H drugs and therefore can only be dispensed on the prescription of a registered medical practitioner, legal and enforcement loopholes allow an almost completely unregulated sale of topical agents containing corticosteroids.

An important reason for such widespread use is the ability of TCs to give relatively quick relief in most unpleasant signs and symptoms of skin diseases. Symptoms such as itch, stinging, and tenderness are rapidly relieved regardless of the underlying cause, as are redness, scaling, and hyperpigmentation. The transient nature of such improvement becomes quickly apparent upon discontinuation of treatment and can lead to a vicious cycle of abuse of TC to control worsening complaints that are only suppressed, not treated.

The increasing popularity of esthetic dermatology has also subtly led to a shift in physician and patient behavior where the former have simply become purveyors of various treatments designed to enhance appearance and the latter into demanding clients or consumers of such services. Patient satisfaction is a very important parameter in this scenario [4], which can lead to diminished importance being given to potential long-term adverse effects of treatments. The pigment-lightening activity of TC is especially pertinent in this scenario, with a lot of Indian clients demanding "fairness treatments" from their esthetic physicians, who advertise such services in contravention of medical ethics and law. This leads to widespread misuse of TC-containing products in the community [5–8]. Even apart from the esthetic dermatology setting, traditional dermatologists are facing increasingly demanding patients who are intolerant of unpleasant symptoms and expect instant gratification in medicine, as in modern life in general. This greatly increases the chances of unethical or irrational use of these agents. This misuse happens due to various errors of omission or commission by patients, pharmacists, and physicians themselves, as several studies have shown [5–8]. Both local and systemic side effects can occur due to such misuse of TC [6].

The extent of damage that is caused by the rampant abuse of TC can be gauged by a recent study of 1000 dermatology outpatients [9] where 51.9% of patients using these agents reported suffering from at least one side effect. In this study, acne was one of the most common reasons for use, an indication of the extent of irrational use of TC in the community. It is perhaps due to such misuse that TCs have acquired a bad reputation in the minds of lay persons, and a small but growing population of patients are becoming TC-phobic, eschewing their use even for legitimate indications [10, 11]. For these reasons, it is absolutely essential that clinicians reacquaint themselves with rational and ethical use of topical corticosteroids.

5.2 What Are the Ethical Issues That Are Relevant to Topical Corticosteroid Use?

Ethical issues in topical corticosteroid use are manifold. From the public health point of view as well as in individual patient-physician interaction, various ethical questions arise vis-à-vis TC use and need to be addressed:

1. Truth telling: Physicians often use TC for symptom relief when they are faced with an irate patient who has severe itching or redness of the skin of unclear etiology, without paying sufficient attention to diagnosing the illness and getting to the root of the problem. The reasons may be multiple, ranging from overcrowded OPDs to a natural human tendency to ease the pain of the patient. However, in most such situations, the patient is not aware that the physician has not been able to arrive at a firm diagnosis and is merely buying time by prescribing something that will give quick relief while planning investigations or a more detailed examination at a subsequent visit. The problem with such an approach is quite evident: the patient happily continues to use the TC for a long time, without bothering to return to the physician for another evaluation or investigations. If the physician honestly confesses to the patient that he is unable to arrive at a firm diagnosis and needs a revisit or investigations to do so, patients can become more amenable to tolerate their unpleasant symptoms while this is done. Quite a few prescriptions of TC can be avoided in this way, thereby minimizing the chances of misuse.

2. Patient autonomy: This refers to respect for the individuals' right to make informed decisions about their personal matters. In other words, the patient has the right to refuse or choose their treatment (*Voluntas aegroti suprema lex*). In direct contrast to this is the concept of paternalistic medicine, where physicians simply order the patients to take a drug, without regard to his personal preferences, beliefs, etc. With regard to TCs, this law applies when we are faced with a steroid-phobic patient. In this situation, "soft paternalism" [12] is often a good approach whereby such a patient should be counselled about the potential benefits of TC use, the harm that can be caused by nonuse, and how common adverse effects can be avoided. However, they should also be informed about alternative therapies, e.g., topical calcineurin inhibitors or calcipotriol and their efficacy vis-à-vis

TCs. After this, whatever their ultimate decision be, it should be respected and a prescription given accordingly.

3. Non-malfeasance: This is the principle of *primum non nocere* (first, do no harm). There are important ramifications of this principle in a TC prescription. A common scenario where non-malfeasance needs to be remembered is a patient who is obsessed with a fair complexion and asks for a TC prescription which he/she may have heard about from a friend. It is absolutely essential to avoid the temptation to give in to the patient's request in this situation. This is especially true in esthetic practice, where healthcare providers are dealing with healthy clients, not sick patients. The desire to give the client what he/she wants can sometimes come into conflict with non-malfeasance in this situation. For example, TC are sometimes used to control redness or post-inflammatory hyperpigmentation caused by a chemical peel or laser resurfacing, which would perhaps not been done if the principle of non-malfeasance had been observed strictly. Non-malfeasance also becomes relevant when we are dealing with an undiagnosed rash and a demanding, distressed patient. Several studies have been reported on the misuse of TCs, especially on the face [6, 7] where the initial prescription was given for an undiagnosed facial rash which then led to prolonged misuse of TCs leading to considerable morbidity. In such a scenario, pending a diagnosis, TCs should be avoided and relief given with safer options like topical antipruritics and oral antihistamines. In the absence of a clear diagnosis and treatment plan, a physician should not hesitate to refer a patient to a senior colleague or an expert instead of using TCs to suppress unpleasant symptoms indefinitely.

4. Beneficence vs. autonomy: This kind of conflict occurs when patients disagree with recommendations that doctors believe are in the patients' best interest. An appropriate example would be a patient with widespread eczema who is applying potent TCs over a large area leading to adverse effects [13]. The appropri-

ate approach in such a situation would be to start a systemic steroid-sparing drug like azathioprine and gradually taper the TC. However, many patients are scared of systemic immunosuppressives and resist such treatment. Appropriate counselling about the dangers of potent TC use over large areas along with laboratory demonstration of adrenal suppression, low serum cortisol levels, etc. will be needed to convince the patient.

In fact, effective communication is the key to resolving almost all ethical dilemmas faced by a physician prescribing TCs. Not only doctor-patient but communication between doctors of different specialties and between doctors and society in general is essential in resolving these ethical issues. This is discussed in greater detail in later sections (*vide infra*).

5.3 Prerequisites for Ethical Use of Topical Corticosteroids [14]

1. The right diagnosis: There are relatively few conditions where there is good evidence of efficacy of TCs. Various eczemas, psoriasis, lichen planus, immunobullous diseases in their localized form, and skin manifestations of collagen vascular diseases like lupus erythematosus or dermatomyositis are the best-established indications. Other conditions where careful, short-term use may be warranted are superficial fungal or bacterial infections associated with significant inflammation, localized itch of any origin, and certain idiopathic diseases characterized by dermal inflammation, e.g., superficial variants of pyoderma gangrenosum. In the absence of a diagnosis, it is very important to avoid TC use so that conditions like tinea incognito and Majocchi's granuloma are not produced [15]. If a patient is already applying TC, thereby obscuring the clinical features of a disease, an appropriate treatment-free interval should be given after explaining to the patient that his/her symptoms may flare up temporarily to facilitate a diagnosis.

2. The right molecule and delivery system: Since they were first introduced in the early 1950s, TCs have grown tremendously as a class, and today, more than 20 different molecules of varying potency are available worldwide, ranging from mild to superpotent. In addition, there are varying concentrations and dosage forms available, viz., creams, gels, lotions, ointments, foams, muco-adherent gels, aerosols, and tapes. It is important for the prescriber to be familiar with at least a few of the molecules, preferably of differing potencies [16]. The characteristics of the various dosage forms should also be thoroughly understood so that the correct drug in the correct vehicle can be given in a particular situation. Although it is generally good to err on the side of caution when prescribing TCs, in many situations, it is better to prescribe a more potent molecule to control the disease quickly and stop treatment fast instead of prolonged treatment with a mild formulation. This is especially true of self-limited conditions like acute irritant dermatitis, paederus dermatitis, etc.

3. The right patient: The age, sex, and occupation of the patient play an important role in determining TC use. Very young and very old patients have impaired epidermal barrier function and relatively thinner skin. In addition, infants have a very high surface area-to-weight ratio that can lead to disproportionately high systemic absorption from topical application [17]. Women who do housework often have damaged skin due to frequent wet-dry cycling. This creates the need for more frequent application, as do certain occupations involving manual labor. Other factors like the anatomical location and extent of the disease also dictate which formulation is optimal. Thin skin areas like the eyelids, face, and scrotum need milder products than the back, palms, and soles. Widespread dermatoses demand easily spreadable dosage forms and milder potencies to guard against undesirable systemic absorption [18]. Cosmetic considerations are paramount when TCs are applied on the face or other visible parts, and creams, gels, and lotions are preferred here due to their elegance.

Intertriginous areas are particularly susceptible to stronger than expected effect due to the occlusion and maceration of the skin, and therefore we should err on the side of caution when deciding the potency on these sites [15].

4. The right amount, frequency, and duration: Perhaps the most common omission in a TC prescription is advice regarding the right amount to be applied in a particular situation. In this regard, the fingertip unit (FTU) devised by Long and Finlay [19] is the simplest way to explain to the patient how much TC is to be applied. An FTU is the amount of ointment that occupies the space from the fingertip to the first skin crease when squeezed out of a 5 mm nozzle. This amount was found to be 0.5 g for most adult-sized hands. This amount is enough to cover a palm-sized area on the skin in the case of creams and about 20% more with ointments due to their increased spreadability. Standard recommendations have been developed to guide how many FTUs are required to cover particular anatomical areas [19]. This should be clearly conveyed to the patient to prevent over- or underuse.

The frequency of application is dependent on patient factors such as site and occupation. The hands and feet often need twice or thrice a day application due to the propensity of being rubbed off. Otherwise, most experts agree that once daily application is optimal for all other sites since more frequent application has shown no added benefit [18, 20–24] and adherence is also expected to be higher with this regimen.

The duration of treatment needs to be clearly told to the patient orally as well as in writing, and he/she should also be apprised of the dangers of overuse at this point. In general, a follow-up visit should be planned after 2–4 weeks to review the progress and institute the exit strategy.

5. The right "exit strategy": It is extremely important to have a clear plan in mind about tapering and stopping TC use after adequate control/remission has been achieved. Except for self-limiting conditions, TC use is often needed for extended periods, much longer than recommended safe durations. This can be done safely by tapering down to progressively less potent preparations or instituting alternate-day or weekends-only treatment [25]. Emollients and/or steroid-sparing drugs like calcineurin inhibitors are prescribed on TC-free days. Finding the right exit strategy can involve a lot of empiricism but is a worthwhile skill to learn for every physician.

6. Focusing on prevention and modifiable factors: In many conditions, lasting remission or cure is only achievable if preventive actions are taken or behavioral modifications are done. TCs can only give temporary relief in these situations. Recurrent irritant hand dermatitis, pseudofolliculitis barbae, and intertrigo are good examples of these conditions. Physicians should ensure that the quick relief provided by TCs does not make them complacent about tackling deeper issues [26]. They should explain to the patients that relief will be transient if preventive actions like skin protection and moisturizing (hand eczema), changing shaving habits (pseudofolliculitis barbae), and keeping the skin dry, losing weight, and wearing loose natural fabrics (intertrigo) are not done.

7. Being aware of corticosteroid allergy: Many times we are faced with a patient who does not show the desired improvement even if appropriate TC is being used. At other times, control is achieved, only to lead to episodes of increased disease activity which are controlled with increasingly higher-potency corticosteroids. In these situations, we should be aware of the possibility of contact dermatitis to topical corticosteroids [25, 27]. This can happen both due to the preservatives/other excipients or the active molecule per se. In these cases, appropriate patch testing followed by prescription of an allergen-free product should be done.

8. Effective communication: Involving and informing the patient at every step of diagnosis and treatment is the key to using TCs safely, ethically, and effectively. A few scenarios are presented below to exemplify this point.

Patients often self-treat themselves with over-the-counter TCs before coming to the physician, altering the appearance of the skin and making diagnosis difficult [15]. In such a situation, it behooves us to explain the situation to the patient and withdraw all TCs while relevant investigations are done. Even if no investigations are done, a steroid-free interval often renders the disease recognizable, allowing proper treatment to be started.

Patients often neglect to come for follow-up when asked to, either due to financial constraints such as loss of wages/inability to pay revisit fees or simply due to negligence. To minimize the chances of adverse effects of TC, partial control of the treatment should be handed over to the patient, thus making them partners in their well-being, not just the recipients of instructions. To this end, they can be told at which point they should start alternate-day treatment, introduce a calcineurin inhibitor, or switch over to a milder TC. With this, they should also be told the warning signs of common adverse effects like folliculitis which would necessitate a revisit immediately.

Many patients are unsure how long it would take for the effect of TCs to start and therefore either become anxious too quickly or continue to use an ineffective TC preparation till the next scheduled visit. To avoid this, patients should be clearly told approximately how long it would take for the beneficial effects of the TC to "kick in." They should be counselled to walk in if they are not feeling substantially better at this point.

Corticosteroid phobia is an increasingly common problem in urban and internet-savvy patients [11]. A lot of counselling and reassurance is needed if these patients or their dependents are not to be denied the benefits of TCs. They also need to be told about the non-TC options available and their relative efficacy. If they still choose not to use TCs, their choice should be respected and an appropriate regimen devised.

Conclusion

Ethical use of corticosteroids demands a sound grasp of dermatotherapeutics and a deep understanding of human behavior. Easy availability of TC and the public perception of topical agents as being harmless are causing a lot of harm to dermatology patients. Many patients are becoming steroid-phobic and are being deprived of the beneficial effects of this class of drugs. It is the need of the hour that dermatologists revisit the ethical aspects of TC use and ensure that they are used effectively and safely by the patients. This can be achieved by adhering to good prescription practices and ensuring effective communication with patients so that they fully understand the nuances of correct use of these agents. It is also our duty to train other physicians who provide basic skin care in the same tenets of safe and effective topical therapy using TC, because it is not possible nor desirable for dermatologists to see to all patients with dermatological complaints.

References

1. Sulzberger MB, Witten VH. The effect of topically applied compound F in selected dermatoses. J Invest Dermatol. 1952;19(2):101.
2. Rathod SS, Motghare VM, Deshmukh VS, Deshpande RP, Bhamare CG, Patil JR. Prescribing practices of topical corticosteroids in the outpatient dermatology department of a rural tertiary care teaching hospital. Indian J Dermatol. 2013;58:342–5.
3. Al Khaja KA, Damanhori AH, Al-Ansari TM, Sequeira RP. Topical corticosteroids in infants: prescribing pattern and prescribing errors in Bahrain. Pharm World Sci. 2007;29:395–9.
4. Prakash B. Patient satisfaction. J Cutan Aesthet Surg. 2010;3:151–5.
5. Kandhari R, Khunger N. Skin-lightening agents-use or abuse? A retrospective analysis of the topical preparations used by melasma patients of darker skin types. Indian J Dermatol Venereol Leprol. 2013;79:701–2.
6. Saraswat A, Lahiri K, Chatterjee M, Barua S, Coondoo A, Mittal A, et al. Topical corticosteroid abuse on the face: a prospective, multicentre study of dermatology outpatients. Indian J Dermatol Venereol Leprol. 2011;77:160–6.
7. Rathi SK, Kumrah L. Topical corticosteroid-induced rosacea-like dermatitis: a clinical study of 110 cases. Indian J Dermatol Venereol Leprol. 2011;77:42–6.
8. Al-Dhalimi MA, Aljawahiri N. Misuse of topical corticosteroids: a clinical study from an Iraqi hospital. East Mediterr Health J. 2006;12:847–52.

9. Nagesh TS, Akhilesh A. Topical steroid awareness and abuse: a prospective study among dermatology outpatients. Indian J Dermatol. 2016;61:618–21.

10. Drake LA, Dinehart SM, Farmer ER, Goltz RW, Graham GF, Hordinsky MK, et al. Guidelines of care for the use of topical glucocorticosteroids. J Am Acad Dermatol. 1996;35:615–9.

11. Bewley A, Berth-Jones J, Bingham A, et al. Expert consensus: time for a change in the way we advise our patients to use corticosteroids. Br J Dermatol. 2008;158:917–20.

12. Hector C. Nudging towards nutrition? Soft paternalism and obesity related reform. Food Drug Law J. 2012;67:103–22.

13. Gilbertson EO, Spellman MC, Piacquadio DJ, Mulford MI. Super potent topical corticosteroid use associated with adrenal suppression: clinical considerations. J Am Acad Dermatol. 1998;38(2 Pt 2): 318–21.

14. Saraswat A. Ethical use of topical corticosteroids. Indian J Dermatol. 2014;59:469–72.

15. Solomon BA, Glass AT, Rabbin PE. Tinea incognito and "over the-counter" potent topical steroids. Cutis. 1996;58:295–6.

16. Ference JD, Last AR. Choosing Topical Corticosteroids. Am Fam Physician. 2009;79:135–40.

17. Chen AY, Zirwas MJ. Steroid-induced rosacea-like dermatitis: case report and review of the literature. Cutis. 2009;83:198–204.

18. Munro DD. The effect of percutaneously absorbed steroids on hypothalamic-pituitary-adrenal function after intensive use in in-patients. Br J Dermatol. 1976;94(Suppl 12):67–76.

19. Long CC, Finlay AY. The finger-tip unit-a new practical measure. Clin Exp Dermatol. 1991;16:444–7.

20. Fisher D. Adverse effects of topical corticosteroid use. West J Med. 1995;162:123–6.

21. Rathi SK, D'Souza P. Rational and ethical use of topical corticosteroids based on efficacy and safety. Indian J Dermatol. 2012;57:251–9.

22. Williams HC. Established corticosteroid creams should be applied only once daily in patients with atopic eczema. BMJ. 2007;334:1272.

23. Lagos B, Maibach H. Frequency of application of topical corticosteroids: an overview. Br J Dermatol. 1998;139:763–6.

24. Giannotti B. Current treatment guidelines for topical corticosteroids. Drugs. 1988;36(Suppl 5):9–14.

25. Saraswat A. Contact allergy to topical corticosteroids and sunscreens. Indian J Dermatol Venereol Leprol. 2012;78:552–9.

26. Saraswat A. Topical corticosteroid use in children: adverse effects and how to minimize them. Indian J Dermatol Venereol Leprol. 2010;76:225–8.

27. Scheuer E, Warshaw E. Allergy to corticosteroids: update and review of epidemiology, clinical characteristics, and structural cross reactivity. Am J Contact Dermat. 2003;14:179–87.

Topical Corticosteroid During Pregnancy: Indications, Safety and Precautions

6

Manas Chatterjee, Manish Khandare, and Vibhu Chatterjee

Abstract

The systemic availability of topical corticosteroids alters during pregnancy due to alterations in the cutaneous hydration and blood flow. Topical corticosteroids are commonly used to treat cutaneous manifestation associated with inflammatory conditions, autoimmune response as well as dermatoses associated with atopy such as atopic dermatitis, contact dermatitis, psoriasis and lichen planus. During the first trimester of pregnancy as per existing data the safety of corticosteroids is difficult to interpret and often conflicting. Due to concerns for possible fetal harm, the pregnant women sometimes get under treated because of 'steroid phobia'.

Keywords

Topical corticosteroids • Orofacial cleft • Fetal growth restriction

Learning Points

1. As compared to high potency corticosteroids, medium potency topical corticosteroids should be used during pregnancy.

2. As second-line therapy, high potency topical corticosteroids can be given to a patient for a short duration, and appropriate obstetric care should be provided because of increased risk of orofacial clefting and intrauterine growth restriction.

3. No data available to determine the association of intrauterine growth restriction and use of newer lipophilic topical corticosteroids with a good therapeutic index such as methylprednisolone aceponate, fluticasone propionate and mometasone furoate.

M. Chatterjee (✉) • M. Khandare
Department of Dermatology, Institute of Naval Medicine, INHS Asvini,
Colaba, Mumbai 400005, India
e-mail: drmanaschatterjee@gmail.com

V. Chatterjee
Department of Obs and Gynae, Command Hospital
(Eastern Command), Kolkata 700027, India

© Springer Nature Singapore Pte Ltd. 2018
K. Lahiri (ed.), *A Treatise on Topical Corticosteroids in Dermatology*,
DOI 10.1007/978-981-10-4609-4_6

6.1   Introduction

Topical therapy constitutes one of the pillars of treatment of dermatological disorders. In 1952, the first report of the successful use of topical corticosteroids in dermatological disorders was published by Sulzberger and Witten [1]. Topical corticosteroids as one of the major components of the dermatologist's therapeutic armamentarium are prescribed to up to 6% of pregnant women for cutaneous manifestations such as chronic cutaneous lupus erythematosus, pemphigoid gestationis, chronic plantar pustulosis, pruritic urticarial papules and plaques of pregnancy (PUPPP), and atopic eruptions [2]. Topical corticosteroids during pregnancy should be used only if the adequate benefit justifies the potential risk to the fetus. The US Food and Drug Administration (FDA) labels topical corticosteroids as pregnancy risk category C [3].

6.2   Cutaneous Absorption and Bioavailability of Topical Corticosteroid in Pregnancy

The percutaneous absorption of topical corticosteroid and its potential for systemic exposure [4] is determined by several factors including:

- Type of vehicle used
- Chemical composition
- Epidermal barrier
- Frequency of application
- Occlusive dressings
- Body surface area involved
- Thickness of the skin as per regional anatomical variation
- Metabolism
- Period of gestation.

Depending on certain pharmacokinetic properties, lipophilicity and degradability, different topical corticosteroids have different systemic bioavailability. In patients suffering from severe skin disease, the least potent corticosteroid hydrocortisone, after percutaneous absorption are capable to suppress the adrenals [5].

Clobetasol propionate ointment which is the most potent topical corticosteroid can result in adrenal insufficiency at doses as low as 2 g daily^{-1} for 1 week [6]. Under extreme conditions adrenal insufficiency can be seen after topical application of lipophilic corticosteroids (i.e., mometasone furoate, fluticasone propionate and methylprednisolone aceponate) [7, 8]. The systemic availability of topical corticosteroids is affected during pregnancy due to alterations in the cutaneous blood circulation and hydration [9].

6.3   Metabolism of Corticosteroid in Pregnancy

Once corticosteroids get absorb, more than 90% of cortisol in plasma is reversibly bound to transcortin or corticosteroid-binding globulin (CBG) which is an α-globulin secreted by the liver and albumin. The corticosteroid effect is mediated by the unbound fraction which enters the cells. Albumin has large binding capacity for corticosteroids and low affinity whereas CBG has relatively low total binding capacity for corticosteroids but high affinity. Most of the hormone gets bound at low as well as normal concentrations of corticosteroids. The protein binding capacity increases due to higher corticosteroid concentrations, and a greater fraction of the corticosteroid exists in the free state. During pregnancy due to physiological hypercorticism, there is increase in the circulating oestrogen levels which induces CBG production, results in increased total plasma cortisone. The synthetic congeners of biologically active adrenocortical corticosteroids gets metabolized in the liver and excreted via kidneys.

The topical corticosteroids effects on fetus also depend on the penetrating efficiency of corticosteroid through placenta. The cortisol (hydrocortisone, the active form) gets converted to cortisone (biologically inactive) by 11β-hydroxysteroid dehydrogenase (11βHSD) which metabolizes corticosteroids in the placenta. Thus, 11βHSD protects the fetus from potential harm by playing an important role in regulating the amount of maternal cortisol that crosses the placenta [10]. In the placenta, because of low potency and high metabolism, hydrocortisone is considered safe for use in antenatal cases, but a study based on maternal–fetal cortisol transfer in the fetal–placental unit before abortion showed that 15% of ^{3}H-cortisol crossed the placenta unmetabolized [11] and another study found a linear relation between maternal and fetal serum cortisol concentrations [12, 13]. Only 1/8th to 1/10th of prednisolone reaches to the fetus by placental transfer [14]. Betamethasone, dexamethasone, and methylprednisolone are less metabolized while fluticasone propionate and budesonide are not metabolized by placental 11βHSD [15, 16] therefore, leads to placental transfer in high concentration. There are no studies available on the other corticosteroids.

6.4   Indications

Topical corticosteroids required to be used during maternal skin conditions in pregnancy:

1. Autoimmune dermatoses such as discoid lupus erythematosus, vesiculobullous disorders such as pemphigoid gestationis, pemphigus vulgaris.
2. Inflammatory dermatoses such as PUPPP, atopic eruption of pregnancy, granuloma annulare, seborrhoeic dermatitis, psoriasis, lichen planus, lichen sclerosus.
3. Other miscellaneous steroid responsive dermatoses.

6.5   Safety Profile

To the best of our knowledge, certain animal studies have found that corticosteroids are present in the fetal blood after topical application, but there are no human studies evaluating the amounts of topical corticosteroids that reach the fetus after topical application. In mice and rabbits, significant amounts of betamethasone 17,21-dipropionate appeared in the fetal blood after topical application to their mothers' skin [17]. Furthermore, corticosteroids are teratogenic not only through systemic administration but also through topical application in animals. For example, diflorasone diacetate

cream on topical application induced cleft palate at a dose of 0.001 mg/kg which is about 30% of the human topical dose, when applied to the chest skin of pregnant rats. The application dose when increased to 0.5 mg/kg per day, the rate of fetal death increased to the untreated controls. It has been observed that rabbits suffered from depressed fetal growth, external anomalies (31.9%), cleft palate (22.2%) and visceral defects (45.5%) on receiving a topical dose of diflorasone diacetate 0.016 mg/kg per day [3]. Taken together, the studies suggest that for pregnant women who need treatment with topical corticosteroids, medium potency topical corticosteroids should be preferred to high potency preparations. If potent or superpotent topical corticosteroids are needed, the amount used should be kept to a minimum and fetal growth should be monitored.

In humans, the available data on the safety of topical corticosteroids in pregnancy are limited and mainly based upon observational studies [2]. The systemic effects of topical corticosteroids depend largely on the extent of skin absorption, which varies from 0.7% to 7% through intact skin [18], which may have an impact on the fetus as well as lead to systemic effects [5]. However, for inflammatory dermatoses where cutaneous absorption is more, topical corticosteroids are often prescribed. Hydrocortisone cream 1% is the low potency corticosteroid, its absorption during exacerbation of atopic dermatitis was 11–31 times that in remission [18]. Although the application of hydrocortisone cream 1% beyond 1 month in patients with severe cutaneous manifestations was shown to suppress the adrenal glands [5]. Administration of hydrocortisone in pregnancy may still affect the fetus and the fetotoxic effects of corticosteroids depend on their ability to cross the placenta [18]. The ability to cross the placental barrier varies among other corticosteroids as stated.

Studies have shown an association between intrauterine growth retardation and the occurrence of chronic diseases during adult life, including coronary artery disease, hypertension and diabetes mellitus [19]. Some studies also indicate the association of effects of corticosteroids in fetus with a higher risk of intrauterine growth retardation [20, 21], congenital malformations such as cleft palate

[22] and cataract [23], and a higher incidence of stillbirth [20, 24]. Though, some studies have failed to confirm this. There is significant difference in the studies suggesting minimal effects on the human fetus as compare to the data derived from animal studies [25]. Inhalational corticosteroid, one of the treatment modalities for asthma may lead to preterm delivery and fetal death [26]. Though, the association between asthma and adverse birth outcomes is because of disease per se or by inhalational corticosteroid therapy, or other unknown factors still to be confirmed.

6.5.1 Orofacial Cleft

Fifth to 12th gestational week is the period for fusion of the lip and palate. [2]. In one of the studies, out of 24 patients composed of women who received a dispensed prescription for topical corticosteroids during the first 12 gestational weeks, eight patients developed orofacial defects [27]. A case-control survey of 48 children with nonsyndromic cleft lip or palate showed a significant increase in the prevalence of maternal use of topical corticosteroid preparations in the first trimester of pregnancy, compared to 58 controls born in the same hospital [28]. In another study, no association of orofacial cleft with early maternal exposure to topical corticosteroids (i.e., receiving one or more prescriptions for topical corticosteroids during the period from 85 days before last menstrual period to gestational week 12) was found. When stratified by corticosteroid potency, no associations of orofacial cleft with exposure to medium potency and high potency topical corticosteroids were found [29].

6.5.2 Fetal Growth Restriction

In a study carried out from data obtained from the NHS in the UK, without stratification for potency, no association was found between maternal exposure to topical corticosteroids and fetal growth restriction. One of these studies showed a significant association of low birth weight with maternal exposure to potent or very potent topical corticosteroids, but not with exposure to mild-to moderate-potency topical corticosteroids and also found that the risk of low birth weight was significantly increased only when the amount of potent or very potent corticosteroids exceeded 300 grams [30]. LBW, lower plasma cortisol levels and a reduced placental weight were noted in babies of mothers who used a very potent topical corticosteroid, clobetasol propionate, at a very high mean quantity of 600 g during the whole pregnancy [31].

6.5.3 Preterm Delivery

No association between maternal exposure to topical corticosteroids and preterm delivery was found. Studies found no associations of preterm delivery with exposure to either mild/moderate or potent/very potent topical corticosteroids. No dose–response relationship between preterm delivery and either medium potency or high potency topical corticosteroids has been found [29–31].

6.5.4 Fetal Death (Miscarriage and Stillbirth)

Stratified analysis found that there is no significant risk for miscarriage on maternal exposure to medium and high potency topical corticosteroids. No associations of stillbirth with exposure to medium and high potency topical corticosteroids were found [29–31].

6.6 Recommendations [32]

1. As compared to more potent corticosteroids, medium potency topical corticosteroids should be used during pregnancy.
2. As second-line therapy, high potency topical corticosteroids can be given to a patient for a short duration, and appropriate obstetric care should be provided because of increased risk of orofacial clefting and intrauterine growth restriction.

3. Topical corticosteroids have lesser bioavailability than that of systemic corticosteroids, therefore topical corticosteroids have lesser potential for fetotoxicity than systemic corticosteroids (systemic corticosteroids are associated with low birth weight and an increase in preterm delivery, and should not be used in preference (grade of recommendation: B).

4. On theoretical grounds there is increased risk of adverse effects on thin skin surface with high absorption like genitals, eyelids, flexures are treated with topical corticosteroids (grade of recommendation: D).

5. No data available to determine the association of intrauterine growth restriction and use of newer lipophilic topical corticosteroids with a good therapeutic index such as methylprednisolone aceponate, fluticasone propionate and mometasone furoate (grade of recommendation: D).

Conclusion

Despite a lack of definitive evidence, topical corticosteroids if used according to guidelines are probably safe during pregnancy [5]. However, findings in the systematic review by Chi et al. should lead physicians to observe the following recommendations:

1. Prescribe topical corticosteroid use prudently between gestational weeks 5–12 (i.e., ask women of childbearing age if a pregnancy is ongoing or is possible) because of a potentially increased risk of orofacial cleft.

2. Consider the possibility of increased risk of fetal growth restriction before prescribing potent or very potent topical corticosteroids to pregnant women.

References

1. Sulzberger MB, Witten VH. The effect of topically applied compound F in selected dermatoses. J Invest Dermatol. 1952;19(2):101–2.
2. Chi CC, Wang SH, Kirtschig G, Wojnarowska F. Systematic review of the safety of topical corticosteroids in pregnancy. J Am Acad Dermatol. 2010;62(4):694–705. Epub 2010 Feb 1
3. Narama I. Reproduction studies of diflorasone diacetate (DDA). IV. Teratogenicity study in rabbits by percutaneous administration. Pharmacometrics. 1984;28(2):241–50.
4. Robertson DB, Maibach HI. Topical corticosteroids. Int J Dermatol. 1982;21:59–67.
5. Turpeinen M. Adrenocortical response to adrenocorticotropic hormone in relation to duration of topical therapy and percutaneous absorption of hydrocortisone in children with dermatitis. Eur J Pediatr. 1989;148:729–31.
6. Sifton DW, editor. Physicians' desk reference. 56th ed. Montvale: Medical Economics Company; 2002.
7. Tschen EH, Bucko AD. Assessment of HPA-axis suppression with fluticasone cream 0.05% in patients with extensive psoriasis or eczema. Clin Drug Investig. 1998;16:111–6.
8. Kecskes A, Heger-Mahn D, Kuhlmann RK, et al. Comparison of the local and systemic side effects of methylprednisolone aceponate and mometasone furoate applied as ointments with equal antiinflammatory activity. J Am Acad Dermatol. 1993;29:576–80.
9. Mattison DR. Transdermal drug absorption during pregnancy. Clin Obstet Gynecol. 1990;33:718–27.
10. Sun K, Yang K, Challis JR. Glucocorticoid actions and metabolism in pregnancy: implications for placental function and fetal cardiovascular activity. Placenta. 1998;19:353–60.
11. Murphy BE, Clark SJ, Donald IR, et al. Conversion of maternal cortisol to cortisone during placental transfer to the human fetus. Am J Obstet Gynecol. 1974;118:538–41.
12. Gitau R, Cameron A, Fisk NM, et al. Fetal exposure to maternal cortisol. Lancet. 1998;352:707–8.
13. Gitau R, Fisk NM, Teixeira JM, et al. Fetal hypothalamic–pituitary–adrenal stress responses to invasive procedures are independent of maternal responses. J Clin Endocrinol Metab. 2001;86:104–9.
14. Beitins IZ, Bayard F, Ances IG, et al. The transplacental passage of prednisone and prednisolone in pregnancy near term. J Pediatr. 1972;81:936–45.
15. Miller NM, Williamson C, Fisk NM, et al. Infant cortisol response after prolonged antenatal prednisolone treatment. BJOG. 2004;111:1471–4.
16. Murphy VE, Fittock RJ, Zarzycki PK, et al. Metabolism of synthetic steroids by the human placenta. Placenta. 2007;28:39–46.
17. Yamada H, Nakano M, Ichihashi T. Fetal concentration after topical application of betamethasone 17,21-dipropionate (S-3440) ointment and teratogenesis in mice and rabbits. Pharmacometrics. 1981;21(4):645–55.
18. Sifton DW. Physicians' desk reference. 6th ed. Medical Economics Company: Montvale; 2002.
19. Seckl JR, Cleasby M, Nyirenda MJ. Glucocorticoids, 11beta-hydroxysteroid dehydrogenase, and fetal programming. Kidney Int. 2000;57:1412–7.
20. Warrell DW, Taylor R. Outcome for the foetus of mothers receiving prednisolone during pregnancy. Lancet. 1968;1:117–8.

21. Pirson Y, Van Lierde M, Ghysen J, Squifflet JP, Alexandre GP, van Ypersele de Strihou C. Retardation of fetal growth in patients receiving immunosuppressive therapy. N Engl J Med. 1985;313:328.

22. Harris JWS, Ross IP. Cortisone therapy in early pregnancy. Relation to cleft palate. Lancet. 1956;267:1045–7.

23. Kraus AM. Congenital cataract and maternal steroid ingestion. J Pediatr Ophthalmol. 1975;12:1107–8.

24. Walsh SD, Clark FR. Pregnancy in patients on long-term corticosteroid therapy. Scott Med J. 1967;12:302–6.

25. Ballard PD, Hearney EF, Smith MB. Comparative teratogenicity of selected glucocorticoids applied ocularly in mice. Teratology. 1977;16:175–80.

26. Wen SW, Demissie K, Liu S. Adverse outcomes in pregnancies of asthmatic women: results from a Canadian population. Ann Epidemiol. 2001;11:7–12.

27. Källén B. Maternal drug use and infant cleft lip/palate with special reference to corticoids. Cleft Palate Craniofac J. 2003;40(6):624–8.

28. Edwards MJ, Agho K, Attia J, et al. Case-control study of cleft lip or palate after maternal use of topical corticosteroids during pregnancy. Am J Med Genet A. 2003;120A:459.

29. Chi CC, Mayon-White RT, Wojnarowska FT. Safety of topical corticosteroids in pregnancy: a population-based cohort study. J Invest Dermatol. 2011;131(4):884–91.

30. Chi C, Wang SH, White RM, Wojnarowska FT. Pregnancy outcomes after maternal exposure to topical corticosteroids. JAMA Dermatol. 2013;149(11):1274–8035.

31. Mahé A, Perret JL, Ly F, Fall F, Rault JP, Dumont A. The cosmetic use of skin-lightening products during pregnancy in Dakar, Senegal: a common and potentially hazardous practice. Trans R Soc Trop Med Hyg. 2007;101(2):183–7.

32. Chi CC, Kirtschig G, Aberer W, Gabbud JP, Lipozencic J, Kárpáti S, et al. Evidence based (S3) guideline on topical corticosteroids in pregnancy. Br J Dermatol. 2011;165(5):943–52. Epub 2011 Sep 29

Pros and Cons of Topical Corticosteroids in Lactating Females

7

Asit Mittal and Sharad Mehta

Abstract

Breastfeeding provides significant advantage to both mother and child. There are many inflammatory dermatoses which can present exclusively over breast and nipple area or can present in generalized form during this period. These dermatoses could be the cause of cessation of breastfeeding in mother. Topical corticosteroid is the mainstay of therapy in such dermatosis. The advantage that topical corticosteroids offer should not be denied to the patient because of fear of their side effects. Using less potent steroid and that too on smaller area can reduce the risk to both mother and breast-fed infant.

Keywords

Topical corticosteroid · Breastfeeding · Safety

Learning Points

1. The use of topical corticosteroid to treat inflammatory dermatosis during breast-feeding should not be withheld due to unwanted fear.
2. Least potent steroid, for the shortest period of time and on limited area only, should be the rule while prescribing topical corticosteroid during breastfeeding.
3. Topical corticossteroid should always be wiped off thoroughly prior to nursing if it is applied over breast or nipple area.

7.1 Introduction

Corticosteroids have been the cornerstone of therapy for a large number of inflammatory skin disorders. Hydrocortisone was the first compound to be used in clinical dermatology. It is a natural glucocorticoid derived from the adrenal cortex. Its basic structure, i.e., cyclopentanoperhydrophenanthrene ring, forms the backbone of most topical corticosteroid molecules [1].

A. Mittal (✉) · S. Mehta
Department of Dermatology, RNT Medical College, Udaipur, Rajasthan, India
e-mail: asitmittal62@gmail.com; drsharadmehta03@gmail.com

© Springer Nature Singapore Pte Ltd. 2018
K. Lahiri (ed.), *A Treatise on Topical Corticosteroids in Dermatology*, DOI 10.1007/978-981-10-4609-4_7

Since their introduction various modifications have been made to this basic structure of hydrocortisone and topical corticosteroids to meet the adequate and safe use of corticosteroids in various inflammatory skin conditions. Numerous topical corticosteroids are now available in different preparations, concentrations, and potencies. Besides the active ingredients, vehicles and formulation also play a very important role in determining the potency of topical corticosteroids. Several formulations of topical corticosteroids are now available, including ointments, creams, gels, lotions, solutions, and newer formulations such as shampoos and foams.

Potency ranking of selected topical corticosteroid preparation [2]

Class	Commonly used topical steroids
Class 1: Superpotent	Clobetasol propionate 0.05% Halobetasol propionate 0.05%
Class 2: Potent	Betamethasone dipropionate 0.05% Mometasone furoate 0.1%
Class 3: Potent upper mid-strength	Betamethasone valerate 0.1% Clobetasone butyrate 0.05%
Class 4: Mid-strength	Fluocinolone acetonide 0.01%, 0.025% Triamcinolone acetonide 0.1% Triamcinolone diacetate 0.1%
Class 5: Lower mid-strength	Betamethasone valerate Fluticasone propionate 0.05%
Class 6: Low potent	Desonide Triamcinolone acetonide 0.025% Triamcinolone diacetate 0.025%
Class 7: Least potent	Hydrocortisone Dexamethasone

Topical steroids produce their effects via local immunosuppressive, antiproliferative, and anti-inflammatory effects. In highly responsive dermatoses, the use of low-to-medium potency corticosteroids is sufficient, while in less responsive ones, higher potency or occlusion is required to achieve an optimal clinical response. In poorly responsive disorders, the use of superpotent or intralesional corticosteroids is often required [3].

7.2 Bioavailability

The systemic effects of topical corticosteroids are generally limited because only about 3% of the medication in topical preparations is absorbed systemically following 8 h of contact with normal skin [4]. Absorption varies with different types and doses of preparations and the nature and extent of underlying skin conditions. When corticosteroids are used for long term or on large areas of the skin, they might have systemic effects [5–9].

7.3 Safety of Topical Steroids During Lactation

Breastfeeding provides many advantages to both mother and infant. One of the major reasons for early cessation of breastfeeding in mother is nipple and breast dermatosis. The use of topical corticosteroids in special circumstances such as breastfeeding is an area, which is filled with uncertainty. The US Food and Drug Administration (FDA) labels topical corticosteroids as pregnancy risk category C, meaning that animal studies have shown adverse fetal effects, but there are no adequate and well-controlled studies in pregnant women [10]. Studies regarding safety of topical corticosteroids in nursing mother are still sparse, but what is certain is that if significant concentration of corticosteroids reaches into systemic circulation of mother, it may lead to adverse effects not only in mother but also in breastfed infants. Nevertheless, topical corticosteroids remain the mainstay of treatment in a number of inflammatory dermatoses, in lactating females. These disorders may be preexisting dermatoses like psoriasis, atopic dermatitis, autoimmune blistering disorders, etc., or they may first appear during pregnancy itself and persist into postpartum period, e.g., pemphigoid gestationis, prurigo of pregnancy. In addition many of these inflammatory conditions may be localized to breast and nipple area only. A number of these disorders require the use of systemic steroids which a physician always feels hesitant to prescribe in a lactating female. In such scenario topical steroids play a very critical role in their management, but lack of information and clarity regarding the risk of topical corticosteroids leads to physician's uncertainty and often results in underprescription, followed by weakened adherence to the regimen and compromised therapeutic effectiveness.

Systemically administered corticosteroids are secreted into breast milk in quantities not likely to have a deleterious effect on the infant [11]. It is therefore unlikely that topical administration of corticosteroids will result in sufficient systemic absorption to produce detectable quantities in the breast. It is for this reason that topical corticosteroids are generally considered safe for use by breastfeeding mothers.

Nevertheless, caution should be exercised when topical corticosteroids are administered to a nursing woman. To minimize the possibility of steroids being absorbed through the skin and passing into the breast milk, one should not use topical corticosteroids on large areas of the skin, underneath airtight dressings, or for prolonged periods of time. Further using less potent or least potent topical corticosteroid and that too only on smaller area of the skin will reduce probability of systemic effects in mother. Also infant's skin should not come directly in contact with the area of the skin that has been treated [12].

Treating any dermatoses on the nipple and areola requires extra caution. Only the lower-potency topical corticosteroids should be applied on the nipple or areola, where infant could directly ingest the drug from the nipple. Clobetasol and other high-potency topical corticosteroids should be avoided on the nipple and areola [12].

Only water-miscible cream or gel products should be applied to the breast, because ointment may expose the infant to a high level of mineral paraffin via licking. Any topical corticosteroids should be wiped off thoroughly prior to nursing if it is being applied to breast or nipple area [13].

Breastfeeding is a special situation where the use of any pharmaceutical product by mother should be with caution and the same holds true for topical corticosteroid also. The adequate knowledge of potency of topical steroid will help the physician in prescribing the safest yet the most effective therapy to his/her patient.

References

1. Katz M, Gans EH. Topical corticosteroids, structure-activity and the glucocorticoid receptor: discovery and development—a process of "planned serendipity". J Pharm Sci. 2008;97:2936–47.
2. Wolff K, Goldsmith LA, Katz SI, Gilchrest BA, Paller AS, Leffell DJ, editors. Fitzpatcrik's dermatology in general medicine. 7th ed. New York, NY: McGraw-Hill; 2006.
3. Lagos BR, Maibach HI. Topical corticosteroids: unapproved uses, dosages, or indications. Clin Dermatol. 2002;20:490–2.
4. Tauscher AE, Fleischer AB Jr, Phelps KC, Feldman SR. Psoriasis and pregnancy. J Cutan Med Surg. 2002;6:561–70.
5. Hardman JG, Limbird LE, Gilman AG. Goodman and Gilman's the pharmacologic basis of therapeutics. 7th ed. New York, NY: McGraw-Hill; 1985. p. 1473.
6. Schaefer H, Zesch A, Stuttgen G. Penetration, permeation, and absorption of triamcinolone acetonide in normal and psoriatic skin. Arch Dermatol Res. 1977;258:241–9.
7. Turpeinen M. Absorption of hydrocortisone from the skin reservoir in atopic dermatitis. Br J Dermatol. 1991;124:358–60.
8. Barnetson RS, White AD. The use of corticosteroids in dermatological practice. Med J Aust. 1992;156:428–31.
9. Melendres JL, Bucks DA, Camel E, Wester RC, Maibach HI. In vivo percutaneous absorption of hydrocortisone: multiple-application dosing in man. Pharm Res. 1992;9:1164–7.
10. Briggs GG, Freeman RK, Yaffe SJ. Drugs in pregnancy and lactation. 8th ed. Philadelphia, PA: Lippincott Williams & Wilkins; 2008.
11. Greenberger PA, Odeh YK, Frederiksen MC, Atkinson AJ Jr. Pharmacokinetics of prednisolone transfer to breast milk. Clin Pharmacol Ther. 1993;53:324–8.
12. Barrett ME, Heller MM, Fullerton Stone H, Murase JE. Dermatoses of the breast in lactation. Dermatol Ther. 2013;26:331–6.
13. Noti A, Grob K, Biedermann M. Exposure of babies to C(15)-C(45) mineral paraffins from human milk and breast salves. Regul Toxicol Pharmacol. 2003;38(3):317–25.

Topical Corticosteroids in Blistering Diseases

8

Swaranjali V. Jain and Dedee F. Murrell

Abstract

The goals of management in autoimmune blistering diseases (AIBDs) are to stop disease progression, alleviate symptoms and minimise adverse effects related to treatment. Although systemic corticosteroids are widely used and effective in many AIBD, serious side effects often limit their use. Consequently, topical corticosteroids have been trialled to determine whether they are effective and safe in treating AIBD. This article will discuss the role of topical corticosteroids in a variety of AIBD and practical considerations for their use.

Keywords

Topical corticosteroids · Autoimmune blistering disease · Bullous pemphigoid · Pemphigus · Clobetasol propionate · Adrenal suppression

Learning Points

1. Superpotent topical corticosteroids are a safe and effective treatment option in a variety of autoimmune blistering diseases.
2. In bullous pemphigoid, clobetasol propionate is the first-line treatment and confers a significant survival advantage compared to oral systemic steroids, particularly in extensive disease.
3. Topical corticosteroids are recommended for mild or localised disease activity in pemphigus, mucous membrane pemphigoid and pemphigoid gestationis.
4. Topical corticosteroids are also useful as adjuvant therapy to reduce the side effects related to systemic therapy.
5. Minimisation of the local and systemic side effects of topical corticosteroids requires careful monitoring and follow-up.

S.V. Jain · D.F. Murrell (✉)
Department of Dermatology, St. George Hospital, and Faculty of Medicine, University of New South Wales, Sydney, NSW 2217, Australia
e-mail: d.murrell@unsw.edu.au

© Springer Nature Singapore Pte Ltd. 2018
K. Lahiri (ed.), *A Treatise on Topical Corticosteroids in Dermatology*, DOI 10.1007/978-981-10-4609-4_8

8.1   Introduction

Corticosteroids are widely used in the management of bullous diseases, particularly autoimmune blistering diseases (AIBDs), in which the immune system becomes dysregulated and produces antibodies against structures in normal skin. Oral corticosteroids along with newer immunosuppressive therapies are effective in attaining disease control, given their critical role in modulating the immune system response. Many of these systemic therapies however have undesirable and potentially serious side effects that can limit their use. Topical corticosteroids have the advantage of acting on local factors of inflammation in the skin while avoiding many of the adverse sequelae caused by the broader actions of systemic therapies. Although the rarity of many AIBD means high-quality evidence derived from large randomised controlled trials is scarce, clinical experience supports the use of potent topical corticosteroids as a treatment option in selected forms of AIBD. This article will discuss the role of topical corticosteroids in a variety of AIBDs and practical considerations for their use.

8.2   Pharmacology of Corticosteroids

8.2.1   Chemical Structure

The endogenous corticosteroid in humans is cortisol (hydrocortisone), which is produced in the adrenal glands through the cholesterol biosynthetic pathway [1]. Hydrocortisone is a 21-carbon corticosteroid arranged in four rings and has a relatively low potency [1, 2]. Most therapeutic corticosteroids are derived from hydrocortisone. These synthetic derivatives have altered chemical structures that increase their glucocorticoid activity and receptor affinity, absorption and duration of action compared to hydrocortisone [2]. Alterations that increase the potency of topical corticosteroids include the addition of a double bond between carbon atoms 1 and 2 (as in triamcinolone and betamethasone), the fluorination of carbon atom 9 (as in clobetasol) and the addition of ester groups (such as propionate and valerate) that increase the lipophilicity and hence epidermal absorption of the drug [1–3]. Clobetasol propionate is the most potent topical corticosteroid (Class I—superpotent) of those currently available, with a potency 1800 times greater than that of hydrocortisone [4]. The vehicle that these are dissolved in also affects their potency, with ointments generally being more effective at drug delivery into the skin than creams.

8.2.2   Mechanism of Action

The anti-inflammatory and immunosuppressive effects of corticosteroids result from the pleiotropic effects of the glucocorticoid receptor on multiple pathways [5]. There are two main modes of action. Corticosteroids act both directly on DNA and indirectly through modulating transcription factors (such as nuclear factor-kB) that control the expression of mediators important in the inflammatory response [1, 5, 6]. In AIBD, topical corticosteroids have the advantage of attaining high concentrations at the site of disease activity, such as the dermoepidermal junction in bullous pemphigoid [7]. They may thus control local inflammatory mediators, such as by inhibiting cytokines, chemokines, proteolytic enzymes, complement activation and the recruitment of inflammatory cells including neutrophils, lymphocytes and eosinophils [6–8].

Recent advances have allowed the postulation of new mechanisms of action of topical corticosteroids in AIBD, particularly in bullous pemphigoid. A bullous pemphigoid experimental model demonstrated that methylprednisolone inhibited the activation of, and signalling pathways in, neutrophils that are known to significantly contribute to autoantibody-induced tissue damage and suggested this pathway may also be affected by topical treatment [9]. Another study observed a rapid reduction in IL-17 expression, known to be produced by neutrophils, and MMP-9 in blister fluid specimens of bullous pemphigoid patients following treatment with superpotent topical corticosteroids. The reduction in IL-17 and MMP-9 mirrored the therapeutic response [10].

In addition to local mechanisms of action, topical corticosteroids may also act systemically. Systemic absorption of topically applied cortico-steroids may be indirectly reflected by suppressed endogenous cortisol levels following treatment [11]. Numerous studies have shown that topical application of clobetasol propionate (0.05%) corresponds with a reduction in morning cortisol levels, even after 1 day and following the first application of 20–30 g of clobetasol propionate [1, 11, 12]. With daily application, 20 mg of clobetasol propionate (40 g of 0.05% cream) may have an effect equivalent to 60 mg of oral prednisone per day [13, 14]. Systemic effects may be even greater in blistering diseases, as corticosteroid absorption is increased by a factor of 16 when skin is blistered [13]. Although a systemic action increases the efficacy of topical corticosteroid treatment, it also increases the likelihood of adverse sequelae related to treatment [15].

8.3   Use of Topical Corticosteroids in AIBD

8.3.1   Bullous Pemphigoid

8.3.1.1 Introduction

Bullous pemphigoid (BP) is the most common AIBD in most countries and is characterised by autoantibodies against BP180 and BP230, components of the dermal-epidermal junction [7]. BP is primarily a disease of the elderly. Consequently, many patients have significant comorbidities and frail general condition in addition to BP, which carries a mortality of up to 40% per year [16, 17].

The treatment of BP has changed significantly in the past decade. Until recently, high-dose systemic corticosteroids were the mainstay of management for BP [3, 7, 8]. Such regimens have been identified as a risk factor for increased mortality in the elderly, particularly as corticosteroids are poorly tolerated in this population [18, 19]. Superpotent topical corticosteroids were first proposed for BP in 1989 [20], with numerous subsequent case reports and uncontrolled trials supporting its use as first-line treatment in mild or limited disease [21]. Table 8.1 summarises the evidence for topical corticosteroid use in a variety of AIBD.

8.3.1.2 Evidence for Topical Corticosteroid Use in BP

Two seminal RCTs conducted by Joly and colleagues with a total of 653 patients confirmed the efficacy and safety of superpotent topical corticosteroids in controlling moderate and severe BP, in addition to improving survival. Joly et al. in 2002 showed that topical clobetasol propionate (0.05%, 40 g/day) cream was significantly superior to oral prednisone (1 mg/kg/day) for extensive disease (more than ten new blisters per day) in terms of overall survival at 1 year (76% vs 58%; $p = 0.02$) [17]. Topical clobetasol propionate cream was applied over the whole body (excluding the face) twice daily until disease control was achieved for 15 days, after which the dose was reduced by 15% every 3 weeks and ceased after 12 months. The topical regimen also had improved rates of disease control at 3 weeks (99% vs 91%; $p = 0.02$), reduced severe side effects (29% vs 54%; $p = 0.006$) and a shorter duration of hospitalisation (mean 17 vs 25 days; $p = 0.002$) compared with oral prednisone. In patients with moderate disease (fewer than ten new blisters per day), no significant differences were found between clobetasol propionate cream (0.05%, 40 g/day) and oral prednisone (0.5 mg/kg/day) regarding overall survival or adverse effects, with excellent disease control in both groups (100% vs 95%, respectively). Importantly, this study had good methodology in terms of adequate power and randomisation. A limitation which may have introduced bias was the non-blinded nature of the study, which potentially could have influenced assessments of disease control, but is likely to have had little impact on the primary endpoint of overall survival [21].

The same group, in 2009, demonstrated the benefits of a milder regimen of clobetasol propionate cream (0.05%, 10–30 g/day based on disease severity and weight) with a shorter duration of treatment (4 months), compared to the standard regimen of 40 g/day tapered over 12 months [22]. The milder regimen, which allowed a reduction in the cumulative dose of corticosteroids of 71%, was efficacious and non-inferior to the standard regimen in terms of disease control (100% vs 98%) for both moderate and severe disease. Significantly, after adjusting for age and

Table 8.1 Evidence for topical corticosteroid use in autoimmune blistering diseases

Type of topical corticosteroid	Level of evidence for use[a]					
	Bullous pemphigoid	Pemphigus	Mucous membrane pemphigoid	Pemphigoid gestationis	Linear IgA disease	Epidermolysis bullosa acquisita
Clobetasol propionate (0.05%)	1 – Generalised disease: superior survival compared to oral systemic steroids in severe disease 3 – Localised disease on lesional skin only	3 – Mild or localised (mucosal) disease	3 – Mild or localised (mucosal) disease	3 – Mild or localised disease	3 – Mild disease	N/A
Betamethasone	N/A	3	3	3	3	N/A
Dexamethasone (mouthwash)	N/A	3	3	N/A	N/A	N/A
Intralesional/ perilesional triamcinolone acetonide (injection)	N/A	3 – Recalcitrant oral lesions	3 – Recalcitrant oral lesions	N/A	N/A	N/A

N/A: data not available

[a]Levels of evidence

- Level 1: Evidence obtained from at least one properly designed randomised controlled trial
- Level 2-1: Evidence obtained from well-designed controlled trials without randomisation
- Level 2-2: Evidence obtained from well-designed cohort or case-control analytical studies, preferably from more than one centre or research group
- Level 2-3: Evidence obtained from multiple time series with or without the intervention. Dramatic results in uncontrolled trials might also be regarded as this type of evidence
- Level 3: Opinions of respected authorities, based on clinical experience, descriptive studies or reports of expert committees

functional status, patients with moderate BP treated with the mild regimen had a twofold decrease in mortality and life-threatening adverse effects (such as sepsis and cardiovascular disorders) during the first year of treatment compared with those on the standard regimen (hazard ratio 0.54, 95% confidence interval 0.30–0.97; $p = 0.039$). This may offset the slightly higher rate of relapse observed in the mild compared with the standard regimen group (43% vs 35%). The study additionally found a reduced basal cortisol response during treatment, supporting the hypothesis that the efficacy of superpotent topical corticosteroids could in part be due to systemic effects. A recent longitudinal study in 100 BP patients potentially supports the systemic role of topical corticosteroids in inducing immune suppression and inhibiting autoantibody synthesis [23]. Treatment with superpotent topical

corticosteroids induced a marked decrease within 60 days in serum levels of anti-BP180 and to a lesser extent anti-BP230, which corresponded with clinical improvement. Given that the RCT in 2002 found topical corticosteroids had fewer side effects but greater efficacy than prednisone, it is possible that systemic steroid levels due to percutaneous absorption are low but have a sustained action [17, 22].

8.3.1.3 Guidelines for the Use of Topical Corticosteroids in BP

The studies above contribute strong evidence of the efficacy and safety of superpotent topical corticosteroids for BP, which is reflected in clinical practice guidelines. Twice-daily whole-body application (excluding the face) of clobetasol propionate 0.05% cream or ointment (10–40 g/day) is recommended by a European consensus as the first-line treatment for both mild and generalised BP [24]. Treatment should begin tapering 15 days after disease control, which has standard definitions according to an international panel of experts (see Murrell et al. for details [25]), with cessation of treatment after 4–12 months. For localised disease, treatment of lesional skin only is recommended, although this regimen has not been validated in controlled studies [24].

The implementation of the above recommendations is potentially limited by practical factors, which are important to consider when choosing treatment. Disadvantages of topical corticosteroid treatment include difficult application in bedridden patients, poor compliance and higher cost (up to 110 times the price of prednisone) [13, 16, 26]. In these cases, systemic steroids are recommended as first-line therapy instead, despite their higher rates of adverse events [16].

Adjuvant therapy with other treatments, for example, with steroid-sparing agents, is recommended for consideration only in patients who are intolerant or resistant to topical corticosteroid treatment [7]. Newer research is investigating the utility of adding adjuvant therapies that are cheap, well-tolerated and also effective in BP to improve the practical use of topical corticosteroids in the future. For example, clobetasol propionate and betamethasone dipropionate have been used to initially induce remission in BP, followed by long-term maintenance with low-dose methotrexate [27, 28].

8.3.1.4 International Management of BP

Internationally, the modes of practice for the management of BP vary, which may be partially explained by the practical considerations discussed above. Some health systems, such as in France and the Netherlands, subsidise the cost of medications and nursing assistance, which may encourage the use of topical corticosteroids in these countries [26]. An international survey found that topical corticosteroid monotherapy was preferred in BP by 52.4% of clinician responders in the Netherlands compared with only 27% in Germany and 14.4% in the UK [29]. A similar survey of dermatologists in the UK

found the majority of responders only used topical corticosteroids for localised BP (98%), rather than generalised BP (34%) [30].

Varying international mortality rates of BP may also influence the relative benefits of topical compared with oral corticosteroids between countries. In the USA, which has a high rate of oral corticosteroid use in BP, a study reported a 1-year survival of 89% [31]. This was significantly higher than the 1-year survival rates reported in the literature, including that of 76% and 58% reported in French patients treated with topical and oral steroids, respectively, in Joly et al.'s 2002 study [13, 17, 18, 26]. These differences may be attributed to the different demographics, patient comorbidities and treatment practices (hospital vs outpatient) of BP between countries, highlighting the need to consider individual circumstances before recommending treatment [13, 26].

8.3.2 Pemphigus Vulgaris/ Pemphigus Foliaceus

Pemphigus vulgaris (PV) and pemphigus foliaceus (PF) are mucocutaneous blistering diseases caused by autoantibodies directed against cellular adhesion molecules, resulting in intraepidermal blistering. In contrast to BP, high-dose systemic corticosteroids are currently the first-line treatment for pemphigus, although adverse side effects may sometimes limit their use [32, 33]. Potent topical preparations are advocated as monotherapy in selected cases of mild or limited (particularly mucosal) disease or as an adjunct to help reduce doses of systemic therapy [32, 33].

Given the rarity of pemphigus, high-quality evidence from large RCTs is scarce. Support for topical corticosteroid use is largely derived from case reports and expert recommendations [3, 33]. Efficacy however appears limited when superpotent topical corticosteroids are used as monotherapy. For example, Dumas et al. in a small study (three PV patients, four PF patients) found that 10 g/day of clobetasol propionate cream 0.05% applied to lesional skin and mucosal lesions (betamethasone valerate 0.1% was used on the face) failed in three patients (two PV patients, one PF patient), necessitating systemic treatment [34]. Treatment efficacy may be increased in patients who at baseline have negative or low levels of autoantibodies [35].

Oral lesions in pemphigus are particularly difficult to treat and slower to heal than skin lesions, given the continuous trauma inherent in the oral environment [36]. Potent topical corticosteroid preparations can be used as adjuvant therapy to limit the systemic side effects of oral corticosteroids [32, 33]. Topical preparations recommended include soluble betamethasone sodium phosphate mouthwashes (0.5 mg tablet in 10 mL water) used four times a day, hydrocortisone (2.5 mg) lozenges and sprayed asthma inhalers (beclomethasone dipropionate 50–200 ug or budesonide 50–200 ug [32]. For isolated mucosal lesions, triamcinolone acetonide (0.1% in adhesive dental paste) and clobetasol propionate can be used [32, 37]. Intralesional/perilesional triamcinolone injections may be effective for recalcitrant oral lesions [36] and were shown in one study in oropharyngeal PV patients who were treated concomitantly with systemic steroids to reduce the total amount of corticosteroids and the time to remission by 27 days [38].

8.3.3 Mucous Membrane Pemphigoid

Mucous membrane pemphigoid (MMP) encompasses a group of inflammatory subepithelial blistering diseases that can affect a variety of mucocutaneous surfaces [39]. Treatment is largely guided by clinical experience and uncontrolled studies, with a paucity of evidence from RCTs demonstrating the efficacy of most interventions in MMP, including topical therapy [40]. Experts recommend consideration of the site and severity of disease to guide treatment. Topical corticosteroids can be used as monotherapy in patients with low-risk disease, defined as disease limited to the oral cavity, or oral mucosa and skin, given these sites are less likely to scar [39, 41]. In severe disease characterised by other mucosal involvement (ocular, pharyngeal, oesophageal and laryngeal mucosae) or in acute exacerbations, systemic corticosteroids are still recommended as the first-line treatment [39, 42, 43].

A variety of moderate-to-high potency topical corticosteroid regimens have been recommended for oral disease. These include clobetasol propionate and betamethasone valerate gels and ointments, which are easy to apply to the mucosa, and dexamethasone mouthwashes (5 mL of 100 g/mL in a 5 min swish-and-spit regimen) used two to four times per day [3, 39–41]. Adherence of medication to the mucosa can be enhanced by drying the mucosa with soft tissue paper before each application, compounding with Orabase [44] and having one application directly before bed, as oral secretions are reduced during sleep [39]. Oral insertable vinyl prosthetic devices made by dentists can also facilitate application and provide some occlusion, which can increase potency of the corticosteroids [37, 39, 41].

Topical corticosteroids may also be beneficial for skin lesions, and steroid sprays and inhalers may be used in nasal, pharyngeal and oesophageal disease [43]. Topical regimens have limited efficacy in controlling ocular disease and should be initiated in consultation with an ophthalmologist [43]. Intralesional triamcinolone acetonide injections every 2–4 weeks have been used for recalcitrant lesions of both the skin and mucosa; however, its use is potentially limited by the lack of long-term benefit and undesirable side effects, such as cataract formation when used near ocular surfaces [39, 41, 43].

8.3.4 Pemphigoid Gestationis

Pemphigoid gestationis (PG) is an autoimmune blistering disease of pregnancy characterised by autoantibodies against BP180 in the dermal-epidermal junction of the skin [45]. As in other AIBD, evidence is limited on corticosteroid use in the disease, particularly as pregnant patients are often excluded from interventional studies.

Systemic therapy is the mainstay of management, although small case studies and retrospective reviews support the use of potent topical corticosteroids in localised PG and mild disease, including those with early urticarial lesions or premenstrual flares [45, 46]. In these studies, clobetasol propionate 0.05% or betamethasone dipropionate 0.05% was applied twice daily. Topical corticosteroid use in pregnancy is safe, with a Cochrane review finding no significant association with congenital abnormalities, preterm delivery or stillbirth [47]. The review did link potent topical corticosteroid use with low birth weight, although the risk may only increase significantly when high doses are used [47–49] or when the amount of potent topical corticosteroid exceeds 300 g [50].

8.3.5 Linear IgA Disease

Linear IgA disease is a mucocutaneous blistering disease which has a long course before undergoing remission. Potent topical corticosteroids such as clobetasol propionate 0.05% have been recommended for mild disease and may be useful in improving symptoms in drug-induced disease following removal of the triggering agent [3, 51, 52]. Most patients however require systemic therapies, such as dapsone, with both oral and topical steroids primarily being used as adjunctive therapy only [3].

8.3.6 Epidermolysis Bullosa Acquisita

Epidermolysis bullosa acquisita (EBA) is an autoimmune blistering disease with two subtypes: an inflammatory type which mimics BP and a noninflammatory mechanobullous type [53]. Unlike most other AIBD, corticosteroids have limited efficacy particularly in the mechanobullous type of EBA, necessitating the use of other systemic therapies [40]. Topical corticosteroids have been used only in two case reports in EBA. In one patient with an inflammatory type of EBA and chronic hepatitis C which contraindicated systemic immunosuppression, daily application of topical clobetasol propionate (total of 40 g) for 2 months induced remission which lasted 8 years [54]. Another case report of EBA

localised to the face found topical corticosteroid initially improved symptom control and, however, was associated with multiple relapses during follow-up [55].

8.4 Side Effects of Topical Corticosteroids

Although topical corticosteroids are generally well-tolerated, they can have a range of local and, less commonly, systemic complications (Table 8.2). Many factors can increase the likelihood of side effects when used in AIBD. These include treatment-related factors, such as high-dose, high-potency and prolonged topical corticosteroid treatment often required in AIBD, and patient-related factors, such as older age, renal and hepatic dysfunction, and those with poor skin integrity [1, 2, 15].

While cutaneous adverse effects such as skin atrophy and purpura are common, they are benign and rarely reported to be a clinical problem [15, 17]. Systemic side effects can be potentially serious but are less common. Transient adrenal suppression was found to occur in up to 48% of patients treated with superpotent topical corticosteroids and can occur with doses as small as 2 g/day

Table 8.2 Side effects associated with topical corticosteroid use [1, 15, 17, 22, 39]

Local (cutaneous)	Systemic
Common	Hyperglycaemia and
Skin	diabetes mellitus
Atrophy	Adrenal insufficiency
Striae	Hypertension
Acne	Glaucoma
Purpura	Severe infection (e.g.
Telangiectasia	pneumonia and
Mucosa	septicaemia)
Atrophy	Cardiovascular diseases
Candidiasis	(MI, cardiac failure,
Dyspepsia	stroke)
Uncommon	DVT/PE
Hypertrichosis	Osteopathy (fractures or
Hypo- or	aseptic osteonecroses)
hyperpigmentation	
Secondary fungal and	
microbial infections	
Allergic contact	
dermatitis	

of clobetasol propionate 0.05% cream [1]. Patients however are usually asymptomatic and cortisol levels recover spontaneously within weeks [56]. In rare cases, topical corticosteroids causing iatrogenic Cushing's syndrome and death due to Addisonian crises have been reported [15].

Optimal management relies on using the minimum effective dose of medication required for disease control and careful monitoring for side effects during therapy. Experts generally recommend using reduced-frequency dosing (such as alternate-day therapy or weekend use) and lower-potency steroids for maintenance to minimise side effects whenever possible [15]; however, these suggestions have not been formally validated in AIBD [24]. Other measures to be considered include monitoring for potential adrenal insufficiency and measuring blood pressure and blood sugar levels, particularly in patients prone to systemic toxicity. Regular follow-up is important to chart progress and also detect relapses of disease, which occur in AIBD particularly after treatment discontinuation [24].

Conclusion

Topical steroids in the form of clobetasol propionate 0.05% cream when applied twice daily all over the body (excluding the face) are effective for patients with bullous pemphigoid. In other blistering diseases, such as pemphigus, they are useful as adjunctive therapies for localised disease outbreaks. Careful monitoring needs to be done to minimise the side effects of use of these therapies, but overall they are much safer than systemically used steroids.

References

1. Burkholder B. Topical corticosteroids: an update. Curr Probl Dermatol. 2000;12(5):222–5.
2. Wiedersberg S, Leopold CS, Guy RH. Bioavailability and bioequivalence of topical glucocorticoids. Eur J Pharm Biopharm. 2008;68(3):453–66.
3. Frew JW, Murrell DF. Corticosteroid use in autoimmune blistering diseases. Dermatol Clin. 29(4):535–44.
4. Olsen EA, Cornell RC. Topical clobetasol-17-propionate: review of its clinical efficacy and safety. J Am Acad Dermatol. 1986;15(2 Pt 1):246–55.
5. Rhen T, Cidlowski JA. Antiinflammatory action of glucocorticoids—new mechanisms for old drugs. New Engl J Med. 2005;353(16):1711–23.
6. Norris DA. Mechanisms of action of topical therapies and the rationale for combination therapy. J Am Acad Dermatol. 2005;53(Suppl 1):S17–25.
7. Fontaine J, Joly P, Roujeau JC. Treatment of bullous pemphigoid. J Dermatol. 2003;30(2):83–90.
8. Di Zenzo G, della Torre R, Zambruno G, Borradori L. Bullous pemphigoid: from the clinic to the bench. Clin Dermatol. 2012;30(1):3–16.
9. Hellberg L, Samavedam UK, Holdorf K, Hansel M, Recke A, Beckmann T, et al. Methylprednisolone blocks autoantibody-induced tissue damage in experimental models of bullous pemphigoid and epidermolysis bullosa acquisita through inhibition of neutrophil activation. J Invest Dermatol. 2013;133(10):2390–9.
10. Le Jan S, Plee J, Vallerand D, Dupont A, Delanez E, Durlach A, et al. Innate immune cell-produced IL-17 sustains inflammation in bullous pemphigoid. J Invest Dermatol. 2014;134(12):2908–17.
11. van Velsen SG, De Roos MP, Haeck IM, Sparidans RW, Bruijnzeel-Koomen CA. The potency of clobetasol propionate: serum levels of clobetasol propionate and adrenal function during therapy with 0.05% clobetasol propionate in patients with severe atopic dermatitis. J Dermatol Treat. 2012;23(1):16–20.
12. van Velsen SGA, Haeck IM, Bruijnzeel-Koomen CAFM. Percutaneous absorption of potent topical corticosteroids in patients with severe atopic dermatitis. J Am Acad Dermatol. 63(5):911–3.
13. Bystryn JC, Wainwright BD, Shupack JL. Oral and topical corticosteroids in bullous pemphigoid. New Engl J Med. 2002;347(2):143–5.
14. McClain RW, Yentzer BA, Feldman SR. Comparison of skin concentrations following topical versus oral corticosteroid treatment: reconsidering the treatment of common inflammatory dermatoses. J Drugs Dermatol. 2009;8(12):1076–9.
15. Hengge UR, Ruzicka T, Schwartz RA, Cork MJ. Adverse effects of topical glucocorticosteroids. J Am Acad Dermatol. 2006;54(1):1–15.
16. Venning VA, Taghipour K, Mohd Mustapa MF, Highet AS, Kirtschig G. British Association of Dermatologists' guidelines for the management of bullous pemphigoid 2012. Br J Dermatol. 2012;167(6):1200–14.
17. Joly P, Roujeau JC, Benichou J, Picard C, Dreno B, Delaporte E, et al. A comparison of oral and topical corticosteroids in patients with bullous pemphigoid. New Engl J Med. 2002;346(5):321–7.
18. Roujeau JC, Lok C, Bastuji-Garin S, Mhalla S, Enginger V, Bernard P. High risk of death in elderly patients with extensive bullous pemphigoid. Arch Dermatol. 1998;134(4):465–9.
19. Rzany B, Partscht K, Jung M, Kippes W, Mecking D, Baima B, et al. Risk factors for lethal outcome in patients with bullous pemphigoid: low serum albumin level, high dosage of glucocorticosteroids, and old age. Arch Dermatol. 2002;138(7):903–8.

20. Westerhof W. Treatment of bullous pemphigoid with topical clobetasol propionate. J Am Acad Dermatol. 1989;20(3):458–61.
21. Kirtschig G, Middleton P, Bennett C, Murrell DF, Wojnarowska F, Khumalo NP. Interventions for bullous pemphigoid. Cochrane Database Syst Rev. 2010;10:CD002292.
22. Joly P, Roujeau JC, Benichou J, Delaporte E, D'Incan M, Dreno B, et al. A comparison of two regimens of topical corticosteroids in the treatment of patients with bullous pemphigoid: a multicenter randomized study. J Invest Dermatol. 2009;129(7):1681–7.
23. Fichel F, Barbe C, Joly P, Bedane C, Vabres P, Truchetet F, et al. Clinical and immunologic factors associated with bullous pemphigoid relapse during the first year of treatment: a multicenter, prospective study. JAMA Dermatol. 2014;150(1):25–33.
24. Feliciani C, Joly P, Jonkman MF, Zambruno G, Zillikens D, Ioannides D, et al. Management of bullous pemphigoid: the European Dermatology Forum consensus in collaboration with the European Academy of Dermatology and Venereology. Br J Dermatol. 2015;172(4):867–77.
25. Murrell DF, Daniel BS, Joly P, Borradori L, Amagai M, Hashimoto T, et al. Definitions and outcome measures for bullous pemphigoid: recommendations by an international panel of experts. J Am Acad Dermatol. 2012;66(3):479–85.
26. Daniel BS, Borradori L, Hall RP, Murrell DF. Evidence-based management of bullous pemphigoid. Dermatol Clin. 2011;29(4):613–20.
27. Du-Thanh A, Merlet S, Maillard H, Bernard P, Joly P, Esteve E, et al. Combined treatment with low-dose methotrexate and initial short-term superpotent topical steroids in bullous pemphigoid: an open, multicentre, retrospective study. Br J Dermatol. 2011;165(6):1337–43.
28. Dereure O, Bessis D, Guillot B, Guilhou JJ. Treatment of bullous pemphigoid by low-dose methotrexate associated with short-term potent topical steroids: an open prospective study of 18 cases. Arch Dermatol. 2002;138(9):1255–6.
29. Meijer JM, Jonkman MF, Wojnarowska F, Wiliams HC, Kirtschig G. Current practice in treatment approach for bullous pemphigoid: comparison between national surveys from the Netherlands and the UK. Clin Exp Dermatol. 2016;41(5):506–9.
30. Taghipour K, Mohd Mustapa MF, Highet AS, Venning VA, Kirtschig G. The approach of dermatologists in the UK to the treatment of bullous pemphigoid: results of a national survey. Clin Exp Dermatol. 2013;38(3):311–3.
31. Colbert RL, Allen DM, Eastwood D, Fairley JA. Mortality rate of bullous pemphigoid in a US medical center. J Invest Dermatol. 2004;122(5):1091–5.
32. Harman KE, Albert S, Black MM. Guidelines for the management of pemphigus vulgaris. Br J Dermatol. 2003;149(5):926–37.
33. Martin LK, Werth V, Villanueva E, Segall J, Murrell DF. Interventions for pemphigus vulgaris and pemphigus foliaceus. Cochrane Database Syst Rev. 2009;1:CD006263.
34. Dumas V, Roujeau JC, Wolkenstein P, Revuz J, Cosnes A. The treatment of mild pemphigus vulgaris and pemphigus foliaceus with a topical corticosteroid. Br J Dermatol. 1999;140(6):1127–9.
35. Muramatsu T, Iida T, Shirai T. Pemphigoid and pemphigus foliaceus successfully treated with topical corticosteroids. J Dermatol. 1996;23(10):683–8.
36. Darling MR, Daley T. Blistering mucocutaneous diseases of the oral mucosa-a review: part 2. Pemphigus vulgaris. J Can Dent Assoc. 2006;72(1):63–6.
37. Lozada-Nur F, Miranda C, Maliksi R. Double-blind clinical trial of 0.05% clobetasol propionate ointment in orabase and 0.05% fluocinonide ointment in orabase in the treatment of patients with oral vesiculoerosive diseases. Oral Surg Oral Med Oral Pathol. 1994;77(6):598–604.
38. Mignogna MD, Fortuna G, Leuci S, Adamo D, Dell'Aversana Orabona G, Ruoppo E. Adjuvant triamcinolone acetonide injections in oro-pharyngeal pemphigus vulgaris. J Eur Acad Dermatol. 2010;24(10):1157–65.
39. Chan LS, Ahmed AR, Anhalt GJ, Bernauer W, Cooper KD, Elder MJ, et al. The first international consensus on mucous membrane pemphigoid: definition, diagnostic criteria, pathogenic factors, medical treatment, and prognostic indicators. Arch Dermatol. 2002;138(3):370–9.
40. Kirtschig G, Murrell D, Wojnarowska F, Khumalo N. Interventions for mucous membrane pemphigoid and epidermolysis bullosa acquisita. Cochrane Database Syst Rev. 2003;1:CD004056.
41. Kourosh AS, Yancey KB. Therapeutic approaches to patients with mucous membrane pemphigoid. Dermatol Clin. 2011;29(4):637–41.
42. Hunzelmann N, Hunzelmann N. Cicatricial pemphigoid (mucous membrane pemphigoid). Am J Clin Dermatol. 2005;6(2):93–103.
43. Fleming TE, Korman NJ. Cicatricial pemphigoid. J Am Acad Dermatol. 43(4):571–94.
44. Gonzalez-Moles MA, Ruiz-Avila I, Rodriguez-Archilla A, Morales-Garcia P, Mesa-Aguado F, Bascones-Martinez A, et al. Treatment of severe erosive gingival lesions by topical application of clobetasol propionate in custom trays. Oral Surg Oral Med Oral Pathol. 2003;95(6):688–92.
45. Semkova K, Black M. Pemphigoid gestationis: current insights into pathogenesis and treatment. Eur J Obstet Gyn R B. 2009;145(2):138–44.
46. Intong LR, Murrell DF. Pemphigoid gestationis: current management. Dermatol Clin. 2011;29(4):621–8.
47. Chi CC, Wang SH, Kirtschig G, Wojnarowska F. Systematic review of the safety of topical corticosteroids in pregnancy. J Am Acad Dermatol. 2010;62(4):694–705.
48. Wan J, Imadojemu S, Werth VP. Management of rheumatic and autoimmune blistering disease in pregnancy and postpartum. Clin Dermatol. 2016;34(3):344–52.
49. Chi CC, Mayon-White RT, Wojnarowska FT. Safety of topical corticosteroids in pregnancy: a population-based cohort study. J Invest Dermatol. 2011;131(4):884–91.

50. Chi CC, Wang SH, Mayon-White R, Wojnarowska F. Pregnancy outcomes after maternal exposure to topical corticosteroids: a UK population-based cohort study. JAMA Dermatol. 2013;149(11):1274–80.

51. Ng SY, Venning VV. Management of linear IgA disease. Dermatol Clin. 2011;29(4):629–30.

52. Culton DA, Diaz LA. Treatment of subepidermal immunobullous diseases. Clin Dermatol. 2012;30(1):95–102.

53. Intong LR, Murrell DF. Management of epidermolysis bullosa acquisita. Dermatol Clin. 2011;29(4):643–7.

54. Abecassis S, Joly P, Genereau T, Courville P, Andre C, Moussalli J, et al. Superpotent topical steroid therapy for epidermolysis bullosa acquisita. Dermatology. 2004;209(2):164–6.

55. Choi GS, Lee E-S, Kim S-C, Lee S. Epidermolysis bullosa acquisita localized to the face. J Dermatol. 1998;25(1):19–22.

56. Walsh P, Aeling JL, Huff L, Weston WL. Hypothalamus-pituitary-adrenal axis suppression by superpotent topical steroids. J Am Acad Dermatol. 1993;29(3):501–3.

Use and Misuse of Topical Corticosteroids in Hair and Scalp Disorders

9

Anil Abraham

Abstract

Topical steroids have been used in the treatment of scalp and hair disorders for several years. The risk and benefit of this use is similar to the use of topical steroids elsewhere. Indications, contra-indications, use in poorly defined conditions with questionable benefit and in formulations which are inappropriate are worth considering in this set of disorders. Rational use of the drug in the correct indication, formulation, strength and duration could avoid the drug acquiring notoriety and unwarranted phobia.

Keywords

Topical • Steroid • Hair • Scalp

Learning Points

1. Topical steroids have been used and misused for scalp and hair disorders.
2. In some conditions, topical or intralesional steroids may be warranted. Alopecia areata and, early cicatricial alopecia and scalp psoriasis are examples of these situations.
3. In most other conditions topical steroids have a doubtful role and should ideally be avoided because they can potentially lead to steroid addiction and abuse with consequent side effects.
4. Even when indicated, an appropriate concentration, potency, duration and formulation should be used on the scalp.
5. Newer non-steroidal options and drug delivery systems that decrease the side-effect profile of topical steroids should be chosen as relevant. For example, tacrolimus instead of steroid or nanoparticle drug delivery of steroid.

9.1 Introduction

The use of steroids in dermatological disease has been traditionally described as a double edged sword. Used sparingly and for the right indications and time period, topical and systemic steroids offer the patient dramatic benefits. On the

A. Abraham
Dermatology, St. John's Medical College,
Bangalore, Karnataka, India
e-mail: docanilabe@yahoo.co.in

© Springer Nature Singapore Pte Ltd. 2018
K. Lahiri (ed.), *A Treatise on Topical Corticosteroids in Dermatology*,
DOI 10.1007/978-981-10-4609-4_9

other hand, used indiscriminately, incorrectly or without medical supervision, steroids can cause more damage than good and lead to an unending cycle of partial remission and relapse [1]. The rules of steroid use and abuse apply equally in the field of trichology and in the management of hair and scalp disorders. This makes it particularly crucial for dermatologists and trichologists to consider utilities of topical steroids against their side effects, and to make informed careful decision regarding their use in each patient based on clinical criteria including age, area involved, indication and chronicity of the hair or scalp disorder.

9.2 Categories of Steroid Use and Misuse in Hair and Scalp Disorders

The use of topical steroids in hair and scalp disorders can be broadly classified into four categories:

1. Conditions of the hair where topical steroids are indicated and approved
2. Conditions of the scalp where topical steroids are indicated and approved
3. Conditions of the scalp and hair where topical steroids have a doubtful role
4. Conditions of the scalp and hair where topical steroids have little or no role.

In each of these the astute clinician may use topical steroids to help the patient, while the less informed dermatologist or physician could misuse topical steroids in a strength or duration that harms the patient.

Similarly the misuse or abuse of topical steroids in this range of disorders can be classified into the following categories:

1. Incorrect dose or duration
2. Incorrect diagnosis or indication
3. Incorrect or inappropriate formulation
4. Prescription from an unqualified person or self-prescription of topical steroid.

Effects and side effects of topical steroids on the skin have been dealt with exhaustively [2]

in other chapters of this compendium. A comprehensive review of hair and scalp disorders and their treatment is also not the aim of this chapter. For purposes of brevity and clarity, the role of topical steroids and the potential for use and abuse will be discussed using an example of relatively common conditions under each category.

9.3 Formulations

Topical steroids used for hair and scalp disorders are usually lotions, gels or shampoos and less commonly ointments, creams, foams or sprays [3].

Ointments are better for lubrication and occlusion than other preparations and improve steroid absorption. But, they should at best be avoided on hairy areas as they may result in folliculitis or maceration.

Creams are cosmetically attractive, but are usually less potent than ointment. Creams are ideally chosen for the scalp margin in conditions like psoriasis when they extend beyond the hairline.

Lotion and gels are the least greasy. There are preferred for hairy areas because they penetrate easily and leave little residue. Gels dry fast and can be applied on the scalp or other hairy areas as they do not result in matting. Foams/mousses and shampoo are effective vehicles for delivering steroid to the scalp but are costly.

Intralesional steroids are often used on the scalp for a local delivery of topical steroid. Steroid shampoos have also been used for conditions including seborrheic dermatitis and scalp psoriasis. Like other body parts topical corticosteroids are the therapeutic backbone for many dermatoses of the scalp and they decrease erythema, scaling and pruritus significantly. Medicated shampoos are a more convenient choice for patients who need topical administration of corticosteroids for the scalp conditions [3]. Tar shampoos are used to treat scalp psoriasis. This preparation is effective for the maintenance of remission in patients who respond to therapy. Antifungal shampoos are useful in seborrheic dermatitis. Fluocinolone acetonide, 0.01% in shampoo formulation has been approved for the treatment of seborrheic dermatitis. Even superpotent corticosteroid shampoo (clobetasol propionate 0.05%) is permitted in the USA for once-daily treatment of scalp psoriasis. It was demonstrated in a pilot study in 2007 that clobetasol propionate shampoo improved the signs and symptoms of seborrheic dermatitis. It is based on these findings we can conclude that high-potency corticosteroid shampoos are considered as an effective therapeutic option for the treatment of scalp dermatoses. The question is not only whether they work or not; the more important question is whether they can be used indiscriminately. There are controversies regarding the efficacy of drug delivery, the relatively short contact time, the potential of over-the-counter misuse and the risk of long-term use by the less informed patient. These need to be addressed and steroid formulations for the scalp have to be chosen considering the hairiness of the anatomical location, the cosmetic importance and visibility of the scalp and hair and the potency and indication for therapy. Other factors like inflammation of the scalp, simultaneous use of oil or gel and frequency of head bath may affect the effectiveness and side effects of these molecules on the scalp.

9.4   Alopecia Areata

Alopecia areata is an example of a hair disorder in which steroids have a significant role, are indicated in select cases and can have a measurable therapeutic benefit. The use of topical steroids in alopecia areata ranges from intralesional injections to potent topical formulations in localized areas.

9.5   Intralesional Steroids in Alopecia Areata

Intralesional corticosteroids is the treatment of choice of Alopecia Areata since 1958. Different studies have reported success rates of 60–75%.

Triamcinolone acetonide (TAC) is the molecule usually preferred. It is to be ideally injected into the deep dermis or upper subcutaneous tissue using a 0.5-inch long 30-gauge needle at multiple sites, 1 cm apart and 0.1 ml into each site, once in 4–6 weeks. Various concentrations (2.5–10 mg/ml) of TAC have been used, but 5–10 mg/ml is preferred for scalp and 2.5 mg/ml for eyebrows and face. The maximum dose per sitting should not exceed 20 mg [4]. Regrowth of hair should be visible in roughly 4 weeks. Discontinuation of intralesional corticosteroids is recommended if there is no significant improvement by the end of 6 months. A subset of patients with decreased expression of thioredoxin reductase 1, an enzyme that activates the glucocorticoid receptor in the outer root sheath of alopecia areata, are resistant to steroid therapy. Atrophy can take place, this can be minimized by avoiding superficial injections, minimizing the volume and spacing the sites of injection. The atrophy, if at all, is usually transient and reversible. Hypopigmentation, telangiectasia and rarely anaphylaxis are reported. Cataract and raised intraocular pressure can occur if intralesional corticosteroids are used near the eyebrows. Hypopigmentation and skin atrophy can occur either when topical corticosteroids are applied/injected topically or locally. Venkatesan and Fangman demonstrated that melanocytes are structurally intact in steroid-induced hypopigmentation. This proposes that topical steroids may disturb melanocyte function more than the structure. Triamcinolone may cause depigmentation as because of its larger size, the greater tendency to aggregate and higher density. Hence for lesions close to the skin surface, particularly in hyperpigmented patient triamcinolone should better be avoided, and topical steroids with smaller particles and less tendency to aggregate may be used [1].

More recently Thappa et al. attempted to classify alopecia areata based on age and percentage of scalp surface involved [5]. Based on this classification topical steroids were used in some patients and intralesional steroids or oral minipulse was chosen for others.

1. *Patients below 10 years of age*: Topical corticosteroid lotion or cream (for example, fluocinolone acetonide 0.05%) is used as second-line therapy. Topical steroids are used overnight on alternate days or on 5 days in a week. This is to prevent atrophy of the skin. Response is expected by 6–8 weeks.
2. *Patients above 10 years, <30% scalp surface involved*: Short contact therapy with anthralin or topical corticosteroids are tried first by Thappa et al. If hair regrowth is not detected in 2–3 months, then intralesional corticosteroids are advised. Injections to be repeated every 4 weeks. Patients should respond by 4–8 weeks. If patients do not show improvement even after 6 months of intralesional corticosteroids, therapy is discontinued and they are termed and classified as non-responders.
3. *Patients above 10 years, >30% scalp involved* or rapid progressive alopecia of less than 1 year duration: The authors recommend the use of dexamethasone pulse therapy as the main line of treatment. If patient is incompatible for intravenous pulse therapy, oral minipulse with 5 mg betamethasone tablets may be given twice weekly for up to 6 months. Patients with alopecia universalis, those having progressive hair loss for more than 2 years or patients not responding to treatment are offered a wig or cap as cosmetic camouflage.

For the apprehension and fear of injections and pain in pediatric population intralesional injections are much less favoured.

9.6 Topical Corticosteroids in Alopecia Areata

Various forms of topical corticosteroids are used for alopecia areata. These include creams, gels, ointments, lotions and foams. Foam forms reported to yield better result that the lotion forms. Folliculitis is a common side effect to topical corticosteroids. Telangiectasia and atrophy may develop rarely. The reported relapse rate is 37–63% [6].

9.7 Seborrhoeic Dermatitis

Malassezia furfur or its yeast form, Pityrosporum ovale, has a contributory role in causing seborrhoeic dermatitis. Malassezia yeasts precipitate the inflammation of seborrheic dermatitis, but the exact mechanism is unknown.

Treatments with antifungal agents such as topical ketoconazole are the mainstay of therapy for seborrheic dermatitis of the face and body. Because of the risk of adverse effects, anti-inflammatory agents such as topical corticosteroids and calcineurin inhibitors are advised to use only for short durations. Various types of medicated shampoos are available for the treatment of seborrheic dermatitis of the scalp. Antifungal shampoos can be used as a long-term and topical corticosteroids for short-term therapeutic planning. These can be used as second-line agents for the treatment of seborrheic dermatitis of the scalp [7].

Exact pathogenesis of seborrheic dermatitis is yet to be ascertained. Till that happens, the choice of therapy will be revolved between antimycotics, topical steroids, medicated shampoos, sebostatics either alone or in combinations.

9.8 Scalp Psoriasis

Almost about 80% of individuals with psoriasis develop scalp involvement. In a majority of these individuals a negative impact on the quality of life has been reported. Topical treatment with corticosteroids with or without vitamin D3 analogues is the basis of treatment in this clinical condition. Utmost appropriate topical therapy for scalp psoriasis is formulated as a solution, lotion, gel, foam, spray, oil or shampoo. Twice in a week application may postpone relapses [8].

Numerous formulations are available for the treatment of psoriasis of the scalp containing high potency steroids, such as clobetasol propionate. These can cause complications and are specially prone to misuse by the uninformed doctor or unwary patient. Variations in formulation and drug delivery are being researched especially for scalp psoriasis. Fluocinolone acetonide (0.01%)

in a newer oil preparation has been classified as low potency (Class 6) steroid. The addition of emollients in the vehicle base helps in softening the stratum corneum and permits infiltration of the steroid component. This makes this preparation an effective treatment for psoriasis of the scalp. A randomized, double-blind, vehicle-controlled multi-centre study demonstrated the improvement in the steroid oil group was significantly greater compared to those in the vehicle-treated group in the question of efficacy and safety. The results of this study were encouraging and showed that low potency steroid in an oil base could be an alternative for the treatment for psoriasis of the scalp [9].

Topical corticosteroids, continued to be the first choice for most physicians in the management of scalp psoriasis. They are quick and effective with limited side effects, when used for a limited period of less than 4 weeks. Topical vitamin D3 analogues are also recommended. Phototherapy or systemic treatment with methotrexate, acitretin and cyclosporin is often either not indicated or not suitable for the treatment of the scalp. Topical corticosteroids are the drugs of choice when the psoriatic lesions are mainly inflammatory. Intermittent use of topical corticosteroids alternating with vitamin D3 derivatives for long-term use proposes to be the most suitable regime for most patients. Because psoriasis of the scalp is a chronic disease, long-term treatment should be economical [10].

9.9   Androgenetic Alopecia

Androgenetic alopecia is caused by interactions between several genetic and environmental factors. Follicular inflammation has been implicated in several studies. The process is slow and sluggish unlike the inflammatory and destructive course in the typical scarring alopecia. Microbial toxins related to *Propionibacterium* sp., *Staphylococcus* sp., *Malassezia* sp. or Demodex may initiate the inflammatory response. Alternatively, keratinocytes respond to chemical stress from cosmetics and grooming agents, pollutants and actinic damage as in UV irradiation

by producing radical oxygen species and nitric oxide [11]. A lymphocytic microfolliculitis targeting the bulge epithelium along with deposits of epithelial basement membrane zone immuno-reactants are common findings in androgenetic alopecia. This points towards an immunologically driven trigger [12]. In the recently defined fibrosing alopecia in a pattern distribution [13], patients with AGA have additional clinical and histological features of inflammation and fibrosis limited to the area of androgenetic hair loss. The preference of this follicular target for the immunologic attack could be explained by the fact that in contrast to the proximal hair follicle, the isthmus and infundibulum area do not have the advantage of any immune privilege [13].

Topical corticosteroids can be used concurrently to help limit irritant dermatitis and pruritus in patients with patterned alopecia.

Minoxidil or its vehicle is known to cause allergic contact dermatitis. A recent paper described a sudden worsening of alopecia due to a telogen effluvium linked to contact dermatitis to minoxidil and propylene glycol. In these cases, use of topical steroid lotions early in the course of disease and patch testing may help to reverse the rapid deterioration of hair loss [14, 15].

9.10   Cicatricial Alopecias

Primary cicatricial alopecias (PCA) are an uncommon and clinically diverse set of disorders in which the hair follicle is irreversibly destroyed leading to permanent alopecia. Clinically, they are characterized by irreversible loss of hair shafts and visible follicular ostia and other perceptible changes in skin surface morphology, while their histopathological hallmark usually (almost always) is the replacement of follicular structures with scar-like fibrous tissue. Early treatment is the key to minimizing the extent of permanent alopecia. Though, unreliable terminology, ill-defined clinical end-points and a lack of good quality clinical trials have plagued the therapeutic part [14, 15]. It is suffice to say that topical steroids in various forms of delivery could have a role during the course of the disease before substantial scarring has set in. Usually the rapid spread and progress warrants treatment with systemic immunomodulators in which case the use of topical steroids becomes redundant. The frustrated clinician and the anxious patient often continue to misuse topical steroids when they are not needed or are unlikely to have any benefit.

Central centrifugal cicatricial alopecia (CCCA) is the commonest scarring alopecia among darker ladies. CCCA has been associated with hot combing and specific hair styling. Well-designed randomized controlled trials are required to determine the ideal management. At this point, patients are advised to avoid traction and chemical treatments; topical and intralesional steroids, calcineurin inhibitors and minoxidil can be helpful in halting the progression. This is an example of relatively random use of steroids in a 'questionable benefit' scenario.

Frontal fibrosing alopecia (FFA) is a type of scarring hair loss mainly seen in postmenopausal women. This pattern is characterized by recession of fronto-temporo-parietal hairline, perifollicular erythema and loss of eyebrows. Management of FFA is not effective as the exact pathogenesis is not properly understood.

Discoid lupus and scarring alopecia: Topical corticosteroids are an essential part of treating all subtypes of CLE including scarring alopecia due to DLE on the scalp. It is surprising that in spite of widespread use there is just one randomized controlled trial, comparing a high potency steroid with a low potency steroid, in the treatment of DLE [16]. DLE may be responsive to intralesional steroids. Though the mainstay of treatment of DLE is topical corticosteroids, it is often ineffectual or invites long-term side effects. Newer therapeutic option with tacrolimus and pimecrolimus has also been tried safely and effectively [17].

9.11   Recent Advances

Newer entities and newer situations that warrant the use of topical steroids are being described as therapy for scalp and hair disorders takes giant technological leaps.

Erosive pustular dermatosis of the scalp (EPDS) is an uncommon inflammatory disease with indefinite etiology that usually occurs in the geriatric age group. EPDS is characterized by numerous sterile pustules, long-lasting crusted erosions, scarring alopecia and skin atrophy. Recently a case of EPDS was reported to be successfully treated with topical corticosteroids [18].

Polyamide hair implants was considered as an effective surgical technique that delivers instant aesthetic results. Safety of this option is questionable as this is often associated with intractable inflammatory reactions. Topical steroids are often used in these patients for a short period to prevent reactions and inflammation of the scalp post-implant [19].

Both non-scarring and scarring alopecia have been reported in patients receiving Epidermal Growth Factor Receptor Inhibitors(EGFRI) therapy. Options for management include topical hydrocortisone 0.2%, steroid shampoos and class 1 steroid lotions [20].

Newer options in the drug delivery of topical steroids are being developed to minimize side effects and retain efficacy. Mometasone furoate hydrogel has been developed recently which might have a better safety profile.

Improving the equilibrium between drug release, interfollicular permeation and follicular uptake may permit diminishing these adverse events and concurrently enhance drug delivery of steroids in hair and scalp ailments. Recently three types of polymeric nanocarriers (nanospheres, nanocapsules, lipid-core nanocapsules) for the potent glucocorticoid clobetasol propionate (CP) were prepared. They all demonstrated a continued release of drug, as was wanted. Nanocapsules formulated as an aqueous dispersion and applied by rubbing to maximize follicular targeting and minimize drug penetration into the interfollicular epidermis. Nanotechnology-based formulations could offer a practical approach for more effective drug delivery to the hair follicle. Moreover, they present a way to diminish adverse effects of potent glucocorticoids by liberating the drug in a measured manner. This could be the compromise solution to make topical steroids effective and safe in the future for scalp and hair disorders [21–26].

References

1. Coondoo A, et al. Side-effects of topical steroids: a long overdue revisit. Indian Dermatol Online J. 2014;5(4):416–25.
2. Abraham A, Roga G. Topical steroid-damaged skin. Indian J Dermatol. 2014;59:456–9.
3. Rathi SK, D'Souza P. Rational and ethical use of topical corticosteroids based on safety and efficacy. Indian J Dermatol. 2012;57(4):251–9.
4. Kircik L. The evolving role of therapeutic shampoos for targeting symptoms of inflammatory scalp disorders. Drugs Dermatol. 2010;9(1):41–8.
5. Seetharam KA. Alopecia areata: an update. Indian J Dermatol Venereol Leprol. 2013;79:563–75.
6. Majid I, Keen A. Management of alopecia areata: an update. BJMP. 2012;5(3):a530.
7. Valia R G. Etiopathogenesis of seborrheic dermatitis. Indian J Dermatol Venereol Leprol 2006;72:253–5
8. Guenther L. Current management of scalp psoriasis. Skin Therapy Lett. 2015;20(3):5–7.
9. Pauporte M, et al. Fluocinolone acetonide topical oil for scalp psoriasis. J Dermatol Treat. 2004;15(6):360–4.
10. van der Vleuten CJ, van de Kerkhof PC. Management of scalp psoriasis: guidelines for corticosteroid use in combination treatment. Drugs. 2001;61(11):1593–8.
11. Kaliyadan F, et al. Androgenetic alopecia: an update. Indian J Dermatol Venereol Leprol. 2013;79:613–25.
12. Magro CM, et al. The role of inflammation and immunity in the pathogenesis of androgenetic alopecia. J Drugs Dermatol. 2011;10(12):1404–11.
13. Trueb RM. Molecular mechanisms of androgenetic alopecia. Exp Gerontol. 2002;37:981–90.
14. Harries MJ, Sinclair RD, Macdonald-Hull S, Whiting DA, Griffiths CE, Paus R. Management of primary cicatricial alopecias: options for treatment. Br J Dermatol. 2008;159(1):1–22.
15. La Placa M, et al. Scalp psoriasiform contact dermatitis with acute telogen effluvium due to topical minoxidil treatment. Skin Appendage Disord. 2016;1(3):141–3.
16. Chang AY, Werth VP. Treatment of cutaneous lupus. Curr Rheumatol Rep. 2011;13(4):300–7.
17. Han YW, et al. Four cases of facial discoid lupus erythematosus successfully treated with topical pimecrolimus or tacrolimus. Ann Dermatol. 2010;22(3):307–11.
18. Shahmoradi Z, et al. Erosive pustular dermatosis of the scalp following hair transplantation. Adv Biomed Res. 2014;22(3):176.
19. Serdev N, et al. Polyamide hair implant (biofibre®): evaluation of efficacy and safety in a group of 133 patients. J Biol Regul Homeost Agents. 2015;29(1 Suppl):103–9.
20. Lacouture ME, et al. Clinical practice guidelines for the prevention and treatment of EGFR inhibitor-associated dermatologic toxicities. Support Care Cancer. 2011;19(8):1079–95.
21. Thappa DM, Vijayikumar M. Alopecia areata. Indian J Dermatol Venereol Leprol. 2001;67(4):188.
22. Alsanatali A. Alopecia areata—a new treatment plan. Clin Cosmet Investig Dermatol. 2011;4:107–1159.
23. Clark GW, et al. Diagnosis and treatment of seborrheic dermatitis. Am Fam Physician. 2015;91(3):185–90.
24. Olsen EA, Bergfeld WF, Cotsarelis G, Price VH, Shapiro J, Sinclair R, et al. Summary of North American Hair Research Society (NAHRS)-sponsored workshop on cicatricial alopecia. J Am Acad Dermatol. 2003;48:103–10.
25. Salgado A, et al. Mometasone furoate hydrogel for scalp use: in vitro and in vivo evaluation. Pharm Dev Technol. 2014;19(5):618–22.
26. Valia RG. Etiopathogenesis of seborrheic dermatitis. Indian J Dermatol Venereol Leprol. 2006;72:253–5.

Use and Misuse of Topical Corticosteroid in Pediatric Age Group

10

Sandipan Dhar, Sahana M. Srinivas, and Deepak Parikh

Abstract

Topical corticosteroid has been used in treatment of various skin disorders from several decades. There are lots of misconceptions among caregivers and parents regarding the use and its adverse effects which have led to steroid phobia. Topical corticosteroid can be used safely in children at the appropriate dose and duration but if misused can lead to local and systemic side effects. Hence it should be carefully prescribed with proper indications and after a thorough counseling to parents regarding application and importance of adherence.

Keywords

Topical • Corticosteroid • Use • Misuse • Children • Counselling

Learning Points

1. Topical corticosteroids, though, a very useful drug in treating various skin disorders in children, if misused, can lead to adverse effects.
2. Even a small amount of potent drugs or prolonged period of treatment with low-potency topical corticosteroids can lead to serious systemic side effects.
3. Iatrogenic Cushing's syndrome is documented more in children than adults.
4. Counselling caregivers about the adverse effects of topical steroids can prevent misuse.
5. Steroid phobia among parents should be dealt cautiously by dermatologists.
6. Advertising about use and misuse of topical corticosteroids in electronic and print media can sensitize parents about the menace caused by it and prevent abuse or misuse.

S. Dhar (✉)
Department of Pediatric Dermatology, Institute of Child Health, Kolkata, India
e-mail: doctorsandipan@gmail.com

S.M. Srinivas
Department of Pediatric Dermatology, Indira Gandhi Institute of Child Health, Bangalore, India

D. Parikh
Department of Pediatric Dermatology, Wadia Hospital for Children, Mumbai, India

© Springer Nature Singapore Pte Ltd. 2018
K. Lahiri (ed.), *A Treatise on Topical Corticosteroids in Dermatology*,
DOI 10.1007/978-981-10-4609-4_10

10.1 Introduction

Topical corticosteroid has been a "boon" in the field of dermatology as it forms the cornerstone of management in several skin disorders. Ever since the first published report of topical hydrocortisone usage by Sulzberger and Witten in 1952, various potent topical corticosteroids have been introduced over the years [1]. Topical corticosteroid has been used in various inflammatory skin disorders in children, providing a rapid symptomatic relief, but over the last decade, it has been misused by dermatologists, non-dermatologists, pharmacists, alternative medicine practitioners, and even nonmedical lay persons (as over-the-counter product) leading to local and systemic adverse effects.

10.2 Topical Corticosteroids in Children

Topical corticosteroids have anti-inflammatory, immunosuppressive, antiproliferative, and vasoconstrictive effects. The efficacy and toxicity are related to their potency and percutaneous absorption. Adverse effects of topical corticosteroid depend on quantity, frequency of application, duration of treatment, vehicle, potency, and site of application. Topical corticosteroids have been ranked in terms of potency into four groups consisting of seven classes as classified in Table 10.1 (mild, moderate, potent, and superpotent) [2]. Potent steroids are generally avoided in children as they cause hypothalamic-pituitary-adrenal (HPA) axis suppression. As compared to adults,

Table 10.1 Classification of topical corticosteroids

Potency	Class	Topical corticosteroid	Formulation
Superpotent	I	Clobetasol propionate	Cream, 0.05%
		Diflorasone diacetate	Ointment, 0.05%
Potent	II	Amcinonide	Ointment, 0.1%
		Betamethasone dipropionate	Ointment, 0.05%
		Desoximetasone	Cream or ointment, 0.025%
		Fluocinonide	Cream, ointment or gel, 0.05%
		Halcinonide	Cream, 0.1%
	III	Betamethasone dipropionate	Cream, 0.05%
		Betamethasone valerate	Ointment, 0.1%
		Diflorasone diacetate	Cream, 0.05%
		Triamcinolone acetonide	Ointment, 0.1%
Moderate	IV	Desoximetasone	Cream, 0.05%
		Fluocinolone acetonide	Ointment, 0.025%
		Fludroxycortide	Ointment, 0.05%
		Hydrocortisone valerate	Ointment, 0.2%
		Triamcinolone acetonide	Cream, 0.1%
	V	Betamethasone dipropionate	Lotion, 0.02%
		Betamethasone valerate	Cream, 0.1%
		Fluocinolone acetonide	Cream, 0.025%
		Fludroxycortide	Cream, 0.05%
		Hydrocortisone butyrate	Cream, 0.1%
		Hydrocortisone valerate	Cream, 0.2%
		Triamcinolone acetonide	Lotion, 0.1%
Mild	VI	Betamethasone valerate	Lotion, 0.05%
		Desonide	Cream, 0.05%
		Fluocinolone acetonide	Solution, 0.01%
	VII	Dexamethasone sodium phosphate	Cream, 0.1%
		Hydrocortisone acetate	Cream, 1%
		Methylprednisolone acetate	Cream, 0.25%

Table 10.2 FDA-approved topical corticosteroid in children

Topical corticosteroid	Age group
Clobetasol propionate 0.05% cream	>12 years
Fluocinonide 0.1% cream	>12 years
Fluocinolone acetonide 0.01% cream	>2 years
Mometasone 0.1% cream	>2 years
Alclometasone 0.05% cream/ointment	>1 year
Fluticasone 0.05% cream/lotion	>1 year
Prednicarbate 0.1% cream/ointment	>1 year
Desonide 0.05% foam/gel	>3 months
Hydrocortisone butyrate 0.1% cream	>3 months

children are more prone for side effects as their skin has poorly developed barrier function and a large surface area-to-weight ratio giving rise to significant absorption of the drug [3]. Topical corticosteroids and their age-related usage are listed in Table 10.2.

10.3 Use of Topical Corticosteroid in Children

Choosing a topical steroid in children depends on type of dermatosis, site, frequency of application, vehicle, duration, and other drug-related factors. Mildly potent topical corticosteroids are used on the face, eyelids, flexures, and diaper region. Moderately to highly potent topical corticosteroids are used in conditions like atopic dermatitis, psoriasis, vitiligo, lichen planus, and lichen planus hypertrophicus (Figs. 10.1, 10.2, 10.3, 10.4, 10.5, and 10.6). Conditions like lichen planus hypertrophicus, lichenified lesions, and prurigo nodularis may require application of topical corticosteroid under occlusion for better absorption, but there is a need to be cautious against side effects, whereas if it is applied on diaper area, it may cause excessive absorption due to occlusive effect leading to adverse effects [4]. Cushing's syndrome has been reported because of use of excess topical corticosteroid in diaper region [5].

Topical corticosteroid plays a vital role in management of atopic dermatitis. The fingertip unit (FTU) can give a guide to the use of topical corticosteroid especially when treating atopic dermatitis. Parents can be counselled about the FTU to prevent excess usage and adverse effects

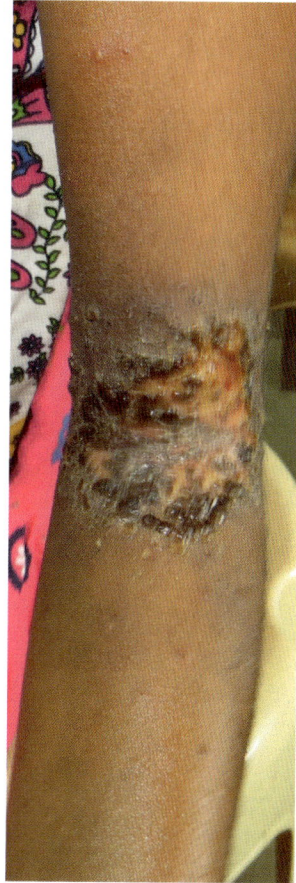

Fig. 10.1 Eczematous lesion of atopic dermatitis on cubital fossa

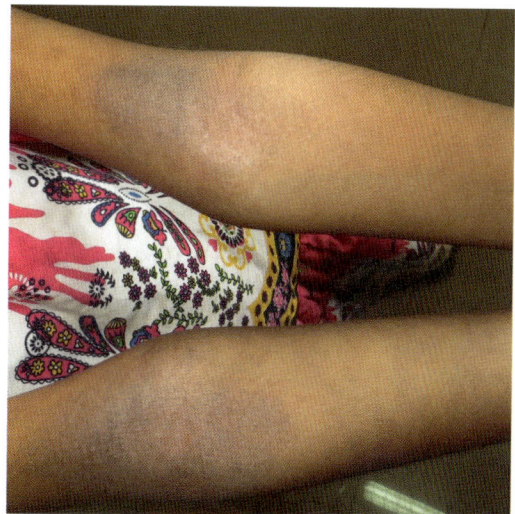

Fig. 10.2 Lichenified lesions present on cubital fossa in atopic dermatitis requiring moderate-potency topical corticosteroid

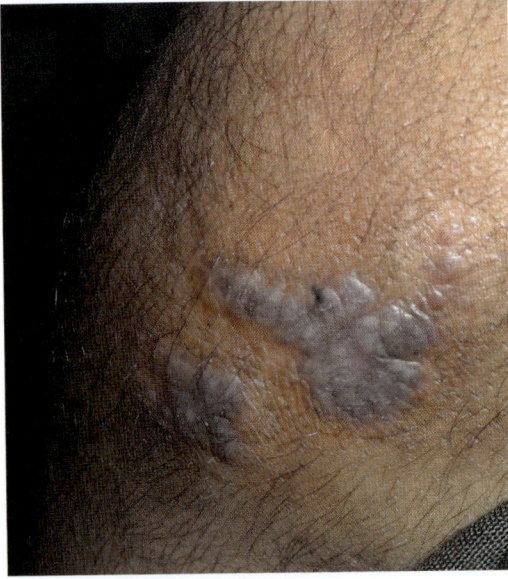

Fig. 10.3 Well-defined violaceous plaque of lichen planus

[6]. Ointment base is used for dry and lichenified lesion, cream base is used for inflamed lesion, and lotion base is appropriate in hairy areas. Ideally topical corticosteroids should be used for localized skin lesions for shorter periods in children. Topical corticosteroids have been used as intermittent therapy, weekend therapy, or intermittent hot spot therapy to prevent tachyphylaxis,

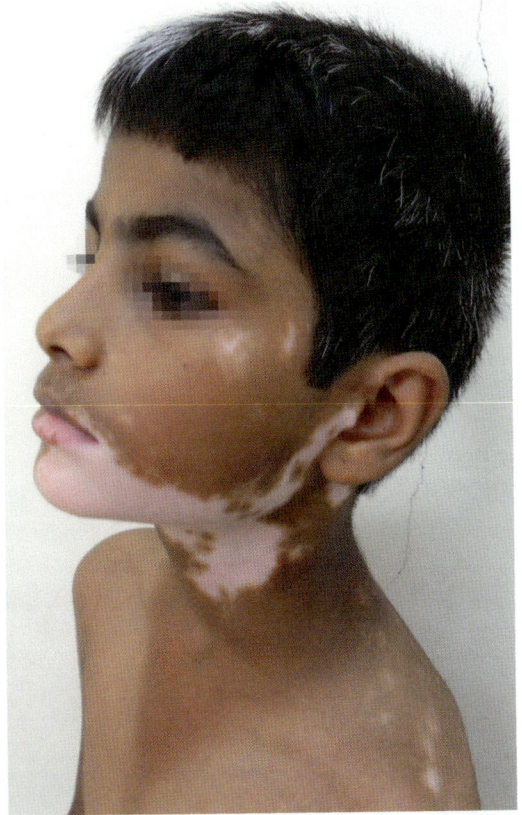

Fig. 10.6 Child with vitiligo associated with leucotrichia

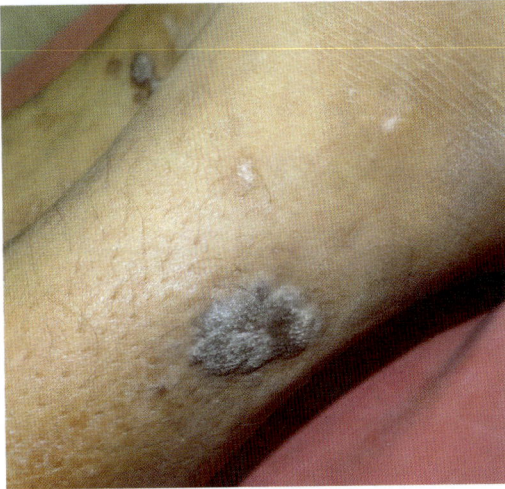

Fig. 10.4 Lichen planus hypertrophicus

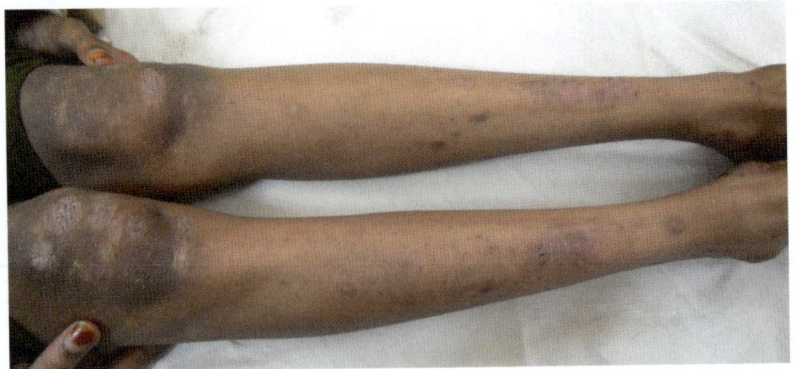

Fig. 10.5 Lesions of chronic plaque psoriasis on the lower limbs

and these types of therapy have been in use mainly for atopic dermatitis [7].

10.4 Adverse Effects of Topical Corticosteroids

Although topical corticosteroids are useful in many dermatoses, it has been extensively abused and misused leading to various local and systemic side effects. Children are more susceptible to local and systemic side effects even with small amount of potent steroids. Adverse effect depends on factors like chemical structure, potency of drug, vehicle, active metabolites, age of child, site of application, quantity of drug, frequency, duration, density of hair follicles, hydration, occlusion, type of dermatosis, or any hepatic or renal involvement [2]. Common local side effects include atrophy, post-inflammatory hypopigmentation or hyperpigmentation, striae, telangiectasias, hemorrhage, purpura, ulceration, hypertrichosis, aggravation of fungal infections, herpes simplex, recurrent furunculosis, tachyphylaxis, and steroid dependency (Figs. 10.7, 10.8, 10.9, 10.10, 10.11, 10.12, and

10.13). In the adolescent age group, topical corticosteroid has been misused for treatment of acne vulgaris leading to steroid acne, perioral dermatitis, rosacea, facial erythema, and folliculitis [8].

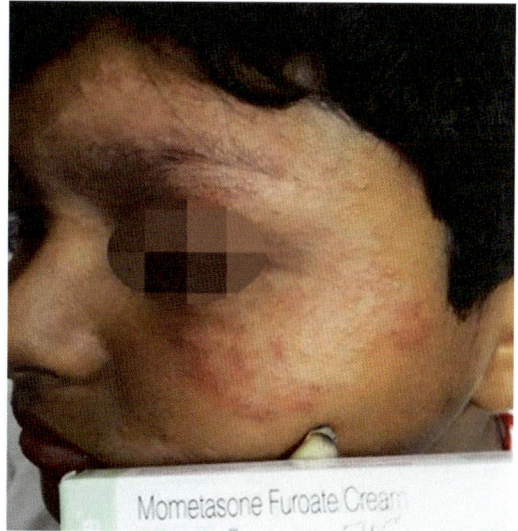

Fig. 10.8 Tinea incognito on the face after using potent steroid (Courtesy of Dr. Koushik Lahiri)

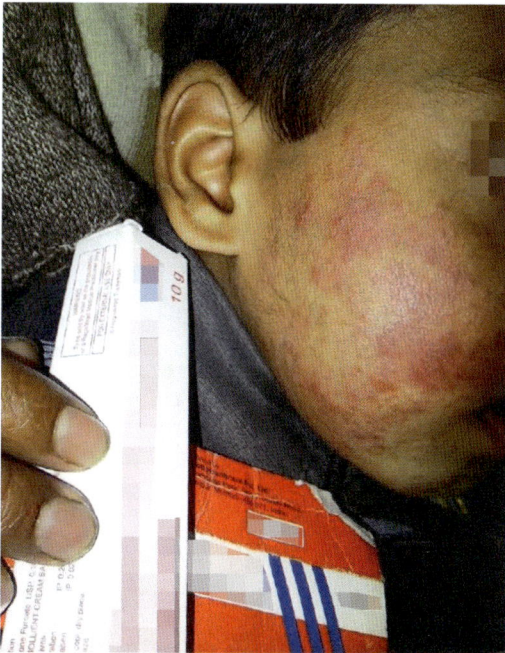

Fig. 10.7 Child with erythema and acneiform eruption on the face after using potent steroids (Courtesy of Dr. Koushik Lahiri)

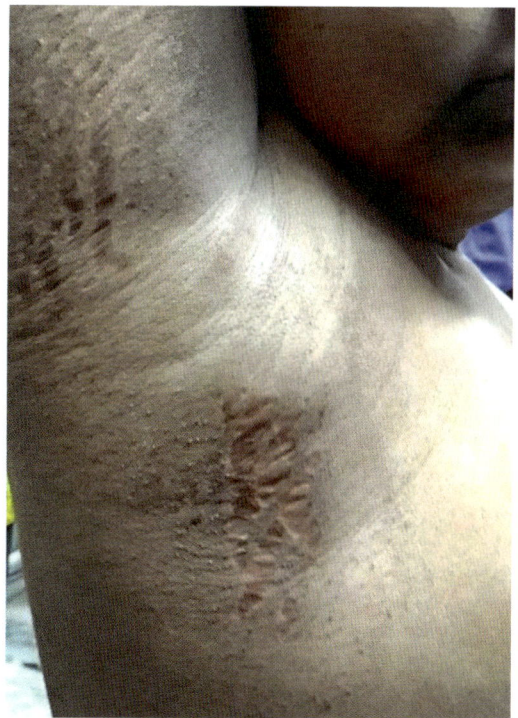

Fig. 10.9 Topical steroid-induced atrophy of the skin (Courtesy of Dr. Koushik Lahiri)

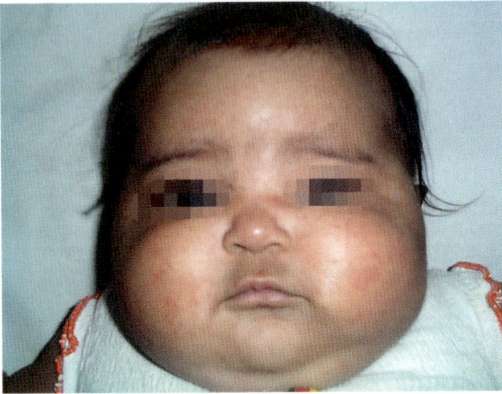

Fig. 10.10 Topical steroid-induced erythema and acneiform eruption with cushingoid features

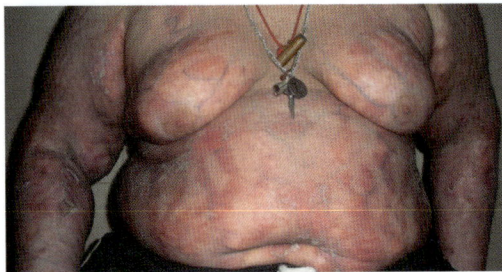

Fig. 10.11 Potent topical steroid-induced striae and atrophy along with telangiectasias and cushingoid features (Courtesy of Dr. Koushik Lahiri)

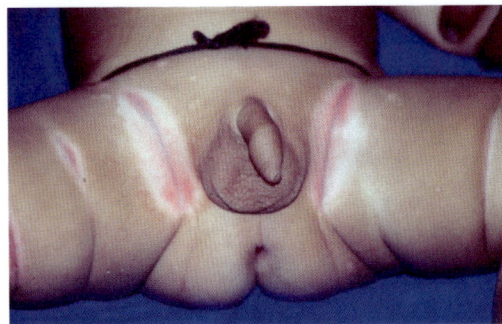

Fig. 10.12 Post-inflammatory hypopigmentation in the flexures after using topical steroid for candidal diaper dermatitis

Prolonged use of topical corticosteroid of low potency, which is commonly used in children, can give rise to allergic contact dermatitis due to instability of the drug. Systemic side effects seen in children are HPA axis suppression, iatrogenic Cushing's syndrome, growth retardation, avascular necrosis of the femoral head, glaucoma due to use of topical steroid on the eyelid, and severe dis-

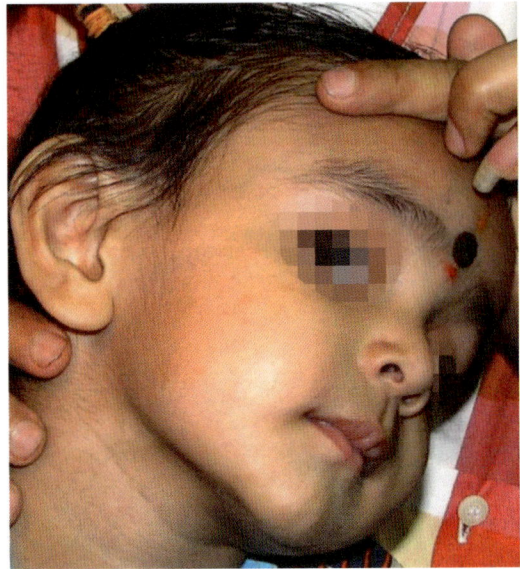

Fig. 10.13 Topical steroid-induced hypertrichosis (Courtesy Dr. Koushik Lahiri)

seminated cytomegalovirus infection resulting in death in infants [9]. Iatrogenic Cushing's syndrome has been documented more in children than in adults. In children it was seen more in infancy group and seen with dermatosis like diaper dermatitis, psoriasis, non-bullous ichthyosiform erythroderma, and xerosis of the skin [10]. Studies have shown that the most common topical corticosteroid associated with iatrogenic Cushing's syndrome in children is clobetasol propionate 0.05% and betamethasone, and the mean duration of application which was from 1 to 17 months with recovery period of HPA axis was 3.49 ± 2.92 months [11]. Slowing of linear growth has been reported in an infant treated with topical corticosteroid [9, 12]. Disseminated cytomegalovirus infection has been reported in two infants after using clobetasol propionate. [5].

10.5 Misuse of Topical Corticosteroid

Use and misuse of topical corticosteroid are the two sides of the same coin. Misuse of topical corticosteroid has been occurring at the level of manufacturing, marketing, prescription (family physician, pediatrician, dermatologist), and sales and through laypersons. There is growing addiction about fair complexion not only in adults but also in parents for their children. Topical corticosteroids have been misused by parents as fairness cream for their children which has either been recommended by friends, relatives, practitioners, and non-dermatologists [13]. Topical steroid along with antibacterial or antifungals has been randomly abused to treat fungal infections. This has led to the emergence of fungal resistance in adults, and this has provided a source of recurrent fungal infection in children also. Combination steroids have been associated with masking of disease, aggravation, or recurrence of the symptoms with stoppage of treatment. Infantile granuloma gluteale is a rare complication seen due to prolonged treatment of diaper dermatitis with topical corticosteroids [14]. On the flip side, adverse effects and rampant abuse of topical corticosteroid which has been advertised in electronic media, the Internet, through mouth-to-mouth word by practitioners and parents have developed steroid phobia which is encountered more in atopic dermatitis [15]. In a study of steroid phobia conducted on caregivers of children with atopic dermatitis, 38.3% were reluctant to use topical corticosteroids [16]. In another study of childhood eczema, 50% of parents preferred nonsteroidal prescriptions [17]. Recently Moret et al. have developed the TOPICOP scale to measure topical corticosteroid phobia [18]. Steroid phobia among parents has compelled them to use alternative medicine products that contain steroids (though not documented) considering them to be safe and indirectly lead to adverse effects on prolonged usage. Lack of awareness of adverse effects by healthcare practitioners in rural areas and their availability over the counter at affordable prices has led to misuse of the same among caregivers [19]. Teenagers and adolescents being preoccupied with their appearance and fairness fall prey to use of potent topical corticosteroids on the face [20, 21].

10.6   Measures to Prevent Misuse of Topical Corticosteroid

Practitioners and dermatologist should be aware of the adverse effects and misuse of topical corticosteroids. Many of the dermatosis not requiring topical steroids should be managed with symptomatic treatment. Potent steroids should be avoided in children unless indicated. Counselling parents plays an important role in preventing adverse effects and misuse. Caregivers should be strictly counselled about the adverse effects of topical corticosteroids and their usage. On the other hand, parents suffering from steroid phobia should be warned about the misinformation and undertreatment of skin disorders. Dermatologists should counsel about the damage caused due to use of over-the-counter medications and alternative medicine products, prescription by non-dermatologists and quacks, and advice given by relatives and friends. Information about combination products and their consequences should be explained to parents.

The role of spreading awareness to school teachers may be of great importance in such situations. Caregivers have the opinion that creams prescribed for them can be used for children also and often misuse these, which should be addressed meticulously. Counselling should be done about the overuse of prescribed cream for faster relief and adverse effects of using same prescription medicines all the time for all skin disorders. FTU of using topical steroids can be taught to parents especially when treating atopic dermatitis to prevent over usage. Prolonged treatment in dermatosis should be substituted with intermittent or weekend therapy or with nonsteroidal therapies [22, 23].

Conclusions

Topical corticosteroid forms the cornerstone of management in various dermatoses. It is safe if used appropriately at proper dose and application. Children are more susceptible to side effects as compared to adults. Counselling caregivers about their use and misuse is a dramatic step to prevent adverse effects. Strict adherence to the prescription given by dermatologists is important. Parents should discuss about their queries with the treating dermatologists to prevent misuse of topical corticosteroids. Dermatologists, practitioners, manufacturers, pharmacist, and caregivers, all of them should join hands to prevent abuse or misuse of topical corticosteroid.

References

1. Sulzberger MB, Witten VH. The effect of topically applied compound F in selected dermatoses. J Invest Dermatol. 1952;19:101–2.
2. Warner MR, Carnisa C. Topical corticosteroid. In: Wolverton SE, editor. Comprehensive dermatologic drug therapy. Philadelphia, PA: Saunders Elsevier; 2007. p. 595–624.
3. Saraswath A. Topical corticosteroid use in children: adverse effects and how to minimize them. Indian J Dermatol Venereol Leprol. 2010;76:225–8.
4. Coondoo A, Chattopadhyay C. Use and abuse of topical corticosteroid in children. Ind J Paed Dermatol. 2014;15:1–4.
5. Semiz S, Balci YI, Ergin S, Candemis M, Polat A. Two cases of cushings syndrome due to overuse of topical steroid in the diaper area. Pediatr Dermatol. 2008;25:544–7.
6. Long CC, Finlay AY. The finger tip unit: a new practical measure. Clin Exp Dermatol. 1991;16:444–7.
7. Dhar S. Current concepts about the management of atopic dermatitis in infants and children. Ann Inst Child Health. 2004;4:19–28.
8. Coondoo A, Phiske M, Verma S, Lahiri K. Side effects of topical steroids. A long overdue visit. Ind Derm onlin J. 2014;5:416–25.
9. Dhar S, Seth J, Parikh D. Systemic side effects of topical corticosteroids. Indian J Dermatol. 2014;59:460–4.
10. Tempark T, Phatarakijnirund V, Chatproedprai S, Watcharasindhu S, Supornsilchai V, Wananukul S. Exogeneous cushing's syndrome due to topical corticosteroid application: case report and review of literature. Endocrine. 2010;38:328–34.
11. Hengee UR, Ruzicka T, Schwartz RA, Cork MJ. Adverse effects of topical glucocorticosteroids. J Am Acad Dermatol. 2006;54:1–18.
12. Wolthers OD, Heuck C, Ternowitz T, Heickendroff L, Nielsen HK, Frystyk J. Insulin like growth factor axis, bone and collagen turnover in children with atopic dermatitis treated with topical glucocorticoids. Dermatology. 1996;192:337–42.
13. Coondoo A. Topical corticosteroid misuse: the Indian scenario. Indian J Dermatol. 2014;59:451–5.
14. Al-Faraidy NA, Al- Natour SH. A forgotten complication of diaper dermatitis: granuloma gluteale infantum. J Family Community Med. 2010;17:107–9.
15. Ghosh A, Sengupta S, Coondoo A, Jana AK. Topical corticosteroid addiction and phobia. Indian J Dermatol. 2014;59:465–8.
16. Kojima R, Fujiwara T, Matsuda A, Narita M, Matsubara O, Nonoyama S, et al. Factors associated with steroid phobia in caregivers of children with atopic dermatitis. Pediatr Dermatol. 2013;30:29–35.
17. Hon KL, Kam WY, Leung TF, Lam MC, Wong KY, Lee KC, et al. Steroid fears in children with eczema. Acta Paediatr. 2006;95:1451–5.
18. Moret L, Anthoine E, Aubert-Wastiaux H, Le Rhun A, Leux C, Mazereeuw-Hautier J, et al. TOPICOP©: a new scale evaluating topical corticosteroid phobia among atopic dermatitis outpatients and their parents. PLoS One. 2013;8:e76493.
19. Sinha A, Kar S, Yadav N, Madke B. Prevalence of topical steroid misuse among rural masses. Indian J Dermatol. 2016;61:119.
20. Saraswat A, Lahiri K, Chatterjee M, Barua S, Coondoo A, Mittal A, Panda S, Rajagopalan M, Sharma R, Abraham A, Verma SB, Srinivas CR. Topical corticosteroid abuse on the face: a prospective, multicenter study of dermatology outpatients. Indian J Dermatol Venereol Leprol. 2011;77:160–6.
21. Jha AK, Sinha R, Prasad S. Misuse of topical corticosteroids on the face: a cross-sectional study among dermatology outpatients. Indian Dermatol Online J. 2016;7:259–63.
22. Bewley A, Dermatology Working Group. Expert consensus: time for a change in the way we advise our patients to use topical corticosteroids. Br J Dermatol. 2008;158:917–20.
23. Rathi SK, D'Souza P. Rational and ethical use of topical corticosteroids based on safety and efficacy. Indian J Dermatol. 2012;57:251–9.

Rational Use of Topical Corticosteroids

11

Paschal D'Souza and Sanjay K. Rathi

Abstract

Topical corticosteroids (TCs) have been the backbone of a dermatologist's therapeutic armamentarium to treat various steroid-responsive dermatoses. They are available in different strengths and molecular and vehicular formulations that give dermatologist great flexibility to treat diseases of varying severity present at different anatomic sites in patients of different age groups.

However, many of these advantages of TCs have been negated by the frequent instances of misuse and abuse of these drugs by dermatologists, general physicians, and patients alike. This has increased cases with known adverse effects of TC as well as revealed unique TC-induced dermatoses among users. The dermatologist owes the society a responsibility to disseminate proper knowledge regarding when, where, and how to use TC and promote their rational and ethical use. The benefits of proper and appropriate use and the harm of unsupervised overuse in correct indications, misuse for cosmetic purposes, and underuse due to incomplete knowledge or irrational fears need to be clearly conveyed using all available medical, legal, and political resources.

Keywords

Topical corticosteroids • Ethical use • Rational use • Abuse • Misuse • Right

P. D'Souza (✉)
Department of Dermatology, ESIC-PGIMSR, New Delhi, India
e-mail: paschaldsouza@yahoo.com

S.K. Rathi
Consultant Dermatologist, Siliguri, West Bengal, India
e-mail: drsrathi2@gmail.com

Learning Points

1. Topical corticosteroids (TCs) are an indispensable group of drugs for the dermatologist; when used correctly, their benefits are far greater than their potential adverse effects.

© Springer Nature Singapore Pte Ltd. 2018
K. Lahiri (ed.), *A Treatise on Topical Corticosteroids in Dermatology*,
DOI 10.1007/978-981-10-4609-4_11

2. Rational and ethical use of TC implies using it for the appropriate dermatoses, in appropriate potency and strength for the site and severity of disease, and for the appropriate duration keeping in mind the patient's age, sex, physiologic state, and to an extent his/her aesthetic needs.

11.1 Introduction

Topical corticosteroids (TCs) have become the cornerstone in managing noninfective inflammatory dermatoses since they were first introduced in the early 1950s [1–3]. TCs are safe and effective drugs when used for the correct indications, in appropriate strength and formulation, and for appropriate stage of disease keeping in mind among other things the age of patient, site, and extent of disease [4].

In recent times TCs have come more in the news for the wrong reasons. Studies from India and around the world have highlighted instances of TC misuse, abuse, and also disuse due to corticosteroid phobia [5–8]. Apart from the standard indications for use in steroid-responsive noninfective inflammatory dermatoses, they are being used for conditions such as melasma, urticaria, tinea, and even undiagnosed skin rash by dermatologists and general physicians (GPs) [4, 7]. The quick masking of clinical signs and symptoms of many skin disorders by the application of TC makes them popular among GPs and quacks. Nonmedical people like friends, neighbors, beauticians, barbers, etc. advise their use as fairness/cosmetic cream, anti-acne, and antifungal therapy and for that matter any skin eruptions [9–11]. Easy availability of TC without valid prescription and use of old TC containing prescriptions for new or recurrent rash are real issues universally including in our country of billion plus people where enough dermatologists are still not available [12–15]. Awareness about TC misuse is being highlighted by dermatologists at various forums in the country and abroad

[5, 16, 17]. In India the campaign by Indian Association of Dermatologists, Venereologists and Leprologists Taskforce Against Topical Steroid Abuse (ITATSA) against over-the-counter (OTC) availability of TCs has finally borne fruit with the Government of India agreeing to the recommendation of IADVL for including it in Schedule "H" list and to ban sale of all TC without valid prescription. However, to see that this becomes a ground reality, the dermatologist has the responsibility to correctly disseminate education to the patient, the caregivers, and the medical fraternity about ethical and rational use of TC [5, 18].

Steps to ensure rational and ethical use of TC would include the various *rights* regarding TC.

11.2 Right Indications for TC Use

The first step is to prescribe TC for the correct indication and ideally for those dermatoses where there is reasonable evidence of efficacy. They are usually effective for hyper-proliferative, inflammatory, and immunologic skin disorders including dermatoses with mucosal involvement [19, 20]. The details of steroid-responsive dermatoses have been covered in a different chapter of this book, hence not being elaborated here.

Highly responsive dermatoses include flexural psoriasis, atopic dermatitis of childhood, seborrhoeic dermatitis, irritant dermatitis, etc. which will quickly respond to even a mild TC. Medium-potency TCs are adequate for psoriasis, adult atopic dermatitis, and nummular eczema. However, long-standing skin diseases having chronic, hyperkeratotic, lichenified, or indurated lesions, such as palmoplantar psoriasis and lichen simplex chronicus, are the least responsive diseases and require high-potency TC [21].

We should also be open to newer unconventional indications of TC. For example, it has been found that prophylactic treatment with a strong TC is effective for the prevention and control of acute radiation dermatitis in breast cancer patients treated with adjuvant radiotherapy (RT) [22]. As a rule, topical corticosteroids are contraindicated in acne, rosacea, perioral dermatitis, and urticarial and untreated bacterial, fungal, or viral skin lesions. The use of TC for unknown rash should be avoided even though this may provide temporary benefits, as subsequently diagnosis may even be more difficult to make. Knowing the correct indication, different strengths of topical steroids may be used to treat different phases of the disease.

11.3 Right Class/Potency/Strength and Formulation of TC

11.3.1 Potency

Vasoconstrictive property of a TC, though an imperfect method, is usually used to measure its potency [23, 24]. This is because clinical efficacy, which ideally should mirror the potency of a TC, depends on many other variables like the vehicle used, frequency and site of application, and the presence of occlusion or additional ingredients, e.g., salicylic acid, lactic acid, and urea [25–27].

There may surprisingly be difference in potency of TC between generic and its brand equivalent [28]. The first clinically effective molecule hydrocortisone has been structurally modified by halogenation, methylation, acetylation, esterification, etc. with the aim to increase potency and reduce adverse effects [28]. For instance, halogenation increases the potency but also the adverse effects, while esterification improves both the safety profile and the efficacy of TC [29, 30].

A variety of structurally distinct TCs are available which are divided into four groups according to their potency in keeping with the British National Formulary (BNF), while the American system classifies them into seven classes, with class I being the superpotent to the class VII representing the least potent [31].

In an ideal condition, the potency of the TC used should match with the severity of the disease. But this does not often happen in clinical practice. In a study in a rural tertiary care teaching hospital, about 94.36% of the

prescriptions contained very potent steroids [32]. Even in the United States, a 3-year study found that dermatologists were 3.9 times more likely to prescribe very-high-potency steroids than were other physicians [1]. The reasons could be that dermatologists are less afraid or know better about dermatological conditions than physicians which enable them to treat skin diseases with appropriate potency of TC. Lack of availability of low-potency TC in government pharmacy was also cited as a cause with dermatologist having limited choice of TC prescription [32].

11.3.2 Vehicle

TC also differs in potency based on the vehicle in which they are formulated, e.g., betamethasone dipropionate 0.05% in ointment form comes in class I (superpotent) category, while the same drug in cream form is a class II (potent) molecule. The formulation to use generally will depend on the type and site of lesions. TCs are available in ointments, creams, gels, lotions, solutions, etc. [33].

Ointments are very effective for treating dry, thick, hyperkeratotic lesions where they provide more lubrication and occlusion, thus increasing steroid absorption. However, in hairy and intertriginous areas, they may cause maceration and folliculitis. Aesthetically, due to their greasy nature, they are less acceptable which may result in poor patient satisfaction and compliance [9].

Creams are generally less potent than ointment, but because of good lubricating, nonocclusive, and drying effect, they are used for acute exudative inflammation and in intertriginous areas. Their ability to vanish into the skin makes them cosmetically appealing, but the preservatives present in creams can cause irritation, stinging, and allergic reaction [9].

Lotion- and gel-based TCs are least greasy and occlusive and so are useful for hairy areas like scalp where they penetrate easily and leave little residue. In addition, gels dry quickly and do not cause matting of hair [34, 35]. Foams, mousses, and shampoo containing TC are also probably equally effective for the same indication but are costly and so ethically debatable.

Newer formulations are continually being explored to improve efficacy and safety of TC. In atopic dermatitis (AD) which is a chronic and relapsing skin disease, betamethasone valerate (BMV)/diflucortolone valerate (DFV)-loaded liposomes (220–350 nm) incorporated into chitosan gel were applied to AD-induced rats. Results showed that liposomes might be an effective and safe carrier for corticosteroids [36].

Occlusion increases steroid penetration and can be used in combination with all vehicles. Simple plastic dressing results in a sevenfold increase in steroid penetration compared with dry skin [28]. Irritation and infection are major problems with occlusion. TC after a shower or bath also improves its efficacy due to hydration [37].

11.4 Right Quantity, Frequency, and Duration of TC

Unless properly advised, patients use TC in different quantities regardless of site, severity, and extent of involvement according to their own perception of what is adequate, thus manifesting differences in the efficacy and harm profile. Rational use with regard to the quantity of TC would include consistently adopting the "fingertip unit" (FTU) method, recommended by Long and Finlay [38]. A FTU is defined as the amount that can be squeezed from the fingertip to the first crease of the finger using a 5 mm diameter nozzle and amounts to 0.5 g cream/ointment [39]. The amount of ointment necessary for a specific anatomic area is specified in terms of number of FTUs. Tables 11.1 and 11.2 mention the amount of ointment needed in adults and children, respectively, based on specific anatomic area. To put it simply, a single adequate application on the whole body of an adult will consume approximately 30 g of TC. An area of the one hand (palm and digits) requires half FTU per application. It is advisable not to exceed

45 g/week of potent or 100 g/week of a moderately potent topical steroid in an adult, while in children, the amounts should be smaller [40]. Try not to mix TC with other topical products and apply it in the direction of hair growth when using on hair-bearing areas to prevent the development of folliculitis. A gap between applications (e.g., 30 min) will help to avoid dilution of the corticosteroid or spreading it to other uninvolved areas [41].

As per conventional practice, once or twice daily application of TC is recommended [28]. Newer formulations requiring only once daily application are available [42]. It is doubtful whether more frequent administration translates into better results [43]. A review of RCTs in atopic dermatitis failed to convincingly establish better results from more frequent application of TC [44]. This instead may lead to several local and systemic side effects. Due to the stratum corneum acting as a reservoir for TC, superpotent drugs such as clobetasol propionate 0.05% cream were found to persist in stratum corneum till day 4 [45]. This may mean that a still lower frequency of an alternate or even twice a week application of TC can be advocated. During remission or in well-controlled disease, weekend TC separated by weekdays of emollients or steroid-sparing agents may suffice [40]. It is wise to tailor the frequency schedule depending on phase of the disease so as to maximize the advantages of adequate disease con-

Table 11.1 FTU guidelines for adults[a]

Guidelines for adults		
Anatomic area	FTU required	Amount needed for twice daily regimen in g
Face and neck	2.5	2.5
Anterior and posterior trunk	7	7
Arms	3	3
Hands (both sides)	1	1
Leg	6	6
Foot	2	2

[a]Adapted from Long and Finlay [38]

Table 11.2 FTU guidelines for children[a]

Guidelines for children				
	FTU required	Amount needed for twice daily regimen in g		
Anatomic area	3–6 months	1–2 years	3–5 years	5–10 years
Face and neck	1/1	1.5/1.5	1.5/1.5	2/2
Arm and hand	1/1	1.5/1.5	2/2	2.5/2.5
Leg and foot	1.5/1.5	2/2	3/3	4.5/4.5
Anterior trunk	1/1	2/2	3/3	3.5/3.5
Posterior trunk and buttocks	1.5/1.5	3/3	3.5/3.5	5/5

[a]Adapted from Long et al. [83]

trol, decrease local and systemic adverse effects, and improve patient compliance [19, 46]. Advise should be given to patients to start treatment as soon as signs of a flare appear and to continue for 48 h after clinical remission [47]. Patients who experience frequent, repeated outbreaks at the same body sites may benefit from the proactive application of TCS once to twice weekly at these locations even when the eczema is quiescent. This can be used safely up to 40 weeks [48].

All TCs, regardless of the potency, should ideally not be used for more than 2–4 weeks duration at a stretch. Superpotent and potent preparations need a relook after continuous use for a maximum duration of only 2 weeks [9, 28]. The absence of clinical response or worsening of lesions calls for discontinuation of TC and reevaluation of the diagnosis. Patients should be reviewed periodically taking into account the severity and site of their initial condition and potency of topical corticosteroid being used. This would mean around 4 weeks for adults and 2 weeks for children [49].

Skin penetration and absorption of drugs in normal healthy skin vary at different anatomic sites depending on the characteristics of the stratum corneum and skin lipid structure, e.g., over the eyelids, it is 300 times more than the sole [50]. The scrotum absorbs up to 40% of applied drugs, while the face and forearms have much lower absorption of 10% and 1%, respectively [40]. It can be two- to tenfold higher in diseased states, due to defective epidermal barrier. Palms

and soles need to be treated with high-potency preparations, while eyelids, the groin, the axilla, and other intertriginous areas can do with medium- to low-potency TC [1, 3, 9]. It is safer to use low- to medium-potency preparation when large surface areas are involved because of the increased risk of systemic absorption.

11.5 Right TC for the Right Kind of Patient

The age, sex, expectation of the patient, and underlying special physiological conditions like pregnancy and lactation are important considerations when choosing a TC [1, 3, 9]. Children have larger surface area to body weight ratio, have difficulty in metabolizing potent corticosteroids, and so may be more sensitive to stronger TC [40, 51]. In them, low-potency corticosteroid for short periods without occlusion is preferable. In the elderly, skin fragility may risk increased adverse effects unless milder TC is used. Though all TCs are classified category C by the US Food and Drug Administration [52], the Australian government's Therapeutic Goods Administration(TGA) classifies some like fluocinolone, betamethasone, triamcinolone, and even halcinonide (though strength not mentioned) as category A [53]. Limited and inconclusive data for humans seems to suggest an association between very potent topical corticosteroids and fetal growth restriction [54]. As of now, there are no reported adverse effects during lactation, though direct application over nipples should be avoided before breastfeeding [40].

11.6 Right Use of TC in Combination with Antibacterials, Antifungals, and Other Agents

Perhaps no other pharmacologically active molecule has been combined in so many combinations and permutations and for so many indications as TC. To mention and discuss all will be beyond the scope of this chapter. Briefly and commonly, TC is prescribed by dermatologist in combination with antibacterials for lesions of atopic dermatitis (AD) [55]; antifungals for inflammatory and very itchy lesions of tinea and even chronic paronychia [56, 57]; emollients, salicylic acid, vitamin D analogs, and tazarotene for psoriasis [58–60]; and hydroquinone and tretinoin for melasma [61]. The rationale behind some of these is as follows:

a. Superantigens produced by *Staphylococcus aureus*, a common colonizer of AD lesions, may perpetuate the eczema and produce steroid insensitivity [62]. The use of topical and/or systemic antibiotics along with TC may reduce colonization of the skin and nasal mucosa and thus improve the eczema [63].
b. Bioavailability and activity of the antimycotic are increased, and inflammatory symptoms are rapidly reduced on adding TC in highly inflammatory tinea [56].
c. Salicylic acid increases penetration of TC, enhancing its efficacy in psoriasis [58].
d. Early and greater efficacy and steroid-sparing effect of vitamin D analogs when combined with TC [59].
e. TC reduces the potential irritancy of tazarotene apart from having a synergistic effect in psoriasis [60].

Caution points and proper measures to be remembered are:

1. Inappropriate use of TC + antimicrobials increases the risk of bacterial resistance and sensitization and can increase the cost of treatment [49]. TC containing antimicrobials should only be used when dermatitis is not responding despite adequate TC alone, for dermatitis associated with mild clinical infection in localized areas and for no longer than 2 weeks. It is felt that combination is more appropriate for treating eczematous lesions close to the anterior nares, flexures, perianal areas, and finger or toe web spaces [64]. They should not be issued as repeat prescriptions.
2. Indiscriminate use of TC+ antifungal is thought to be one of the reasons for increasing incidence of difficult to treat tinea infections which is being experienced by almost all dermatologists in India. Complete avoidance of this combination, using them only for the first week in inflammatory or severely symptomatic patients, and using topical antifungals with additional anti-inflammatory properties may be a way forward.
3. Patients should be advised to continue using their emollient while using TC [47]. It is recommended to apply the emollient before the TC, though there is no hard and fast rule [65].
4. To prevent steroid toxicities when adding salicylic acid to TC, it is recommended that this combination be limited to no more than medium-potency (class 3–4) TC.
5. Combination therapies including TC for melasma should not be used for more than 4 weeks. In Indian scenario, it is better to opt for safer alternative due to prevalence of more abuse than proper use [66].
   In the 1980s, triple combinations of TC, antibacterial, and antifungal were very popular and apparently very effective [67, 68]. Presently these unethical and irrational fixed drug combinations (FDC) containing 3–4 active ingredients are among the top sellers in the market [15]. Today, there is no doubt in the

fraternity that they were more of a way to escape from committing to a diagnosis while offering temporary relief and have caused terrible harm over the years. They should be a strict *no* for the dermatologist.

11.7 Right Choice of TC When Multiple Choices Are Available

There will be times when there are many TCs available of the same class which are likely to be effective for the stage and extent of disease in a case. In this case, ethics call for prescribing the product with the lowest acquisition cost, taking into account pack size, extent of disease, and frequency of application required. It is better to be familiar with few drugs in each class rather than be swayed by the temptation to try newer things each time as per the persistence of the pharmaceutical executives who visit our hospitals and clinics. Disproportionately costly drugs offering no clinical advantage should be avoided [49]. Efficacy between generic and branded drugs even of the same compound may differ and so may their cost which should be kept in mind [28, 32]. TCs in combination packs are fairly costly and should not be used unless there is appropriate justification [5]. The only probable reason for choosing a costlier of the equipotent clinically effective TC would be the patient preference in terms of its aesthetic quality, all other things being equivalent.

11.8 Right Knowledge of Adverse Effects of TC

Details of the well-known cutaneous and systemic adverse effects [52, 69–73] are covered in other chapters of this book and will be omitted here. Reversible suppression of the hypothalamic–pituitary–adrenal axis has been described in children with TC doses as little as 14 g per week [40].

The phenomena of steroid addiction, tachyphylaxis, and contact dermatitis (CD) due to TC are issues to be aware of while treating the patient for a dermatoses or encountering one in a grip of steroid abuse. The adverse effects increase with potency of steroid, duration of use, amount applied, site of application, age of the patient, and conditions of application like hydration, occlusion, combination with salicylic acid, etc. TC addiction is an underreported entity caused due to inappropriate use of TC and probably includes several erythema syndromes such as red face syndrome, post-peel erythema, red scrotal syndrome, vulvodynia, perianal atrophoderma, chronic actinic dermatitis, and chronic recalcitrant eczemas [69, 70]. A recent systemic review of TC withdrawal revealed 34 studies involving TC addiction mostly on the face and genital area (99.3%) of women (81.0%) due to long-term inappropriate use of potent TCS [6]. Burning and stinging were the most frequently reported symptoms (65.5%) with erythema being the most common sign (92.3%). TC abuse on the face manifests as "topical corticosteroid-induced rosacea-like dermatitis" (TCIRD) or "topical steroid-dependent face" (TSDF) [17, 74]. It is very difficult to manage due to a compromised epidermal barrier as well as due to a rebound flare-up of skin lesions on attempting withdrawal of TC [17, 74].

11.9 Right Education Regarding the Use of TC

It is known that peer pressure, rapid feel good effect, and ignorance about harmful effects lead to TC abuse [16]. The excessive obsession with fairness has led to the unprecedented, unsupervised use of triple combination creams containing TC which are approved primarily as a short-term treatment for melasma and other hyperpigmented disorders. Time spent in educating on these points will hopefully prevent mishaps. It will also take care of the other extreme of excessive fear of using TC which leads to inadequate usage and poor clinical results.

Perhaps the beginning can be done by proper education of ourselves and our residents in medical colleges to write out a proper prescription especially when TC is prescribed. It should contain relevant information regarding diagnosis, site, frequency, and duration of treatment, something glaringly missing in most prescriptions [3]. From the patients' point of view, they need to be counseled about having realistic expectations regarding outcomes: "control not cure" of the underlying disease needs to be stressed. In long-standing disease like childhood atopic dermatitis, patients and caregivers should be actively involved in disease management [48, 75].

On the other hand, topical corticosteroid concerns (TCC)/corticosteroid phobia has become an important issue in patients, parents of children with atopic dermatitis, clinicians, dermatologist, and pharmacist leading to nonadherence involving TC use, with poor disease control and increased healthcare costs [8, 76–78]. The prevalence of TCC was 41.5% among patients in a questionnaire-based study [8], while clinicians showed minor TCC themselves in 74% in another study [77]. Corticophobia among parents continues to be high resulting in undertreating their children especially in cases of AD [18]. The source of negative attitude about TC was found to be the Internet, media, family, friends, and also pharmacist and doctors. Confusing information is being received many times by parents and care-givers accessing online discussion forums regarding the use of TC [77]. Proper education about safe and rational use of TC and provision of written and oral information have led to positive change in attitude of pharmacist [76] and significant reduction in TCC in patients [8].

11.10 Right Administrative Measures Regarding the Use of TC

According to Drugs and Cosmetics (D and C) Act 1940, the TC falls under the category of Schedule H drugs, to be sold only on the valid prescription of a qualified doctor [79]. This had never been seriously implemented due to prevailing confu-sions [15]. Lack of qualified dermatologists, more so in rural areas, is also compounding the problem of irrational use of TC [5]. Presently more than 119 FDC formulations are available in Indian market, though only 60 are featured among the Central Drugs Standard Control Organization's (CDSCO's) approved list of FDCs permitted for continued manufacturing and marketing in respect of the applicants under 18-month policy decision in India (as of December 16, 2016) [81]. For the pharmaceutical companies that are marketing non-approved FDCs, the regulator needs to take stern steps to enforce law of the land by putting in place improved surveillance mechanisms. More than 7.5 lakh chemists in India, who are the point of first contact for majority of Indian population for minor healthcare ailments, need to be involved in fight against menace of TC abuse [5]. The Medical Council of India is also encouraging addition of postgraduate seats in all medical specialties in both government and private medical colleges to improve doctor/patient ratio.

Conclusions

TCs are a wonderful group of drugs in the correct hands. This implies that their benefits are far greater than their potential adverse effects when used for the appropriate dermatoses, in appropriate potency and strength for the site and severity of disease, for the appropriate duration keeping in mind the patient's age, sex, physiologic state, and to an extent his/her esthetic needs. Awareness of TC-related adverse effects helps to put in place urgent preventive and therapeutic measures. Temptation to use TC for undiagnosed rash or in combination therapies which are expensive and of unproven additional advantage should be resisted. To ensure that rational and ethical use of TC percolates to the ground level, an ongoing multipronged approach involving medical fraternity, pharmaceutical industry, and political and legal establishment should be undertaken [16].

The commendable work of Indian Association of Dermatologists, Venereologists and Leprologists to increase awareness about

TC misuse/abuse at every available forum needs to be appreciated. Political leaders and government officials should be repeatedly apprised of the prevailing situation and the need to curb this menace. The use of media for public education on topical steroid misuse is warranted, and the involvement of general practitioners, nurses, and pharmacists is needed. The legal approach should include the enforcement of the existing legislation related to the control of these drugs, so that TCs are not sold without proper prescriptions. Pharmaceutical companies could play their part by including package inserts containing clear "fingertip unit" instructions on TC application [82].

References

1. Stern R. The pattern of topical corticosteroid prescribing in the United States 1989–1991. J Am Acad Dermatol. 1996;35:183–96.
2. Sulzberger MB, Witten VH. The effect of topically applied compound F in selected dermatoses. J Invest Dermatol. 1952;19:101–2.
3. Kumar AM, Noushad PP, Shailaja K, Jayasutha J, Ramasamy C. A study on drug prescribing pattern and use of corticosteroids in dermatological conditions at tertiary care teaching hospital. Int J Pharm Sci Rev Res. 2011;9:132–5.
4. Rathi SK, D'Souza P. Rational and ethical use of topical corticosteroids based on safety and efficacy. Indian J Dermatol. 2012;57:251–9.
5. Kumar S, Goyal A, Gupta YK. Abuse of topical corticosteroids in India: concerns and the way forward. J Pharmacol Pharmacother. 2016;7(1):1–5. doi:10.4103/0976-500X.179364.
6. Hajar T, Leshem YA, Hanifin JM, Nedorost ST, Lio PA, Paller AS, et al. (The National Eczema Association Task Force); A systematic review of topical corticosteroid withdrawal ("steroid addiction") in patients with atopic dermatitis and other dermatoses. J Am Acad Dermatol. 2015;72(3):541–549.e2. doi:10.1016/j.jaad.2014.11.024.
7. Shakya Shrestha S, Bhandari M, Shrestha R, Thapa SR, Karki A, Prajapati M, et al. Study on corticosteroids use pattern in dermatological practice and investigating adverse effect of corticosteroids including its associated factors. Kathmandu Univ Med J (KUMJ). 2015;13(51):261–7.
8. Müller SM, Tomaschett D, Euler S, Vogt DR, Herzog L, Itin P. Topical corticosteroid concerns in dermatological outpatients: a cross-sectional and interventional study. Dermatology. 2016;232(4):444–52.
9. Ference JD, Last AR. Choosing topical corticosteroids. Am Fam Physician. 2009;79:135–40.
10. Jha AK, Sinha R, Prasad S. Misuse of topical corticosteroids on the face: a cross-sectional study among dermatology outpatients. Indian Dermatol Online J. 2016;7(4):259–63.
11. Rathi S. Abuse of topical steroid as cosmetic cream: a social background of steroid dermatitis. Indian J Dermatol. 2006;51:154–5.
12. Bhat YJ, Manzoor S, Qayoom S. Steroid induced rosacea: a clinical study of 200 patients. Indian J Dermatol. 2011;56:30–2.
13. Al-Dhalimi MA, Aljawahiri N. Misuse of topical corticosteroids: a clinical study from an Iraqi hospital. East Mediterr Health J. 2006;12:847–52.
14. Solomon BA, Glass AT, Rabbin PE. Tinea incognito and "over the-counter" potent topical steroids. Cutis. 1996;58:295–6.
15. Verma SB. Sales, status, prescriptions and regulatory problems with topical steroids in India. Indian J Dermatol Venereol Leprol. 2014;80:201–3.
16. Malangu N, Ogunbanjo G. Predictors of topical steroid misuse among patrons of pharmacies in Pretoria. SA Fam Pract. 2006;48:14.
17. Saraswat A, Lahiri K, Chatterjee M, Barua S, Coondoo A, Mittal A, et al. Topical corticosteroid abuse on the face: a prospective, multicentre study of dermatology outpatients. Indian J Dermatol Venereol Leprol. 2011;77:160–6.
18. Lee JY, Her Y, Kim CW, Kim SS. Topical corticosteroid phobia among parents of children with atopic eczema in Korea. Ann Dermatol. 2015;27(5):499–506.
19. Giannotti B. Current treatment guidelines for topical corticosteroids. Drugs. 1988;36(Suppl 5):9–14.
20. Gonzalez-Moles MA, Scully C. Vesiculo-erosive oral mucosal disease management with topical corticosteroids: (1) fundamental principles and specific agents available. J Dent Res. 2005;84:294–301.
21. Valencia IC, Kerdel KA. Topical corticosteroids. In: Goldsmith LA, Katz SI, Gilchrest BA, Paller AS, Leffell DJ, Wolff K, editors. Fitzpatrick's dermatology in general medicine. 7th ed. New York, NY: McGraw-Hill; 2008.
22. Ulff E, Maroti M, Serup J, Nilsson M, Falkmer U. Prophylactic treatment with a potent corticosteroid cream ameliorates radiodermatitis, independent of radiation schedule: a randomized double blinded study. Radiother Oncol. 2017;122:50–3. doi:10.1016/j.radonc.2016.11.013.
23. Mc Kenzie AW, Stoughton RB. Method for comparing percutaneous absorption of steroids. Arch Dermatol. 1962;86:608–10.
24. Goa KL. Clinical pharmacology and pharmacokinetic properties of topically applied corticosteroids. A review. Drugs. 1988;36(Suppl 5):51–61.
25. Mc Kenzie AW. Comparison of steroids by vasoconstriction. Br J Dermatol. 1966;78:182–3.

26. Olsen EA. A double-blind controlled comparison of generic and trade-name topical steroids using the vasoconstriction assay. Arch Dermatol. 1991;127:197–201.

27. MeReC. Using topical corticosteroids in general practice. MeReC Bull. 1999;10(6):21–4.

28. Drake LA, Dinehart SM, Farmer ER, Goltz RW, Graham GF, Hordinsky MK, et al. Guidelines of care for the use of topical glucocorticosteroids. J Am Acad Dermatol. 1996;35:615–9.

29. Epstein NN, Epstein WI, Epstein JH. Atrophic striae in patients with inguinal intertrigo. Arch Dermatol. 1963;87:450–5.

30. Mukhopadhyay AK, Baghel V. A study to evaluate the efficacy and safety of hydrocortisone aceponate 0.127% lipophilic cream in steroid responsive dermatoses in Indian patients. Indian J Dermatol Venereol Leprol. 2010;76:591.

31. Jacob SE, Steele T. Corticosteroid classes: a quick reference guide including patch test substance and cross-reactivity. J Am Acad Dermatol. 2006;54:723–7.

32. Rathod SS, Motghare VM, Deshmukh VS, Deshpande RP, Bhamare CG. Prescribing practices of topical corticosteroids in the outpatient dermatology Department of a Rural Tertiary Care Teaching Hospital. Indian J Dermatol. 2013;58(5):342–5.

33. Lee NP, Arriola ER. Topical corticosteroids. Back to basics. West J Med. 1999;171:351–3.

34. Sheman AJ. Proper use of topical corticosteroids. In: Frankel DH, editor. Field guide to clinical dermatology. 2nd ed. Northvale, NJ: LWW; 2006. p. 3.

35. Maibach HI. In vivo percutaneous penetration of corticosteroids in man and unresolved problems in the efficacy. Dermatologica. 1976;152(Suppl 1):11–25.

36. Eroğlu İ, Azizoğlu E, Özyazıcı M, Nenni M, Gürer Orhan H, Özbal S, et al. Effective topical delivery systems for corticosteroids: dermatological and histological evaluations. Drug Deliv. 2016;23(5):1502–13.

37. Pariser DM. Topical steroids: a guide for use in the elderly patients. Geriatrics. 1991;46:51–4. 57–60

38. Long CC, Finlay AY. The finger-tip unit-a new practical measure. Clin Exp Dermatol. 1991;16:444–7.

39. Tadicherla S, Ross K, Shenefelt PD, Fenske NA. Topical corticosteroids in dermatology. J Drugs Dermatol. 2009;8:1093–105.

40. Carlos G, Uribe P, Fernández-Peñas P. Rational use of topical corticosteroids. Aust Prescr. 2013;36:5–61.

41. National Institute for Health and Care Excellence, Clinical Knowledge Summaries. Corticosteroids–topical (skin), nose, and eyes. Last revised August 2010 quoted in NHS Prescqipp Bulletin 116: Topical corticosteroids. 2015. Accessed via https://www.prescqipp.info/topical-corticosteroids/category/228-topical-corticosteroids.

42. Brazzini B, Pimpinelli N. New and established topical corticosteroids in dermatology: clinical pharmacology and therapeutic use. Am J Clin Dermatol. 2002;3:47–58.

43. du Vivier A. Tachyphylaxis to topically applied steroids. Arch Dermatol. 1976;112:1245–8.

44. NICE. Appraisal consultation document of application of topical corticosteroids for atopic eczema. National Institute for Health and Clinical Excellence. 2004.

Available from https://www.nice.org.uk/guidance/ta81/documents/appraisal-consultation-document-frequency-of-application-of-topical-corticosteroids-for-atopic-eczema. Accessed 19 Jan 2017.

45. Abidi A, Ahmad F, Singh SK, Kumar A. Study of reservoir effect of clobetasol propionate cream in an experimental animal model using histamine-induced wheal suppression test. Indian J Dermatol. 2010;55:329–33.

46. Lagos B, Mibach H. Frequency of application of topical corticosteroids: an overview. Br J Dermatol. 1998;139:763–6.

47. National Institute for Health and Care Excellence (NICE): Atopic eczema in children—Management of atopic eczema in children from birth up to the age of 12 years. [CG57] London: National Collaborating Centre for Women's and Children's Health; 2007. http://www.nice.org.uk/guidance/CG57/chapter/1-Guidance. Accessed 19 Jan 2017.

48. Sathish Kumar D, Moss C. Topical therapy in atopic dermatitis in children. Indian J Dermatol. 2016;61(6):656–61.

49. NHS Prescqipp Bulletin 116: Topical corticosteroids. 2015. Accessed via https://www.prescqipp.info/topical-corticosteroids/category/228-topical-corticosteroids. Accessed 12 Jan 2017.

50. Feldmann RJ, Maibach HI. Regional variation in percutaneous penetration of 14C cortisol in man. J Invest Dermatol. 1967;48:181–3.

51. Saraswat A. Topical corticosteroid use in children: adverse effects and how to minimize them. Indian J Dermatol Venereol Leprol. 2010;76:225–8.

52. Hengge UR, Ruzicka T, Schwartz RA, Cork MJ. Adverse effects of topical glucocorticoids. J Am Acad Dermatol. 2006;54:1–15.

53. Prescribing medicines in pregnancy database: Australian Government-Department of health Therapeutic goods administration via https://www.tga.gov.au/prescribing-medicines-pregnancy-database#searchname. Accessed 15 Jan 2017.

54. Chi CC, Wang SH, Kirtschig G. Safety of topical corticosteroids in pregnancy. JAMA Dermatol. 2016;152(8):934–5.

55. Khobragade KJ. Efficacy and safety of combination ointment fluticasone propionate 0.005% plus mupirocin 2% for the treatment of atopic dermatitis with clinical suspicion of secondary bacterial infection: an open label uncontrolled study. Indian J Dermatol Venreol Leprol. 2005;71:92–6.

56. Havlickova B, Friedrich M. The advantages of topical combination therapy in the treatment of inflammatory dermatomycoses. Mycoses. 2008;51(Suppl 4):16–26.

57. Rigopoulos D, Larios G, Gregoriou S, Alevizos A. Acute and chronic paronychia. Am Fam Physician. 2008;77(3):339–46.

58. Koo J, Cuffie CA, Tanner DJ, Bressinck R, Cornell RC, DeVillez RL, et al. Mometasone furoate 0.1%-salicylic acid 5% ointment versus mometasone furoate 0.1% ointment in the treatment of moderate-to-severe psoriasis: a multicenter study. Clin Ther. 1998;20:283–91.

59. Papp KA, Guenther L, Boyden B, Larsen FG, Harvima RJ, Guilhou JJ, et al. Early onset of action and efficacy of a combination of calcipotriene and betamethasone dipropionate in the treatment of psoriasis. J Am Acad Dermatol. 2003;48:48–54.

60. Koo JY, Martin D. Investigator-masked comparison of tazarotene gel q.d. Plus mometasone furoate cream q.d. vs. mometasone furoate cream b.i.d. in the treatment of plaque psoriasis. Int J Dermatol. 2001;40:210–2.

61. Rajaratnam R, Halpern J, Salim A, Emmett C. Interventions for melasma. Cochrane Database Syst Rev. 2010;7:CD003538.

62. McFadden JP, Noble WC, Camp RD. Superantigenic exotoxin secreting potential of staphylococci isolated from eczematous skin. Br J Dermatol. 1993;128:631–2.

63. Dhar S, Kanwar AJ, Kaur S, Sharma P, Ganguly NK. Role of bacterial flora in the pathogenesis and management of atopic dermatitis. Indian J Med Res. 1992;95:234–8.

64. Dhar S. Should topical antibacterials be routinely combined with topical steroids in the treatment of atopic dermatitis? Indian J Dermatol Venereol Leprol. 2005;71:71–2.

65. Guidelines for the management of atopic eczema. Primary Care Dermatology Society & British Association of Dermatologists . Available from https://www.nice.org.uk/guidance/ta81/resources/primary-care-dermatology-society2. Accessed on 22 Jan 2017.

66. Kandhari R, Khunger N. Skin lightening agents-use or abuse? A retrospective analysis of topical preparations used by melasma patients of darker skin type. Indian J Dermatol Venereol Leprol. 2013;79(5):701–2.

67. Pellerano S. Use of a combination of an anti-inflammatory steroid, an antibacterial agent and an antifungal in dermatological practice. Int J Clin Pharmacol Ther Toxicol. 1985;23(4):215–8.

68. Pazzaglia A. Clinical results obtained with a combination of an anti-inflammatory steroid, an antibacterial agent and an antifungal in dermatological outpatient practice. Int J Clin Pharmacol Ther Toxicol. 1985;23(7):367–72.

69. Katz HI. Topical corticosteroids. Dermatol Clin. 1995;13:805–15. 6055

70. Keipert JA, Kelly R. Temporary Cushing's syndrome from percutaneous absorption of betamethasone 17-valerate. Med J Aust. 1971;1:542–4.

71. Gilbertson EO, Spellman MC, Piacquadio DJ, Mulford MI. Super potent topical corticosteroid use associated with adrenal suppression: clinical considerations. J Am Acad Dermatol. 1998;38(2 Pt 2):318–21.

72. Ohman EM, Rogers S, Meenan FO, Mckenna TJ. Adrenal suppression following low-dose topical clobetasol propionate. JR Soc Med. 1987;80:422–4.

73. Munro DD. The effect of percutaneously absorbed steroids on hypothalamic-pituitary-adrenal function after intensive use in inpatients. Br J Dermatol. 1976;94(Suppl 12):67–76.

74. Rathi SK, Kumrah L. Topical corticosteroid-induced rosacea like dermatitis: a clinical study of 110 cases. Indian J Dermatol Venereol Leprol. 2011;77:42–6.

75. Tollefson MM, Bruckner AL. Section on dermatology. Atopic dermatitis: skin-directed management. Pediatrics. 2014;134:e1735–44.

76. Smith SD, Lee A, Blaszczynski A, Fischer G. Attitudes of Australian dermatologists to the use and safety of topical corticosteroids in paediatric atopic dermatitis. Australas J Dermatol. 2015;57:278–83. doi:10.1111/ajd.12402.

77. Mueller SM, Tomaschett D, Vogt DR, Itin P, Cozzio A, Surber C. Topical corticosteroid concerns from the clinicians' perspective. J Dermatolog Treat. 2016:1–5. doi:10.1080/09546634.2016.1255307.

78. Teasdale E, Muller I, Santer M. Carers' views of topical-corticosteroid use in childhood eczema: a qualitative study of online discussion forums. Br J Dermatol. 2016; doi:10.1111/bjd.15130 [Epub ahead of print].

79. The Drugs and Cosmetics Rules. Ministry of Health and Family Welfare, Government of India. 1945. Available from: http://cdsco.nic.in/html/copy%20of%201.%20dandcact121.pdf. Last accessed on 19 Jan 2017.

80. Petitioning the Drug Controller of India-Stop indiscriminate OTC sale of topical steroid without prescription, most are Schedule H drugs. Available from: http://www.change.org/p/the-drug-controller-of-india-stop-indiscriminate-otc-sale-of-topicalsteroid--without-prescription-most-are-schedule-h-drugs. Accessed on 21 Jan 2017.

81. FDCs permitted for continued manufacturing and marketing in respect of the applicants under 18 months policy decision. Central Drugs Standard Control Organization, India. As on 16 Dec 2016. Available from: http://cdsco.nic.in/writereaddata/Final%20Rational%20list%20as%20on%2021_12_2016.pdf. Accessed on 22 Jan 2017.

82. Bewley A. Expert consensus: time for a change in the way we advise our patients to use corticosteroids. Br J Dermatol. 2008;158:917–20.

83. Long CC, Mills CM, Finlay AY. A practical guide to topical therapy in children. Br J Dermatol. 1998;138:293–6.

Abuse of Topical Corticosteroid as Cosmetic Cream: A Social Background of Steroid Dermatitis

12

Sanjay K. Rathi and Paschal D'Souza

Abstract

Topical corticosteroids (TC) are used frequently for approved and non-approved indications in dermatology. This improper use and misuse has now also spilled over to TC being used for cosmetic purpose as fairness cream which is accepted fairly well in the society with recommendations originating from relatives, friends, neighbour, beautician, chemists, etc. This addiction and abuse of TC particularly on the face as cosmetic cream has led to development of unique 'steroid dermatitis', manifesting as perioral, diffuse, centrofacial and malar variants. Rapid effect, cheap, easy availability, ignorance of adverse effects, inappropriate marketing and society's attitude towards fair skin colour are few reasons which tempt patients (mostly females) to start TC as cosmetic creams. TC-damaged face is really difficult to treat which therefore calls for measures preventing its development in the first place. Proper education regarding TC needs to be imparted at individual and community levels using all available resources to prevent its misuse as cosmetic creams. Administrative, regulatory and enforcement measures need to be strengthened to ensure that TC are only available through proper channel of prescription by authorised specialists.

Keywords

Topical corticosteroid • Abuse • Cosmetic cream • Steroid dermatitis • Social background • Cause • Management

Learning Points

1. Topical corticosteroid abuse as a cosmetic in the social context has its genesis in the elevation of status of some topical corticosteroids as beautifying creams which are apparently effective, have instantaneous results and are cheap, easily available, socially acceptable and popular.

S.K. Rathi (✉)
Consultant Dermatologist,
143, Hill Cart Road, Siliguri 734 001, West Bengal,
India
e-mail: drsrathi2@gmail.com

P. D'Souza
Department of Dermatology, ESIC-PGIMSR,
New Delhi, India
e-mail: paschaldsouza@yahoo.com

© Springer Nature Singapore Pte Ltd. 2018
K. Lahiri (ed.), *A Treatise on Topical Corticosteroids in Dermatology*,
DOI 10.1007/978-981-10-4609-4_12

2. This has led to the development of unique 'steroid dermatitis' due to the so-called steroid addiction and inability to withdraw the drug on account of extreme discomfort in attempting to do so.

workers: light-sensitive seborrheic dermatitis, perioral dermatitis, rosea-like dermatitis, steroid rosacea, steroid dermatitis resembling rosacea, steroid-induced rosacea-like dermatitis, topical corticosteroid-induced rosacea-like dermatitis (TCIRD) and topical steroid-dependent face (TSDF) [5–14].

12.1   Introduction

Since hydrocortisone was first introduced in 1951 and modifications over subsequent years of the primary molecule led to birth of new molecules with different potencies, efficacy and safety profile, dermato-therapeutics has undergone a tremendous revolution [1]. It has never been easier to treat a variety of dermatoses in such an effective manner and bring quick relief to patients suffering with them for months or several years. With prudence over time, the ethical dermatologist used it mainly for non-infective inflammatory conditions and as per certain guidelines [2]. Sadly, TC started being used for improper indications like acne, tinea, urticaria, non-specific pruritus, etc. by general practitioners (GP), registered medical practitioners (RMP), practitioners of alternate medicine, quacks, chemists and homemade doctors (parents, siblings, neighbours) [3]. Due to the prolonged or improper use of TC in approved and non-approved indications, some well-defined adverse effects of TC came to be known [4]. Simultaneously, there came a time when the use of these wonder drugs spilled into the cosmetic realm where some of the pharmacological and adverse effects of TC, e.g. vasoconstrictive and melanopenic effects, were perceived as boom for people hungry to look fair. This was more apparent specially in those of brown and dark races. Here was a situation where people of 'no skin disease' preferred to use TC over safe cosmetic creams to look fair or hide their blemishes. With this, a new dermatosis emerged due to long and improper use and for obvious reasons was mainly confined to the face. This dermatosis was named variously by different

12.2   Epidemiology of TC Abuse as a Cosmetic

Abuse of TC as a cosmetic probably must be as old as the discovery of TC itself. Almost all dermatologist encountered patients revealing inappropriate use of TC but very few documented it and brought it up to the level of published literature [9–12, 15, 16]. It is only in the last two decades when it has assumed epidemic proportion and unusual steroid induced difficult to treat dermatitis started appearing, that the community has been jolted to actively survey prevalence of the problem in the society resulting in many recent studies to this effect [8, 14, 17–20].

The phenomenon of TC abuse as a cosmetic is universal with reports appearing across the world [21–26]. Due to the society's increased preference for fairness which is a commonplace in Caucasian American and European skin, the abuse appears to be more in races that have constitutive brown or black skin. Although generally not mentioned, one study found that frequency of patients with TC-related adverse effects amounted to 5.63% of all the dermatology patients seen during the period [26]. It is seen more often in the younger age group of 21–30 years, probably because they are socially more active [19, 24–27]. A strong female preponderance is seen in almost all studies. This may be because of their quest to look pretty and because in our society 'a fair bride' is always preferable. Most studies have found an urban preponderance though some reported it more in rural areas [24, 27]. Individuals are usually of poor socioeconomic background with surprisingly good educational level [25, 26, 28]. Majority of them were students or housewives [24–28]. The problem of TC abuse as a cosmetic is not limited to lay people alone. In a study, 31% of nursing students were using face creams containing steroid alone or in combination, of which 64% were of potent category [29].

Among the TC involved, betamethasone valerate appears to be the commonest followed variably by different steroid + antibacterial + antifungal combinations, clobetasol propionate, fluocinolone acetonide and mometasone furoate creams [8, 14, 19, 24–28]. It is a fact that there is hardly any household in India which has not heard of the brand name Betnovate cream (containing betamethasone valerate) by Glaxo. Duration of use of TC was usually for less than 12 months in most studies before patient presented with evidence of steroid dermatitis though TC applications up to 20 years have been documented [14]. Steroid dermatitis usually starts appearing within 6 months of continuous TC abuse [8].

Among the common cosmetic reasons for the use of TC are to look fair and beautiful; for acne, blemishes, suntan and dry skin; and as general skin care purpose [8, 14, 19, 24–28]. The suggestion to start TC as cosmetic cream comes from many quarters including friends, relatives, chemists and beauticians.

12.3 Reason for Popularity of TC as Cosmetic Cream

Among the factors responsible for the commonplace use of TC as a cosmetic cream by so many individuals are:

1. *Rapid effect*: Most patients cite the instant magical effect of TC as one of the commonest reasons for its use in their common day-to-day perceived problems on their skin [8, 14]. This is also the reason of their repetitive and prolonged use in many instances which ultimately bring them to the dermatologist with frank steroid dermatitis.
2. *Cheap*: Compared to the regular standard fairness and beauty creams in the market, some of the brands regularly used by the patients are very cheap as they come under government DPCO (Drug Control Price Order) [1]. A simple example is of a 20 gm of betamethasone valerate cream which would cost 18.63 rupees compared to a Fair & Lovely brand of cosmetic cream containing niacinamide which costs around 45 rupees for 25 gm. This cost comparison may not always be in favour of TC particularly when it comes to TC containing triple combinations which can be costlier.
3. *Easy availability*: As of today, TC are available for the asking in both cities and villages. The disturbing part is that even the most potent TC like clobetasol propionate especially in combination creams are available over the counter and are among the top-selling brands in India [30].
4. *Ignorance about adverse effects of TC*: Most patients are blissfully unaware of the adverse effects of TC abuse [26]. Even when they start noticing the adverse effects of TC on their skin, they continue to use them due to the rebound phenomenon they experience on attempting to withdraw the drug [8]. This cycle continues for some time before they are forced to ask for help from a specialist.
5. *Inappropriate counselling by healthcare workers when prescribing TC for appropriate indications*: Some of the social problem of TC abuse is because of failure of the dermatologist to explain in a balanced way the potential dangers of not following the advice given when patients are being treated for proper steroid-responsive dermatoses [31]. Patients tend to self-medicate frequently once they get good response and don't bother to return to their doctor. They frequently experiment with TC for imagined similar-looking skin conditions including on the face. The vasoconstrictive, anti-inflammatory and melanopenic effects are noticed by them and used later to lighten their skin for cosmetic use.
6. *Inappropriate marketing strategies of pharmaceutical firms*: A recent report appeared of illegal sale of steroid-laden creams by Himachal Pradesh-based manufacturer

Torque Pharma [32]. The two products U-B Fair for men and No Scars cream for women contained TC like fluocinolone acetonide and mometasone along with skin bleaching agents. Maharashtra FDA seized them on the premise that products have been advertised as beauty treatments in contravention to the provisions of Schedule J of Drugs and Cosmetics Act 1940 and Drugs and Magic Remedies Act. Many times drugs are positioned as fairness creams through companies' advertisements to mislead the public with false claims on enhancing skin complexion and treatment, whereas ideally they are supposed to be advertised or positioned as a drug which requires a prescription for its use as indicated clinically and not to be sold to be used as a cosmetic under the provisions of the law of the land.

7. *Availability of inappropriate TC combinations*: The Kligman formula using TC along with tretinoin and hydroquinone was helpful for the dermatologist in treating melasma aggressively who at the appropriate time switched over to a non-TC maintenance regime. Very soon triple combination including modified Kligman formula containing mid-potency steroids started being misused by physicians and patients alike for various types of hyperpigmentation and as anti-blemish and fairness creams and that too for prolonged period resulting in adverse effects [1, 33].

8. *Social attitudes to skin colour*: As mentioned earlier, the preference in the society for fair people particularly females has been omnipresent [34]. This has been further fuelled by cosmetic companies promoting "fairness" and by beauty parlours who have been selling TC-containing creams illegally which has also led to widespread TC abuse as a cosmetic [1, 25].

9. *Lack of availability of qualified dermatologist*: As India has a very poor dermatologist vs general population ratio of approximately 1 dermatologist for 176,000 citizens (7500 dermatologists [30]:1.32 billion population [35]), most of the people do not have access to a specialist to address their queries and guide them appropriately. They then have to fall back upon RMP, GP, chemists, pharmacist, relatives and family elders who may dole out completely inappropriate and many times harmful advise. This 'falling in the wrong hands' has also led to TC abuse as a cosmetic. Thus, easy availability of TC and poor access to dermatologists make the situation in India ripe for their misuse in the community [1].

12.4 Hidden Danger of TC Abuse

So far we have been dealing with the overt use of TC as a cosmetic. It may very well be possible the other way too, i.e. the so-called purely cosmetic creams, apparently benign skin products, may contain TC as one of the many hidden ingredients. Cosmetics are not governed as stringently as drugs and are not subject to extensive premarketing trials [36]. The aggravated and misleading claims of advertisements about cosmetics changing the look and even the inherent skin type of the patient for the better are often overlooked. In a study involving 150 patients, it was found that 25 patients who used only fairness creams experienced adverse effects almost similar to steroidal dermatitis resembling rosacea (SDRS) seen in 85 patients who used fairness creams in combination with TC [28].The authors suspected that fairness creams could themselves be deliberately contaminated with steroids which could explain the similar adverse effect profile. In a significant study, Agarwal et al. tested face creams commonly used by Indian population on regular basis for moisturisation, sunscreen, fairness and anti-ageing effect and found that 13 of 23 creams/lotion tested contained steroids [37]. Many of them claimed to be herbal and devoid of any harmful effects and included some well-known brands like Fair and Handsome Cream, Ayur Cream, Garnier Fairness and Vaseline-SPF. They concluded that many marketed preparations which promise instant fairness, glowing, bright skin could have serious side effect due to presence of steroid in them.

12.5 Clinical Manifestations of TC Abuse

The dermatoses happen to be due to addiction and abuse/misuse of TC on the face.

In this so-called steroid dermatitis, initially patient gets wonderful and almost magical response for whatever cosmetic reason they have started the TC. But on continuous application, they start developing rashes and features of rebound phenomenon, which is the initiation of this problem. Subsequently they continue to use their cosmetic cream (TC) to prevent rebound effects; once the magical response of their cosmetic cream ceases they consult a doctor.

The primary lesions in the eruption are small red- and skin-coloured papules, which slowly subside and are replaced by more diffuse redness over the course of time. Further, the continuous use of TC finally leads to a diffusely inflamed thickened oedematous skin [14]. A recent systemic review of the current literature regarding steroid addiction yielded 34 studies [38]. Burning and stinging were the most frequently reported symptoms (65.5%), and erythema was the commonest sign (92.3%). TC addiction could be either the commoner erythematoedematous variant or the papulopustular subtype. Apart from this, there may be telangiectasia and acneiform lesions.

Depending upon their clinical presentations, four types of manifestations of steroid dermatitis have been described in the literature: (1) perioral, (2) diffuse, (3) centrofacial and (4) malar [6, 14]. The malar variant appears to be unique to Indian skin [14].

These patients may notice exacerbation of symptoms after sun exposure and hair epilation, probably due to atrophy and vasodilatation of the facial skin after prolonged use of TC. Many of these patients notice subjective symptoms like itching, burning sensation, dryness and sensation of tightness of skin, mostly corresponding to period of abstinence from TC use. This causes rebound phenomenon effects due to addictive features. An accumulation of the nitric oxide (potent vasodilator) due to prolonged use of TC may be one of the speculative reasons for the cutaneous manifestations in these patients like erythema, burning sensation and pruritus [39].

12.6 Response to TC Abuse as a Cosmetic

As dermatologists, our response can be at two levels:

A. *Patient level*: The suffering patient needs to be treated for the steroid dermatitis and at the same time counselled to not go back into addiction. This requires a lot of patience, skill and persuasion, and it is likely that the patient shows poor compliance initially and consults many dermatologists before agreeing to follow the desired instructions

  I. *Treatment of steroid dermatitis*: A red TC-damaged face in dermatology is one of the most difficult therapeutic challenges to a dermatologist [14]. The damaged cutaneous barrier makes the patient intolerant to any topical treatment. Although discontinuation of TC is essential, it is easier said than done. Rebound flare up is extremely distressing to patient [5]. Switching slowly to milder TC before complete withdrawal has been advocated [40, 41]. Patients with severe symptoms are usually given oral azithromycin 500 mg in the form of weekly pulse therapy (three tablets per week for 8 weeks) or oral doxycycline/minocycline 100 mg once daily for 6–8 weeks [27, 42]. Topical metronidazole, calcineurin antagonists such as tacrolimus and pimecrolimus have been used in the treatment for milder cases alone or as adjuvant with systemic drugs for severe cases [43–45].

  II. *Educating the patient*: The patient should be made to realize the difficult situation he or she has landed into due to TC abuse. They have to be told about the difficulties with treatment and importance of persistence with withdrawal therapy despite initial rebound phenomenon. Use of gentle cleansers, liberal application of bland emollients and avoidance of sun exposure should be explained. Potential risks of using TC based on advice from non-dermatologist need to be emphasized.

B. *Society level*: Media, print and electronic, should be made use consistently to put across the message that TC are drugs which should be used only for medical reasons and under instructions of a dermatologist. The harm that they are capable of causing when used as a cosmetic should be prominently highlighted at every interaction with the public. The recent efforts by IADVL to use social networking sites like Facebook and roping in Bollywood celebrities are commendable. Though it is a wishful thinking to change completely the society's attitude to fair skin, the protective attributes of pigmented skin should be put across to encourage individuals to accept their constitutive skin colour. Continuing medical education programs targeting medical, paramedical personnel and pharmacists are also needed to create awareness about the hazards of misuse of topical corticosteroids as they are many times the first contact persons of end users [26].

In addition, tireless efforts should continue to engage the administrative and regulatory authorities to enforce the laws in place and to curb unrestricted and unethical sale of TC without valid prescription. A constant watch is also to be kept on the jumbo cosmetic industry so that unscrupulous companies may not peddle TC under garb of benign looking, instantly working fairness creams and lotions. Even though it is an uphill task, hopefully it is achievable with the combined efforts of all.

References

1. Coondoo A. Topical corticosteroid misuse: the Indian scenario. Indian J Dermatol. 2014;59(5):451–5. doi:10.4103/00195154.139870.
2. Drake LA, Dinehart SM, Farmer ER, Goltz RW, Graham GF, Hordinsky MK, et al. Guidelines of care for the use of topical glucocorticosteroids. J Am Acad Dermatol. 1996;35:615–9.
3. Rathi SK, D'Souza P. Rational and ethical use of topical corticosteroids based on safety and efficacy. Indian J Dermatol. 2012;57:251–9.
4. Hengge UR, Ruzicka T, Schwartz RA, Cork MJ. Adverse effects of topical glucocorticosteroids. J Am Acad Dermatol. 2006;54:1–18.
5. Ljubojeviae S, Basta-Juzbasiae A, Lipozeneiae J. Steroid dermatitis resembling rosacea: aetiopathogenesis and treatment. J Eur Acad Dermatol Venereal. 2002;16:121–6.
6. Chen AY, Zirwas MJ. Steroid-induced rosacealike dermatitis: case report and review of the literature. Cutis. 2009;83(4):198–204.
7. Wilkin J, Dahl M, Detmar M, Drake L, Liang MH, Odom R, et al. Standard grading system for rosacea: report of the National Rosacea Society Expert Committee on the classification and staging of rosacea. J Am Acad Dermatol. 2004;50(6):907–12.
8. Rathi S. Abuse of topical steroid as cosmetic cream: a social background of steroid dermatitis. Indian J Dermatol. 2006;51(2):154–5.
9. Frumess GM, Lewis HM. Light sensitive seborrheid. Arch Dermatol. 1957;75:245–8.
10. Mihan R, Ayres S Jr. Perioral dermatitis. Arch Dermatol. 1964;89:803–5.
11. Sneddon I. Iatrogenic dermatitis. Br Med J. 1969;4:49.
12. Leyden S, Thew M, Kligman AM. Steroid Rosacea. Arch Dermatol. 1974;110:619–22.
13. Zmegac lurin Z, Zmegac Z. So-called perioral dermatitis. Lijec Vjesn. 1976;98:629–38.
14. Rathi SK, Kumrah L. Topical corticosteroid-induced rosacea like dermatitis: a clinical study of 110 cases. Indian J Dermatol Venereol Leprol. 2011;77:42–6.
15. Burry JN. Topical drug addiction: adverse effects of fluorinated corticosteroid creams and ointments. Med J Aust. 1973;1:393–6.
16. Kligman AM, Frosch PJ. Steroid addiction. Int J Dermatol. 1979;18:23–31.
17. Rapaport AMJ, Rapaport V. Eyelid dermatitis to red face syndrome to cure: clinical experience in 100 cases. J Am Acad Dermatol. 1999;41:435–42.
18. Nnoruka E, Okoye O. Topical steroid abuse: its use as a depigmenting agent. J Natl Med Assoc. 2006;98:934–9.
19. Saraswat A, Lahiri K, Chatterjee M, Barua S, Coondoo A, Mittal A, et al. Topical corticosteroid abuse on the face: a prospective, multicentre study of dermatology outpatients. Indian J Dermatol Venereol Leprol. 2011;77:160–6.
20. Hameed AF. Steroid dermatitis resembling rosacea: a clinical evaluation of 75 patients. ISRN Dermatol. 2013;2013:491376. doi:10.1155/2013/491376.
21. Mahe A, Ly F, Aymard G, Dangou JM. Skin diseases associated with the cosmetic use of bleaching products in women from Dakar, Senegal. Br J Dermatol. 2003;148:493–500.
22. Al-Dhalimi MA, Aljawahiri N. Misuse of topical corticosteroids: a clinical study from an Iraqi hospital. East Mediterr Health J. 2006;12:847–52.
23. Lu H, Xiao T, Lu B, Dong D, Yu D, Wei H, Chen HD. Facial corticosteroid addictive dermatitis in Guiyang City, China. Clin Exp Dermatol. 2010;35(6):618–21.

24. Bhat YJ, Manzoor S, Qayoom S. Steroid—induced rosacea: a clinical study of 200 patients. Indian J Dermatol. 2011;56:30–2.

25. Chohan SN, Suhail M, Salman S, Bajwa UM, Saeed M, Kausar S. Facial abuse of topical steroids and fairness creams: a clinical study of 200 patients. J Pak Assoc Dermatol. 2014;24(3):204–11.

26. Dey VK. Misuse of topical corticosteroids: a clinical study of adverse effects. Indian Dermatol Online J. 2014;5:436–40.

27. Inakanti Y, Thimmasarthi VN, Anupama, Kumar S, Nagaraj A, Peddireddy S, Rayapati A. Topical corticosteroids: abuse and misuse. Our Dermatol Online. 2015;6(2):130–4.

28. Reddy NK, Siddarama R, Hari SH, Anjum BB, Subbaiah VM. Topical corticosteroids and fairness creams abuse on face, causing steroidal dermatitis resembling rosacea (sdrr). Int J Dev Res. 2015;5(12):6334–8.

29. Shashikumar BM, Harish MR, Kavya M, Deepadarshan K. Assessment of over the counter topical steroid use among the nursing students in Mandya District. Sch J App Med Sci. 2016;4(7A):2357–60.

30. Verma SB. Sales, status, prescriptions and regulatory problems with topical steroids in India. Indian J Dermatol Venereol Leprol. 2014;80:201–3.

31. Kumar MA, Noushad PP, Shailaja K, Jayasutha J, Ramasamy C. A study on drug prescribing pattern and use of corticosteroids in dermatological conditions at a tertiary care teaching hospital. Int J Pharm Sci Rev Res. 2011;9:132–5.

32. Nautiyal S. Maha FDA to test leading cosmetic brands to probe marketing of steroid laden cream. Available http://www.pharmabiz.com/NewsDetails. aspx?aid=90618&sid=1. Accessed on 3 Feb 2017.

33. Majid I. Mometasone based triple combination therapy in melasma: is it really safe? Indian J Dermatol. 2010;55:359–62.

34. Shankar PR, Subish P. Fair skin in South Asia: an obsession. J Pak Assoc Dermatol. 2007;17:100–4.

35. India guide: Population of India 2017. Available at www.indiaonlinepages.com/india-current-population.html. Accessed on 8 Feb 2017.

36. Newburger AE. Cosmeceuticals: myths and misconceptions. Clin Dermatol. 2009;27:446–52.

37. Agarwal A, Singhvi IJ, Bele D. Evaluation of steroids in face creams of different marketed brands. Int J Pharm Technol. 2011;3:2480–6.

38. Hajar T, Leshem YA, Hanifin JM, Nedorost ST, Lio PA, Paller AS, Block J, Simpson EL; (The National Eczema Association Task Force). A systematic review of topical corticosteroid withdrawal ("steroid addiction") in patients with atopic dermatitis and other dermatoses. J Am Acad Dermatol. 2015 72(3):541–9.e2. doi: 10.1016/j.jaad.2014.11.024.

39. Rapaport M, Rapaport V. Serum nitric oxide levels in "red" patients: separating corticosteroid-addicted patients from those with chronic eczema. Arch Dermatol. 2004;140:1013–4.

40. Uehara M, Mitsuyoshi O, Sugiura H. Diagnosis and management of the red face syndrome. Dermatol Ther. 1996;1:19–23.

41. Bikowski JB. Topical therapy for perioral dermatitis. Cutis. 1983;31:678–82.

42. Kaur Brar B, Nidhi K, Kaur Brar S. Topical corticosteroid abuse on face: a clinical, prospective study. Our Dermatol Online. 2015;6(4):407–10.

43. Veien NK, Munkvad JM, Neilsen AO, Niordson AM, Stahl D, Thormam J. Topical metronidazole in the treatment of perioral dermatitis. J Am Acad Dermatol. 1991;24:258–60.

44. Goldman D. Tacrolimus ointment for the treatment of steroid induced rosacea: a preliminary report. J Am Acad Dermatol. 2001;44:995–8.

45. Chu CY. An open-label pilot study to evaluate the safety and the efficacy of topically applied pimecrolimus cream for the treatment of steroid-induced rosacea-like eruption. J Eur Aca Dermatol Venereol. 2007;21:484–90.

Topical Steroid Damaged/Dependent Face (TSDF)

13

Arijit Coondoo and Koushik Lahiri

Abstract

Topical steroid damaged/dependent face (TSDF) is a syndrome complex first described by Lahiri and Coondoo in 2008. It is caused by unsupervised application of topical corticosteroids (TCs) of the wrong potency over a prolonged period of time on the face. This abuse, misuse or overuse results in damage to the skin of the face as well as a severe pharmacodependence on the TC. The combined effect of this damage and dependence severely affects the quality of life (QoL) of the patient. Management of TSDF is difficult and necessitates both physical treatment of the skin and psychological counselling to improve the psyche of the patient.

Keywords

Topical corticosteroid • Face • Abuse • Misuse • Dependence

Learning Points

1. Topical corticosteroids were introduced in 1952 and since then have been used extensively in various inflammatory disorders.
2. Physical side effects and addiction to topical corticosteroids may occur due to overuse and misuse of the drug.
3. The phenomenon of "TSDF" which is an acronym for "topical steroid damaged/dependent face" has been recently described.
4. TSDF is a disease entity which encompasses a plethora of physical signs and symptoms as well as steroid addiction due to unsupervised overuse and misuse of the drug for an unspecified period of time.
5. The drug is easily available in India over the counter and is often applied on the advice of people who are unaware of the ill effects of such misuse.
6. Withdrawal of the drug is a physical and psychological challenge.

A. Coondoo (✉)
Department of Dermatology, K.P.C Medical College and Hospital, Raja S.C Mullick Road, Jadavpur, Kolkata, West Bengal 700032, India
e-mail: acoondoo@gmail.com

K. Lahiri
Department of Dermatology, Apollo Gleneagles Hospitals and WIZDERM,
Kolkata, West Bengal, India

© Springer Nature Singapore Pte Ltd. 2018
K. Lahiri (ed.), *A Treatise on Topical Corticosteroids in Dermatology*,
DOI 10.1007/978-981-10-4609-4_13

13.1 Definition

Topical steroid damaged/dependent face (TSDF) is defined as the semi-permanent or permanent damage to the skin of the face precipitated by the irrational, indiscriminate, unsupervised or prolonged use of topical corticosteroids (TC) resulting in a plethora of cutaneous signs and symptoms and psychological dependence on the drug [1].

13.1.1 Historical Perspective

Sulzberger and Witten introduced the first TC in the form of compound F (hydrocortisone) topical corticosteroids in 1952 [2]. Though this drug caused a complete revolution in the treatment of dermatological disorders particularly inflammatory diseases, reports of side effects of TC gradually started appearing in the world literature since 1963 [3]. A decade later, Burry in 1973 and Kligman in 1976 reported cases of addiction to TC [4, 5]. Reports of TC addiction on the face were subsequently published, and various names such as dermatitis rosaeciformis steroidica [6], red skin syndrome [7] and steroid-induced rosacea-like dermatitis [8] were assigned to these entities. The first report of TC misuse on the face was published in 2006 [9]. Subsequently, a proposal named "Stop OTC supply of potent topical steroids" was submitted by Lahiri K and Coondoo A to the General Body of the Indian Association of Dermatologists, Venereologists and Leprologists (IADVL) and was passed unanimously at Chennai in January, 2007. This entity of damage due to TC application on face and the resultant dependence on the drug was labelled as "Topical steroid damaged/dependent face" (acronym TSDF) by one of us (Lahiri K) in March 2008 [10]. From April through July 2008, a multicentric study that year under the aegis of IADVL, a pan-Indian multicentric study on TSDF, was conducted in 12 centres. The results of this study was presented at the national conference of IADVL (DERMACON) at Bengaluru in January 2009 and subsequently published in 2011 [11].

13.2 The Facial Skin

The facial skin has some special characteristics which makes it more vulnerable to the ill effects of sunlight, pollution, friction, cosmetics, drugs and comments from onlookers. Percutaneous absorption of cosmetics and drugs occurs more rapidly because of the thinness of the skin of this region. Secretion of sebum (due to larger sebaceous glands) and sweating occur more on the face resulting in frequent rubbing in hot and humid climates. The skin of the face being visible to the whole world is the most important part of a person's body image, a fact that is enhanced by the damaging effect of frequently looking into the mirror and comments and advice from assorted laymen. This beauty consciousness makes it vulnerable to the ill effects of injudicious use of cosmetics and drugs such as TC [1] (Figs. 13.1, 13.2, 13.3, 13.4, 13.5, 13.6, 13.7, 13.8, 13.9, 13.10, 13.11, 13.12 and 13.13).

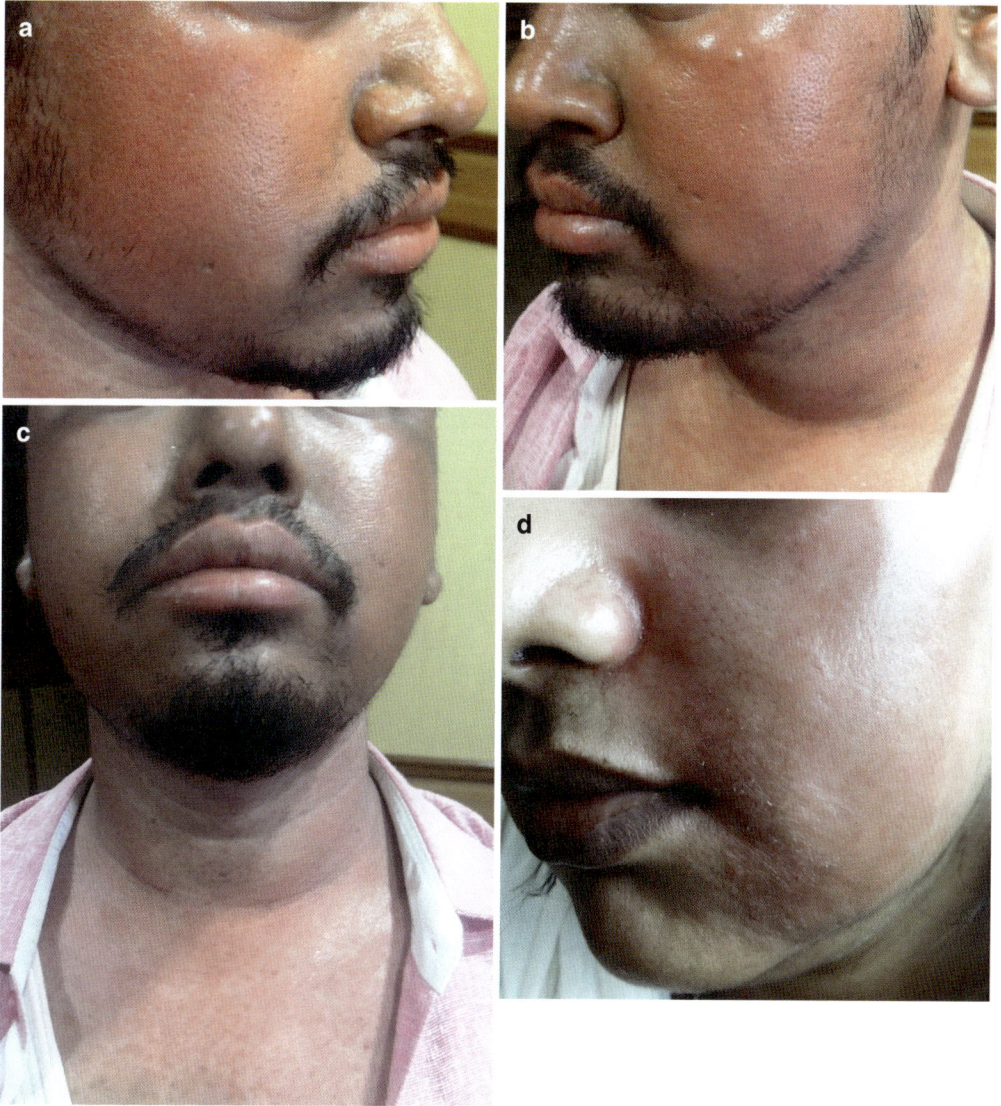

Fig. 13.1 (**a–d**) Erythema due to topical steroid abuse

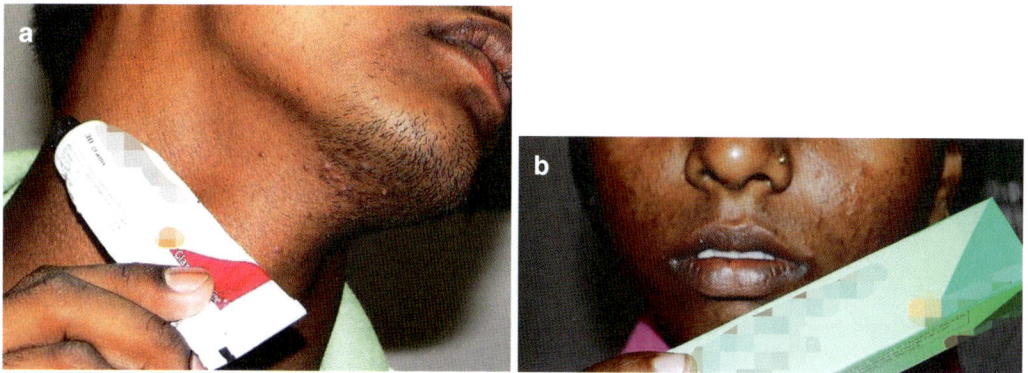

Fig. 13.2 (**a, b**) Papules due to topical steroid abuse

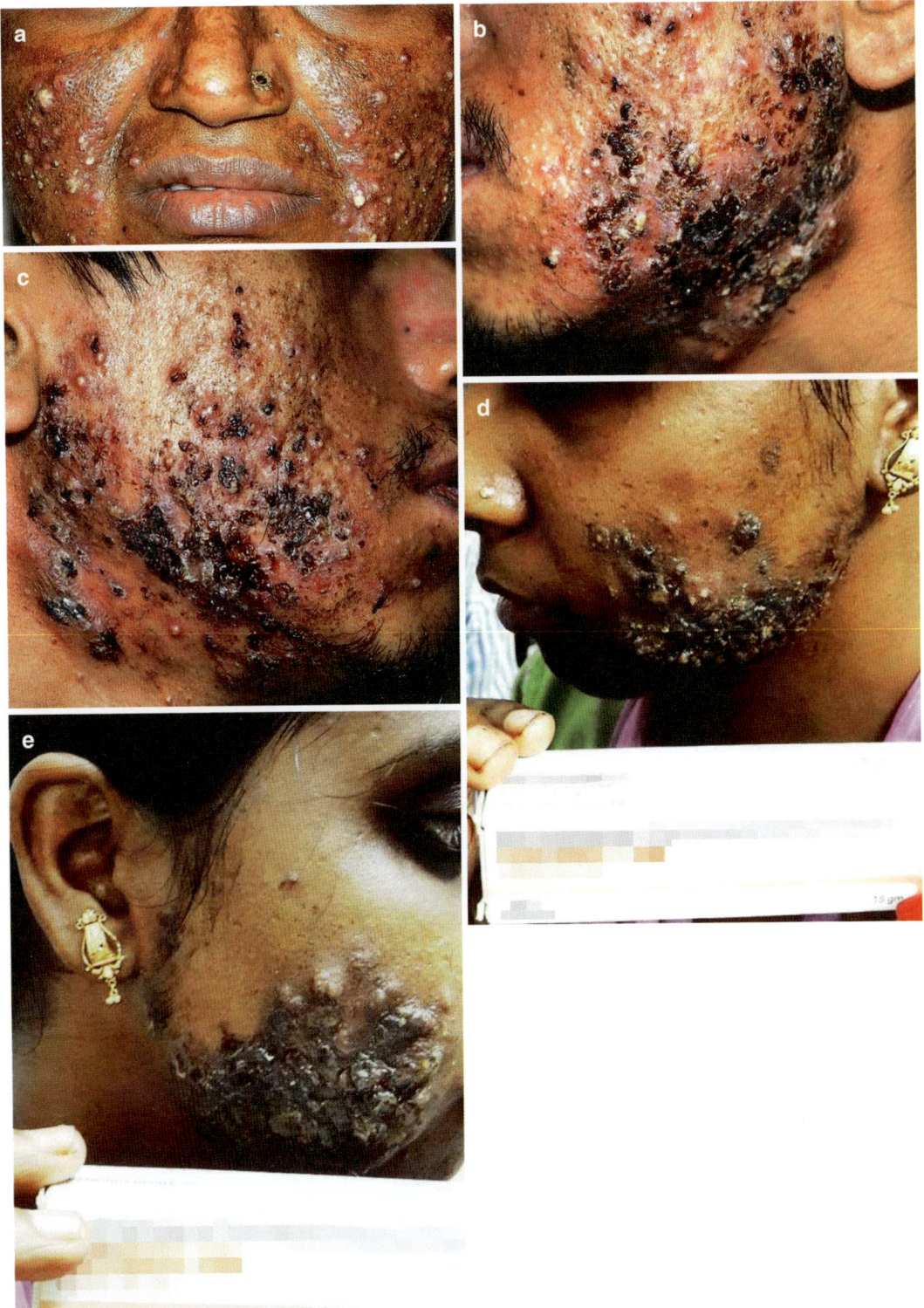

Fig. 13.3 (**a–e**) Pustules (secondary bacterial infections) due to topical steroid abuse

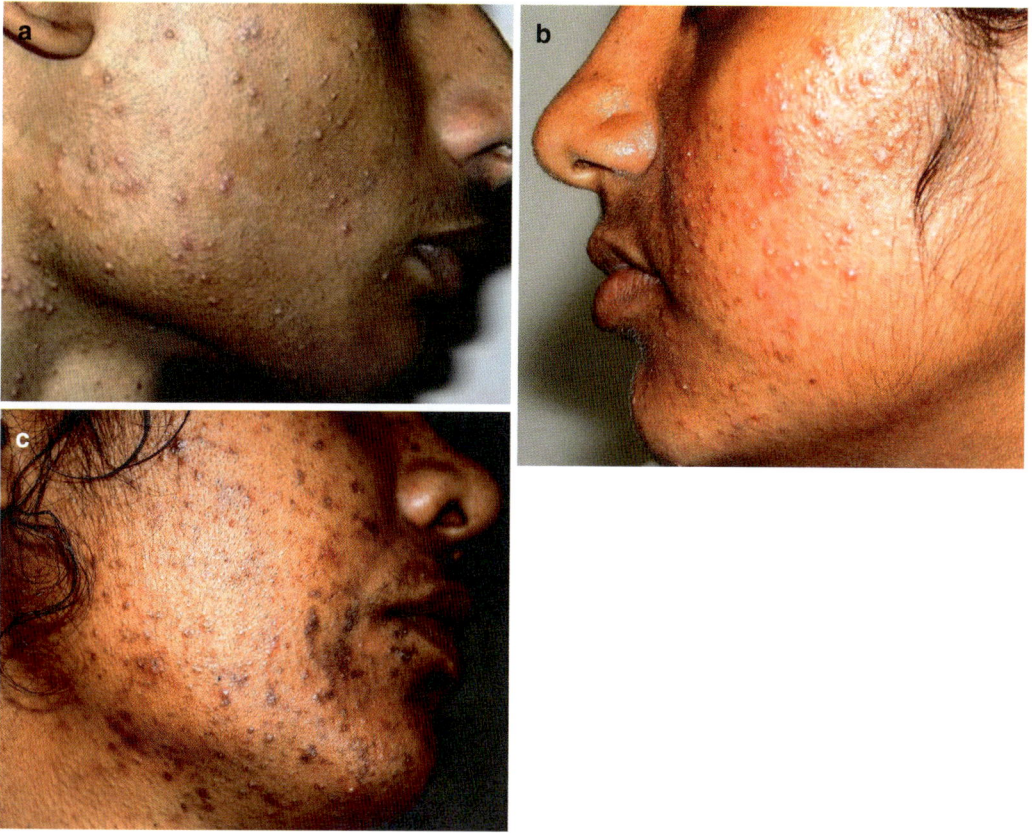

Fig. 13.4 (**a–c**) Acneiform eruptions due to topical steroid abuse

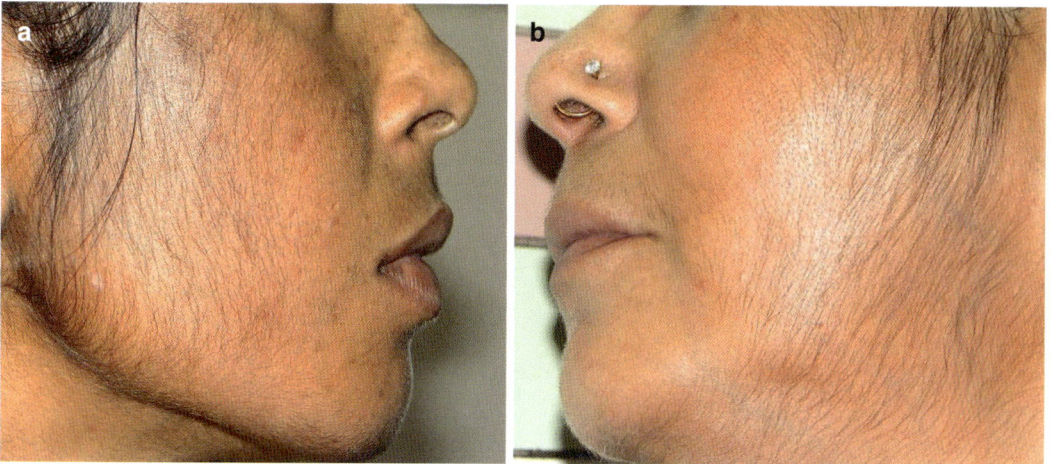

Fig. 13.5 (**a–d**) Hirsutism due to topical steroid abuse

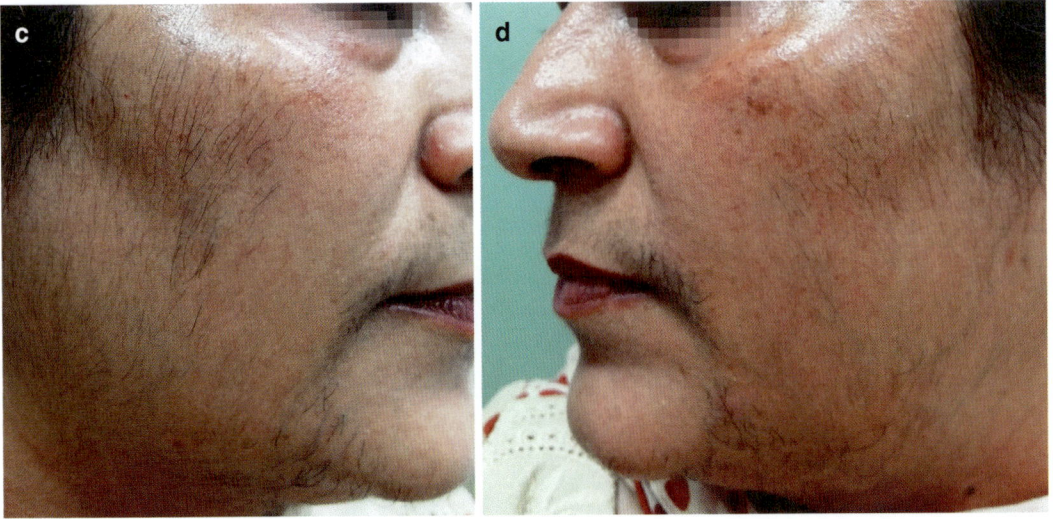

Fig. 13.5 (continued)

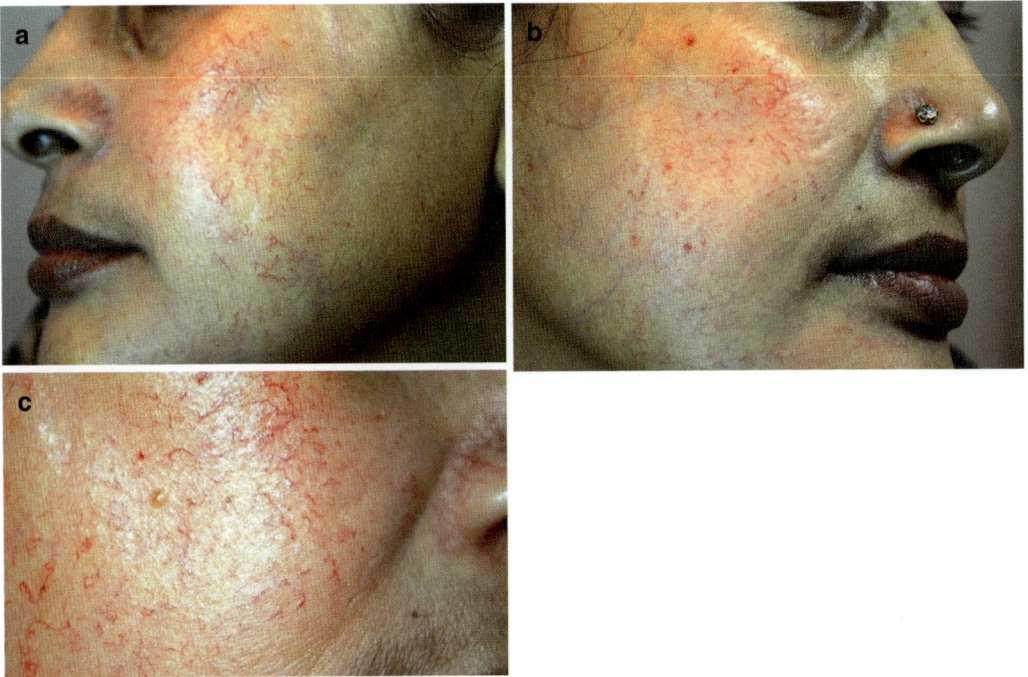

Fig. 13.6 (**a–c**) Telangiectasia due to topical steroid abuse

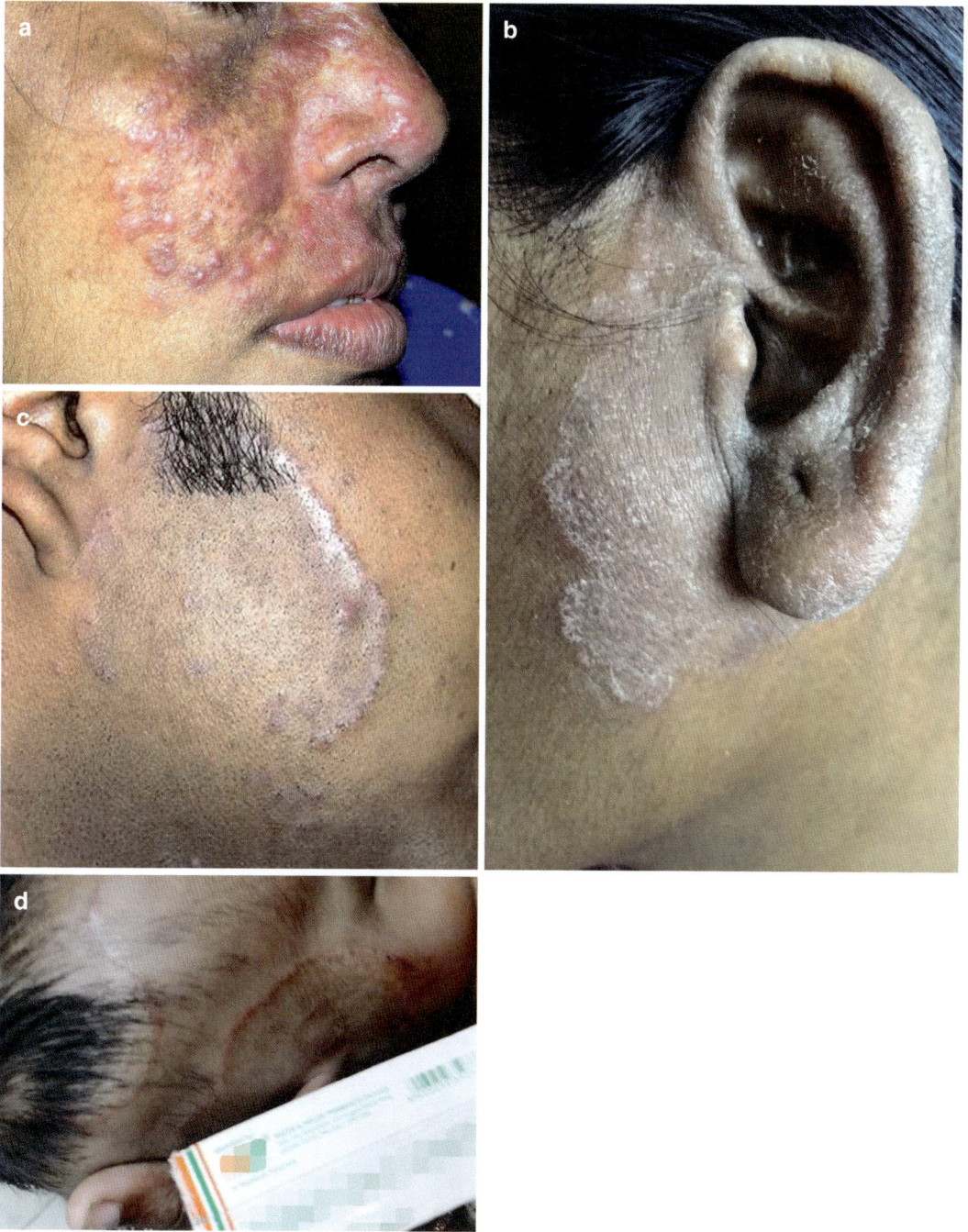

Fig. 13.7 (**a–d**) Tinea incognito due to topical steroid abuse

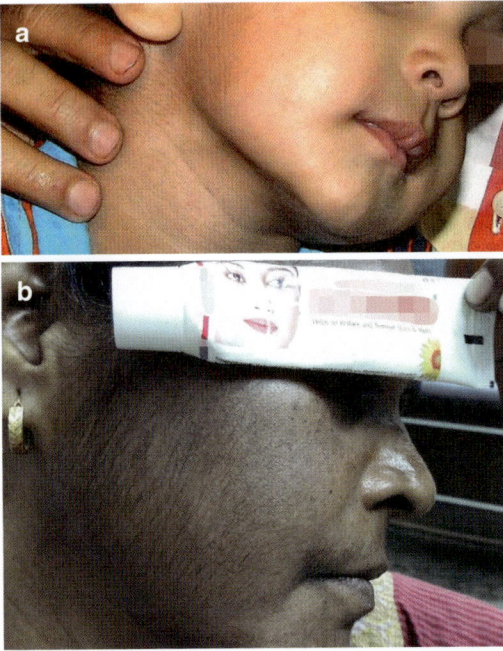

Fig. 13.8 (**a**, **b**) Hypo- and hyperpigmentation due to topical steroid abuse

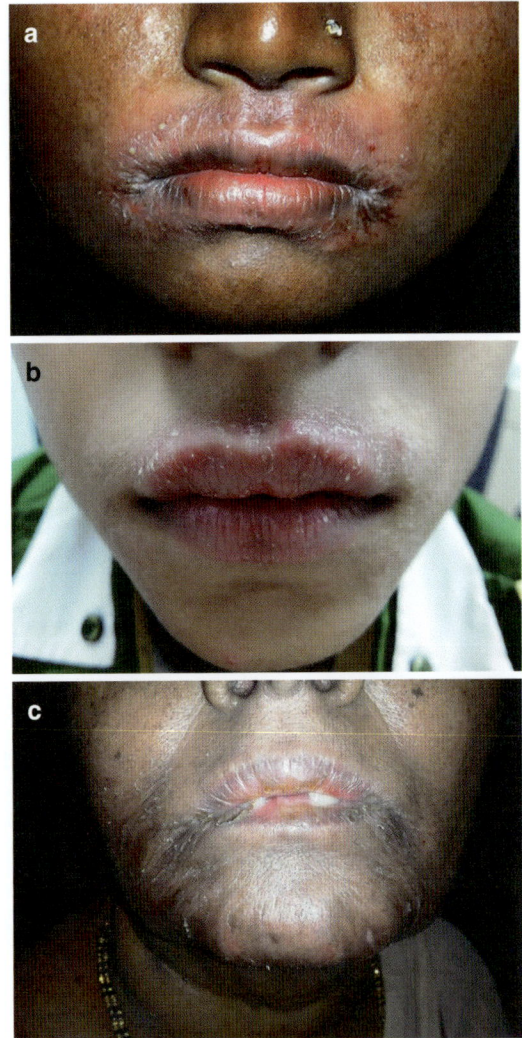

Fig. 13.9 (**a–c**) Perioral dermatitis due to topical steroid abuse

Fig. 13.11 (**a**, **b**) Allergic contact dermatitis due to topical steroid abuse

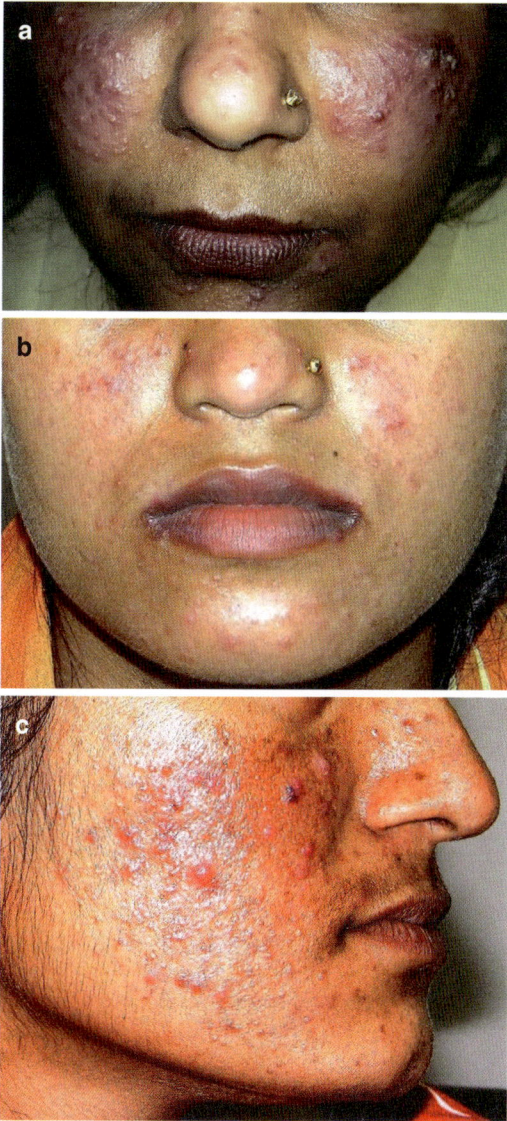

Fig. 13.10 (**a–c**) Rosacea-like features due to topical steroid abuse

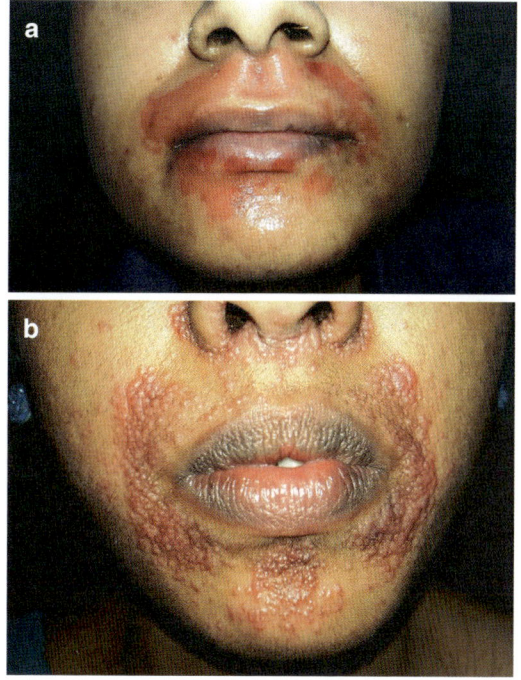

Fig. 13.13 (a, b) Atrophy and striae due to topical steroid abuse

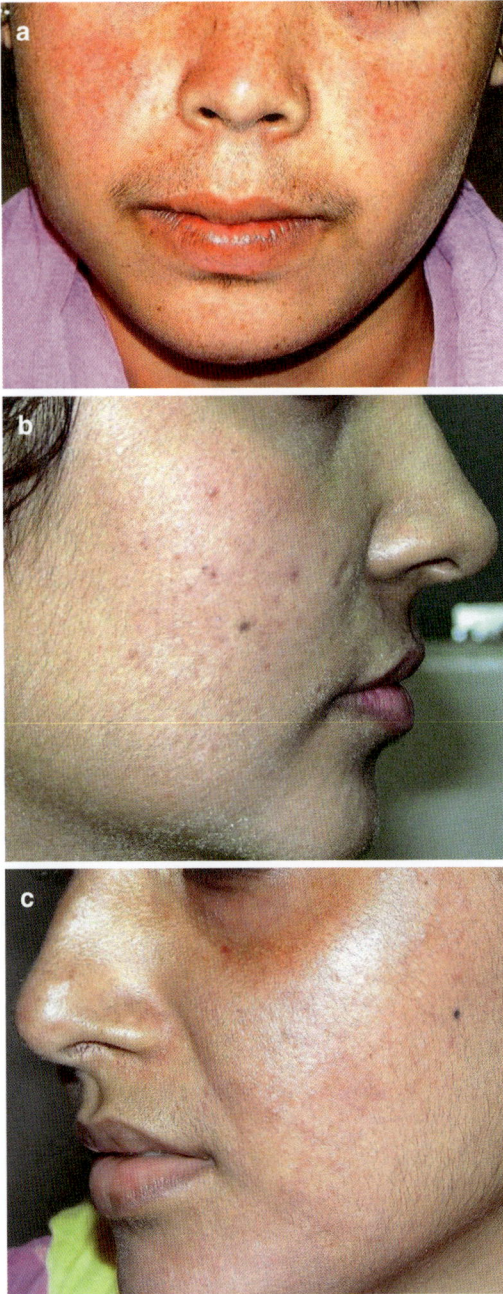

Fig. 13.12 (a–c) Photosensitivity due to topical steroid abuse

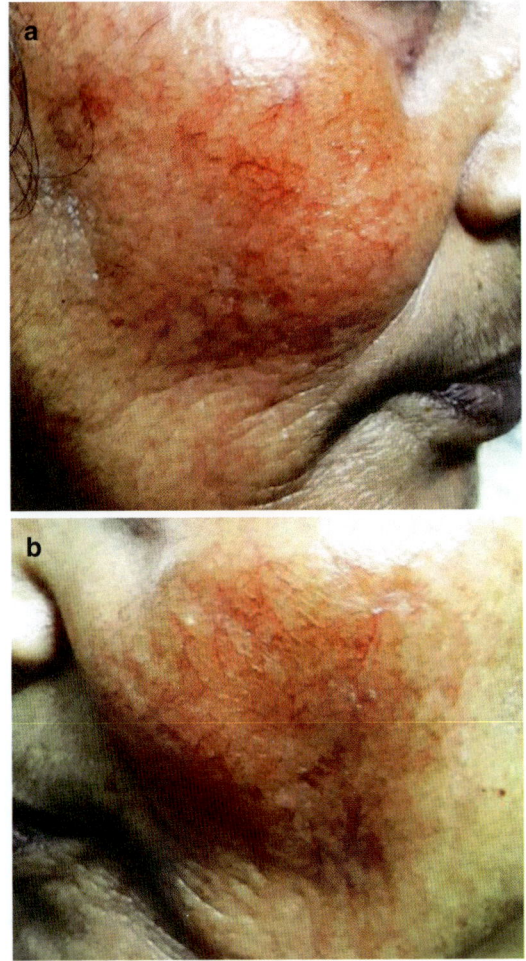

13.3 Ethical Use of TC on Face

Judicious use of TC on face depends on a number of factors such as indication, potency of the drug, age of the patient and duration, amount and frequency of application [12]. TCs have various therapeutic effects on the skin and hence are useful in hyperproliferative, inflammatory and immunologic disorders [11]. However, application of TC in diseases which are not steroid responsive or where TCs are contraindicated may lead to the catastrophic effects enumerated later [13]. The penetrability of the skin of the face is much higher than the skin of the other parts of the body because of its inherent thinness. Hence, TCs of higher potency should be avoided, and TCs of least potency should be applied on the skin of the face [12]. The age of the patient also determines the thickness of the skin of the face, e.g. children have even thinner skin than adults. Hence, TCs should preferably be avoided in this age group, and only TCs of least potency should be used if absolutely necessary [14, 15]. The duration of application is also important. It has been recommended that irrespective of the potency, TCs beyond a period of 2 weeks on the face should not be applied [11]. In fact most experts recommend once daily application of the proper amount of TC based on FTU [16] (Tables 13.1, 13.2, 13.3, 13.4 and 13.5).

Table 13.1 Major indications of topical corticosteroids

Eczematous diseases	Atopic dermatitis, seborrhoeic dermatitis, contact dermatitis
Papulosquamous diseases	Psoriasis, lichen planus, erythroderma
Bullous diseases	Pemphigus foliaceus, bullous and cicatricial pemphigoid
Connective tissue disease	Discoid lupus erythematosus, morphoea
Pigmentary disorders	Vitiligo, melasma (Kligman's formula)
Neutrophilic diseases	Behcet's syndrome, Sweet's syndrome
Cutaneous malignancies	Cutaneous T cell lymphoma, lymphocytoma cutis, lymphomatoid papulosis
Miscellaneous	Papular urticaria, alopecia areata, lichen sclerosus et atrophicus

Table 13.2 Contraindications of topical corticosteroids

Absolute	Relative
Hypersensitivity to TC	Infections (fungal, bacterial, viral)
Hypersensitivity to vehicle	Parasitic infestations
	Ulcerated skin

Table 13.3 Side-effects of TC

Local	Systemic
Acneiform eruptions	Adrenal suppression
Atrophy, striae	Hypopigmentation
Hypopigmentation	Growth retardation in children
Hypertrichosis	Glaucoma/Cataract
Erythema (hallmark of TSDF)	
Telangiectasia	
Infections (fungal, bacterial and viral)	
Purpura, bruising and ulcerations	
Allergic contact dermatitis	

Table 13.4 Methods of abuse of topical corticosteroids

Sources of abuse	Methods
Bureaucratic red tape	Approval of multiple drug combinations containing TCs Inability to stop indiscriminate sale of TCs as OTC products at chemists
Pharmaceuticals	Marketing scientifically unethical combinations Advertisement of TC containing products as fairness creams
Pharma salesmen	Marketing of TCs to non-dermatologists and quacks
Prescribers	Dermatologists: incomplete prescriptions or counselling Non-dermatologists: not aware of norms of TC use Quacks: no knowledge about TCs
Chemists	All TCs are sold as OTC products Salesmen considered by patients as medical advisors Sell TCs of all potencies for wrong indications Promote TCs as fairness creams

(continued)

Table 13.4 (continued)

Sources of abuse	Methods
Patients	Apply TCs on advice of friends, neighbours or relatives Apply TCs in diseases which are not steroid responsive or may be aggravated by TCs Repeat TC prescriptions indefinitely Apply potent TCs of all potencies for melasma
Laymen other than patients	Misuse of TCs as fairness creams

Table 13.5 Commonly abused TC molecules

Betamethasone valerate
Mometasone furoate
Clobetasol propionate
Fluticasone pivalate
Beclomethasone

13.4 TSDF: Aetiology and Precipitating Factors

TSDF is a symptom complex of various side effects of TC applied on the facial skin resulting in total dependence on the TC applied. Hence, TSDF is basically a form of drug dependence. This dependence results in addiction to the drug and withdrawal upon stopping the TC. Addiction to TC is caused by chronic misuse and overuse of the drug. The commonest site of TC addiction is the face [17]. TSDF occurs when it is used on the face in the wrong indication (usually acne vulgaris or melasma) or by prescription misuse in the proper indication, for a prolonged period, in the wrong age group (children and geriatric patients) or in the wrong potency (mid- or super-potent TC on face). Such usage is usually unsupervised [11].

A series of factors have contributed to the phenomenal increase in the misuse of TC on the face in India. Over the years, an apathetic and ill-informed bureaucracy has failed to realise the implications of this abuse [18]. Taking advantage of this laxity, pharmaceutical companies market unethical combinations containing

TCs—e.g. the so-called modified Kligman's formula and other two, three, four or five drug combinations—to boost sales [10]. Further down the line, salesmen of pharmaceutical concerns market these unethical combinations to non-dermatologists, alternative medicine practitioners and quacks without proper detailing of TC usage [10]. Even in the case of dermatologists, prescriptions may not contain proper or adequate directions about the amount, frequency and duration of use of TC [11]. Salesmen in the chemist shops further contribute to the problem by selling TCs of all potencies to patients and laymen irrespective of the disease or prescriptions for the same [10]. Patients with lesions on the face may also apply TCs for nonsteroid responsive diseases or diseases which may be aggravated by steroids on the recommendation of friends, neighbours and relatives without consulting doctors at all [11]. Finally, the greatest (mis)users of TCs are laymen who rampantly apply TCs either singly or as components of the "modified Kligman's formula" as fairness creams [19]. In its totality, the Indian scenario regarding misuse of topical steroid on face is very dismal and disturbing [20].

As mentioned earlier, a multicentric study on TSDF was planned under the aegis of Indian Association of Dermatologists, Venereologists and Leprologists (IADVL) as a follow-up of the proposal of "Stop OTC supply of potent topical steroids" approved by IADVL General Body in 2007 (vide supra) and was conducted at 12 centres spread across India [11]. It was conducted on 2926 cases of facial dermatoses out of which 433 cases (14.33%) were found to be applying TC on the face. TC was found to be used more by semi-literate, urban patients in their third decade of life. Fifty percent of patients were using a brand of betamethasone valerate followed by mometasone furoate (17.8%) and clobetasol propionate (12%). Two or more combinations with antibacterials, antifungals, hydroquinone, retinoids, etc. were being used by 59.6% cases. Potent steroids (halobetasol propionate, clobetasol propionate, betamethasone dipropionate, beclomethasone dipropionate and betamethasone valerate) were being in semiurban areas by patients who were in their second decade of life on the recommendation of non-dermatologists (relatives, friend, peers, pharmacist or beauticians). Of the remainder, 55.7% were from dermatologists, 26.7% from MBBS doctors, 11.3% from other specialists and 6.3% from practitioners of alternate medicine. Inappropriate TC usage was found in 403(93%) cases. Unfortunately, TCs were being used as fairness creams by 29% patients and as a skin-lightening agent in hyperpigmentary disorders such as melisma in a further 28% cases. Other diseases where TCs were being used inappropriately were acne vulgaris (24%), rosacea, tinea, facial dermatitis, etc. (14%). The duration of usage of TC varied from 1 week to 30 years [11].

13.5 Clinical Features

TSDF is caused by patients and laymen applying TCs of wrong potency on the face usually for the wrong indication [11]. Due to this TC misuse on the face either on the diseased skin (e.g. melisma, acne vulgaris, etc.) or normal skin (as fairness creams), the skin develops various types of lesions such as acneiform eruptions, erythematous papules, pustules, perioral dermatitis, dryness, telangiectasia, rosacea-like features, hyperpigmentation, hypopigmentation, photosensitivity or allergic contact dermatitis [21–24]. When the TC is withdrawn, the facial skin develops erythema (red face) for about 2 weeks. This is followed by desquamation. The flare resolves but reappears within 2 weeks if the patient does not use the TC again (rebound phenomenon) [21]. This cycle of flare and resolution continues for some time with flares of decreasing intensity and resolutions of prolonged duration prolonged till the patient becomes completely cured. The rebound phenomenon sometimes occurs in an area which is larger than the original site of TC misuse or even at distant locations [7]. Symptoms similar to status cosmeticus or chronic actinic dermatitis might occur in some patients [7]. However, the principal clinical feature and hallmark of TSDF are a diffuse erythema, a manifestation which was initially noted as red face syndrome [7].

In the pan-Indian multicentric TSDF study mentioned earlier, 90.2% cases had adverse effects with more than one type of lesion seen in 32.6% cases. The most common lesions seen were acneiform lesions either arising de novo or occurring as aggravation due to misuse in acne vulgaris. Other significant adverse effects were telangiectasia, atrophy, hypopigmentation, perioral dermatitis, rosacea, tinea incognito and hirsutism [11].

13.6 Management of TSDF

Management of TSDF is difficult involving both counselling of the patient regarding the ill effects of TC application and treatment of both the rebound phenomenon as also damage caused by the TC. Victims of TSDF need a substantial amount of psychological support. Counselling needs to be done regarding the ill effects of the TC used as self-medications and also its overuse and misuse. Cosmetics, soap and emollients containing glycolic acid, lactic acid etc. should be avoided during flares. The face must be washed with warm water only [7]. The patient must be advised that on stoppage of the TC, the disease for which the TC is being applied may worsen at first but improve later [17].

As a first step of treatment, the TC needs to be withdrawn, but the mode of withdrawal of TC remains a matter of controversy. Some workers advocate gradual withdrawal to minimise the symptoms of the rebound phenomenon [6]. However, others favour sudden complete stoppage of TC immediately upon starting therapy to prevent further damage to the facial skin [7]. Calcineurin inhibitors have been used as replacement therapy by some workers [25, 26]. However, Rapaport et al. observed that many patients complained of a burning sensation on application of the drug. Pale sulphonated shale oil cream 4% has been reported to be a safe alternative to TC in cases of atopic eczema affecting the face since it has both anti-inflammatory and antibacterial properties [27, 28]. Other drugs such as doxycycline, minocycline and metronidazole have also been used to alleviate the symptoms of rebound phenomenon with varying effects [17]. Oral antihistamines have been recommended to control the pruritus associated with the rebound phenomenon [7]. Oral antifungals have also been used to control the resulting demodex/pityrosporum folliculitis in most of the cases.

References

1. Lahiri K, Coondoo A. Topical steroid damaged/dependent face (TSDF): an entity of cutaneous pharmacodependence. Indian J Dermatol. 2016;61:265–72.
2. Sulzberger MB, Witten VH. The effect of topically applied compound F in selected dermatoses. J Invest Dermatol. 1952;19(2):101–2.
3. Epstein NN, Epstein WL, Epstein JH. Atrophic striae in patients with inguinal intertrigo. Arch Dermatol. 1963;87:450–7.
4. Burry JN. Topical drug addiction: adverse effects of fluorinated corticosteroid creams and ointments. Med J Austr. 1973;1:393–6.
5. Kligman AM. Topical steroid addicts. JAMA. 1976;235:1550.
6. Juzbasić A, Subić JS, Ljubojević S. Demodex folliculorum in development of dermatitis rosaceiformis steroidica and rosacea-related diseases. Clin Dermatol. 2002;20(2):135–40.
7. Rapaport MJ, Rapaport V. The red skin syndromes: corticosteroid addiction and withdrawal. Expert Rev Dermatol. 2006;1:547–61.
8. Rathi SK, Kumrah L. Topical corticosteroid-induced rosacea-like dermatitis: a clinical study of 110 cases. Indian J Dermatol Venereol Leprol. 2011;77:42–6.
9. Rathi S. Abuse of topical steroid as cosmetic cream: a social background of steroid dermatitis. Indian J Dermatol. 2006;51:154–5.
10. Coondoo A. Topical steroid misuse: the Indian scenario. Indian J Dermatol. 2014;59:451–5.
11. Saraswat A, Lahiri K, Chatterjee M, Barua S, Coondoo A, Mittal A, et al. Topical corticosteroid abuse on the face: a prospective, multicentre study of dermatology outpatients. Indian J Dermatol Venereol Leprol. 2011;77:160–6.
12. Rathi S, D'Souza P. Rational and ethical use of topical corticosteroids based on safety and efficacy. Indian J Dermatol. 2012;57(4):251–9.
13. Ambika H, Sujatha VC, Yadalla H, et al. Topical corticosteroid abuse on face: a prospective study on outpatients of dermatology. Dermatol Online. 2014;5(1):5–8.
14. Saraswat A. Topical corticosteroid use in children: adverse effects and how to minimize them. Indian J Dermatol Venereol Leprol. 2010;76:225–8.
15. Coondoo A, Chattopadhyay C. Use and abuse of topical corticosteroids in children. Indian J Paediatr Dermatol. 2014;15:1–4.
16. Saraswat A. Ethical use of topical corticosteroids. Indian J Dermatol. 2014;59:469–72.
17. Ghosh A, Sengupta S, Coondoo A, Jana AK. Topical corticosteroid addiction and phobia. Indian J Dermatol. 2014;59:465–8.
18. Verma SB. Sales, status, prescriptions and regulatory problems with topical steroids in India. Indian J Dermatol Venereol Leprol. 2014;80:201–3.
19. Dey VK. Misuse of topical corticosteroids: a clinical study of adverse effects. Indian Dermatol Online J. 2014;5:436–40.
20. Verma SB. Topical corticosteroid misuse in India is harmful and out of control. BMJ. 2015;351:h6079.
21. Fisher M. Steroid-induced rosacealike dermatitis: case report and review of the literature. Cutis. 2009;83:198–204.
22. Abraham A, Roga G. Topical steroid damaged skin. Indian J Dermatol. 2014;59(5):456–9.
23. Coondoo A, Phiske M, Verma S, Lahiri K. Side-effects of topical corticosteroids. A long overdue revisit. Indian Dermatol Online J. 2014;5:416–25.
24. Saraswat A. Contact allergy to topical corticosteroids and sunscreens. Indian J Dermatol Venereol Leprol. 2012;78:552–9.
25. Goldman D. Tacrolimus ointment for the treatment of steroid-induced rosacea: a preliminary report. J Am Acad Dermatol. 2001;44:995–8.
26. Chu CY. An open-label pilot study to evaluate the safety and the efficacy of topically applied pimecrolimus cream for the treatment of steroid-induced rosacea-like eruption. J Eur Aca Dermatol Venereol. 2007;21:484–9.
27. Warnecke J, Wendt A. Anti-inflammatory action of pale sulfonated shale oil (ICHTHYOL pale) in UVB erythema test. Inflamm Res. 1998;47(2):75–8.
28. Korting HC, Schöllmann C, Cholcha W, Wolff L, The Collaborative Study Group. Efficacy and tolerability of pale sulfonated shale oil cream 4% in the treatment of mild to moderate atopic eczema in children: a multicentre, randomized vehicle-controlled trial. J Eur Acad Dermatol Venereol. 2010;24:1176–82.

Topical Corticosteroid Modified Superficial Dermatophytosis: Morphological Patterns

14

Shyam Verma

Abstract

There are a myriad clinical patterns that one commonly sees in the current scenario of a veritable "steroid-modified tinea epidemic" that India is witnessing. This chapter attempts to give an in-depth insight into the morphological nuances of tinea cruris, tinea corporis, and male genital dermatophytosis recently highlighted by the author.

Keywords

Steroid-modified tinea • Superficial dermatophytosis • Topical steroid antifungal combination creams • Morphological patterns of tinea cruris et corporis

Learning Points

1. There is a veritable epidemic of superficial dermatophytosis, especially tinea cruris et corporis, on the Indian subcontinent.
2. A vast majority of these patients apply topical steroid, antifungal, and antibacterial combination creams bought without a valid prescription.
3. This practice along with erratic use or even absence of oral antifungal agents has led to alteration of morphology of what we have learnt to call "typical lesions of dermatophytosis."
4. "Steroid-modified tinea" seems to be more common than treatment of naive tinea cruris et corporis.

[This chapter is largely reproduced from an invited review article on steroid-modified dermatophytosis due to appear in the May–June 2017 issue of *Indian Journal of Dermatology*. I dedicate this chapter to the editor of the journal as well as this book.]

S. Verma
Nirvan Skin Clinic,
Makarpura Main Road, Vadodara 390009, India
e-mail: skindiaverma@gmail.com

14.1 Introduction

Indian dermatological outpatient departments in private as well as public hospitals are reeling under the heavy burden of superficial dermatophytosis, i.e., predominantly tinea corporis et cruris. A very frequent and relatively uncommonly noticed accompaniment is male genital tinea. These age old and generally easily treatable diseases have now become a dermatologist's nightmare because a majority of patients presenting to dermatologists come with steroid-modified tinea. India has a lax drug licensing policy which has resulted in uncontrolled production and sales of irrational combinations containing potent topical steroids with antifungal and antibacterial agents. This class of topical drugs has been largely responsible for the altered morphological patterns of dermatophytosis seen in India in the past few years. Dermatologists are seldom seeing treatment-naive cases of read tinea cruris et corporis. Most of them have been treated by general practitioners by these irrational combination creams or have bought the creams themselves or upon the recommendation of the pharmacist. This chapter deals with the various features of steroid-modified tinea which we commonly see.

14.2   The Problem

A veritable epidemic of steroid-modified tinea has been going on in India and other developing countries. Topical antifungals used for this condition are most often in combination with potent topical steroids and antibacterials [1, 2]. Such formulations account for about 50% of the sales of all topical steroids. The most common combination in India at present is clobetasol propionate, ornidazole, ofloxacin, and terbinafine [1, 2]. This speaks volumes about the inadequate understanding of the drug control authorities of India who issue permissions to companies manufacturing them. It is a common observation that severity of changes in the clinical pattern correlates with the duration of the abuse of topical steroids. The following are observations regarding the most common patterns occurring in India, namely, tinea cruris et corporis. Memories of didactic lectures during our undergraduate days linger where we were taught that a typical lesion of tinea corporis et cruris was circinate and had

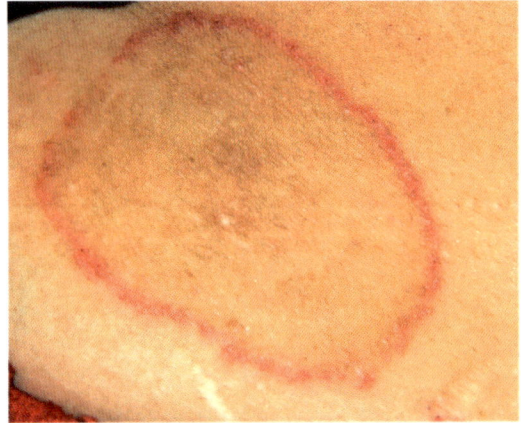

Fig. 14.1 Classic presentation of tinea corporis with an annular appearance and erythematous, scaly border

an active erythematous well-defined border with central clearing (Fig. 14.1).

With the increasing, widespread, unsupervised, and self-prescribed application of steroids, we are noticing the sea change that tinea cruris et corporis have gone through and the way they are presenting now [3]. We are seeing an increasing number of atypical presentations, cases that have been vitiated by topical steroids due to the adverse reactions over the treated and surrounding areas and cases with chronic and widespread lesions many of who do not respond to standard protocols of therapy. This trend is evident both in private practice and in large teaching hospitals. Some tertiary care academic departments report a prevalence of about 5–10% of all new cases, many presenting with recurrent, chronic dermatophytosis with varied clinical presentations [3].

14.3   Clinical Presentations

Larger-sized lesions and *more number of lesions* in individual patients are being observed now with increasing frequency (Fig. 14.2). It is now more common to see patients with more than one lesion of tinea in more than one anatomical location. Tinea cruris et corporis is getting more common.

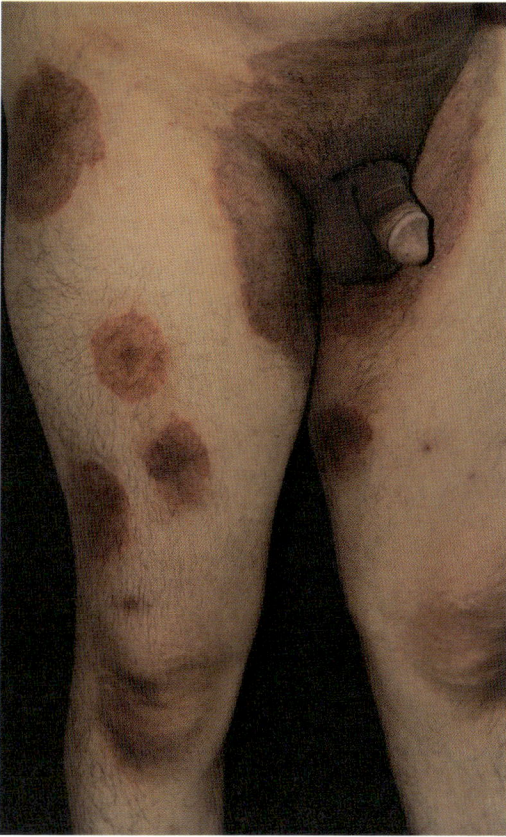

Fig. 14.2 A Tinea cruris and corporis with multiple large lesions

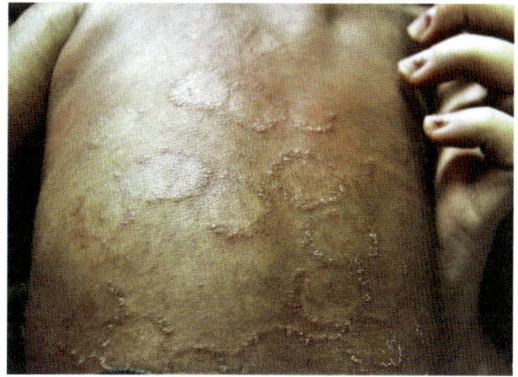

Fig. 14.3 Infant with multiple lesions of tinea corporis

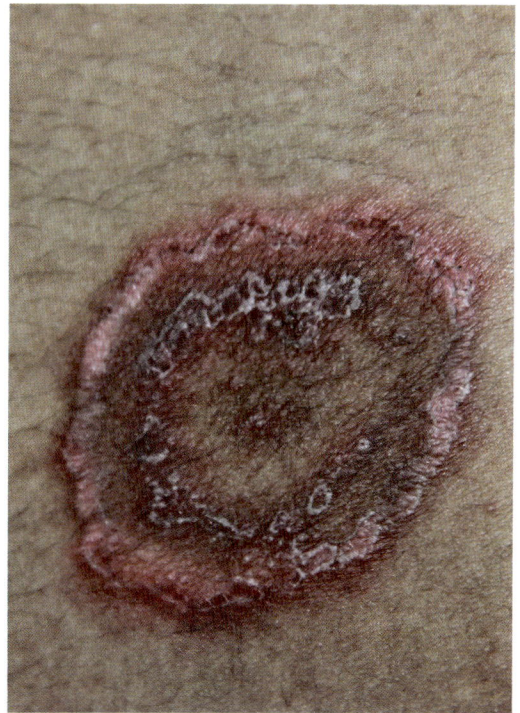

Fig. 14.4 Tinea pseudoimbricata

More women patients *with active tinea corporis, tinea cruris, et corporis et cruris* are being encountered now. These women very often present secondary to the index case that is most often male. A large number of women present with a submammary location of the disease that involves the inframammary fold more than the skin of the breasts. This underscores the role of friction and maceration resulting from moisture of perspiration. We are also seeing *more children afflicted* by dermatophytosis (Fig. 14.3). In the author's experience, obese children are afflicted more. Sharing of bed linen and towels is fairly common in this group of patients.

Dermatologists are observing an increasing number of lesions with *multiple concentric circles* (Fig. 14.4). It has also been described as

tinea pseudoimbricata because it is reminiscent of tinea imbricata which is characterized by multiple concentric rings and has been explained to be occurring due to partial immune response. It has been seen in persons with immune suppression and those applying corticosteroids [4]. This has been described in India too after associating its appearance with the use of topical corticosteroid combinations [5]. The authors have suggested that this be included as a manifestation of tinea incognita induced by topical steroids. The formation of concentric circles can be explained by the local TCS-induced immunosuppression and also its anti-inflammatory effect. The centrifugal spread of dermatophytosis is because of the cell-mediated immunity clearing the fungus in the center of the lesion and the dermatophyte moving further out at a rate that is faster than the rate of shedding of the outer corneocytes in order to survive [6]. It is felt that the use of TCS, especially intermittently used, would lead to suppression of inflammation and therefore promote survival of the dermatophyte which spreads centrifugally but also remains in the center due to inadequate clearance. If this happens repeatedly, it would lead to multiple active borders with intermittent clearing in areas where the organism has been cleared circles concentrically leading to "tinea pseudoimbricata." Though we have used the term *tinea incognito and tinea pseudoimbricata* in our report, I feel the need to propose two easier and more accurate terms. Looking carefully at lesions of tinea pseudoimbricata, one observes that the lesions of tinea incognito do not always have multiple concentric rings but very commonly have two lesions, and in those too, the rings are not always complete. Therefore, I propose the term *double-edged tinea* which is an important clinical pointer to diagnosis of corticosteroid modified tinea (Fig. 14.5). There is also a difference between the terms "tinea incognito" and "steroid-modified tinea." Though we ourselves have used it in the past, the term tinea incognito should be used only in cases where the disease is rendered unrecognizable due to its altered appearance, most commonly due to topical corticosteroids [7]. However it is possible to recognize tinea in most cases of topical steroid abuse where topical steroids and their irrational combinations have been used. Therefore "steroid-modified tinea" is a more inappropriate term [7]. And finally an appeal has also been made as an afterthought that grammatically the phrase "tinea incognito" is incorrect and should actually be "tinea incognita" [7].

As mentioned earlier a large number of *lesions do not show central clearing*. Instead there are *eczematized areas*, often circular, within the circinate lesions (Fig. 14.6). As explained in the pathogenesis of tinea pseudoimbricata, the central eczematization could be due to inadequate clearing of the dermatophytes owing to topical steroid application.

We see *arciform lesions* and an increasing number of *two annular lesions showing confluence, dumbbell-shaped tinea* (Fig. 14.7a, b). Sometimes a curious *clustering of multiple small annular lesions* with active erythematous scaly borders is seen, often in areas prone to friction (Fig. 14.7c). Some *lesions show pustular borders* (Fig. 14.7d). This phenomenon has been attributed to a probable higher virulence of the organism promoting a higher inflammatory response.

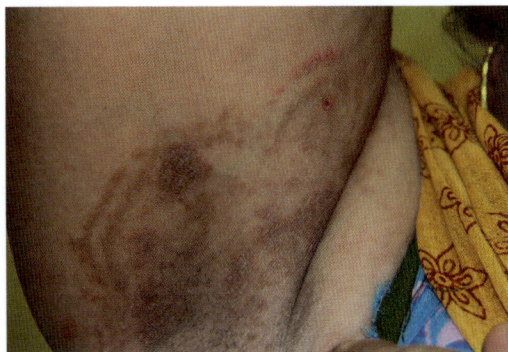

Fig. 14.5 "Double-edged tinea"

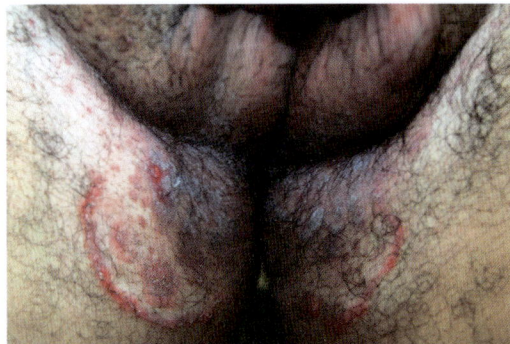

Fig. 14.6 Eczematous lesions in place of expected central clearing

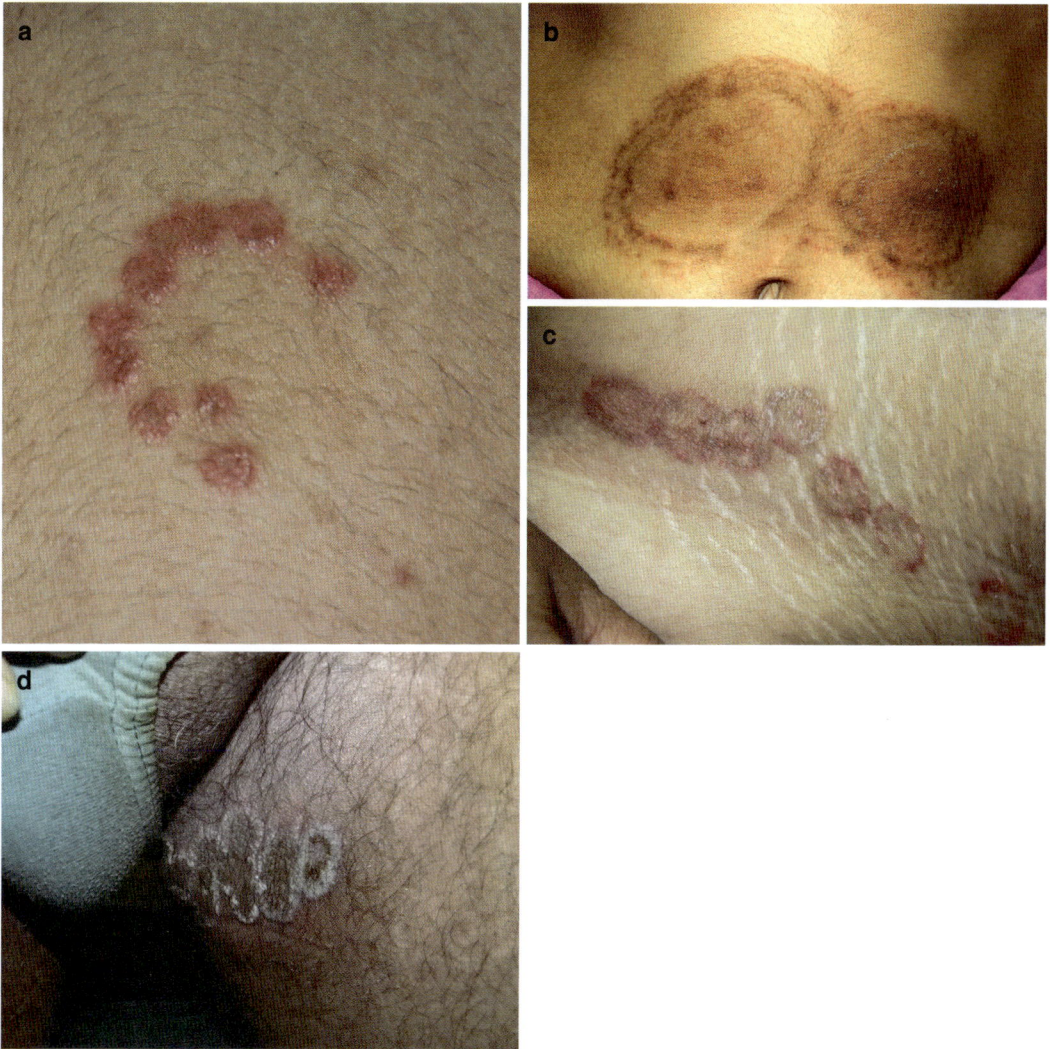

Fig. 14.7 (a) Arciform lesions. (b) Dumbbell-shaped large annular lesions on trunk. (c) Multiple small annular lesions in areas of friction. (d) Multiple annular lesions with pustular borders

A distinct variant of dermatophytosis which seems to have been partially obscured and buried under the more visible rubble of tinea cruris is *male genital tinea*. There have been earlier reports of genital tinea written over two decades ago where Indian authors have observed it frequently, whereas there have been scattered reports of the entity from the West [8–12]. There has been a paucity of recent literature from India on genital dermatophytosis barring one written by the author and Vasani which represents the current scenario against the backdrop of steroid abuse [13]. Genital dermatophytosis is more common in males and occurs more commonly on the penis rather than the scrotum. When it occurs in women, it usually affects the mons pubis and labia majora. De novo appearance of genital tinea is not common and is usually secondary to tinea cruris or tinea cruris et corporis. While classic active borders may be seen on the penile shaft, some variants like areas of ill-defined scaly lesions and powdery scaling are also seen (Fig. 14.8). Often these patients have lesions

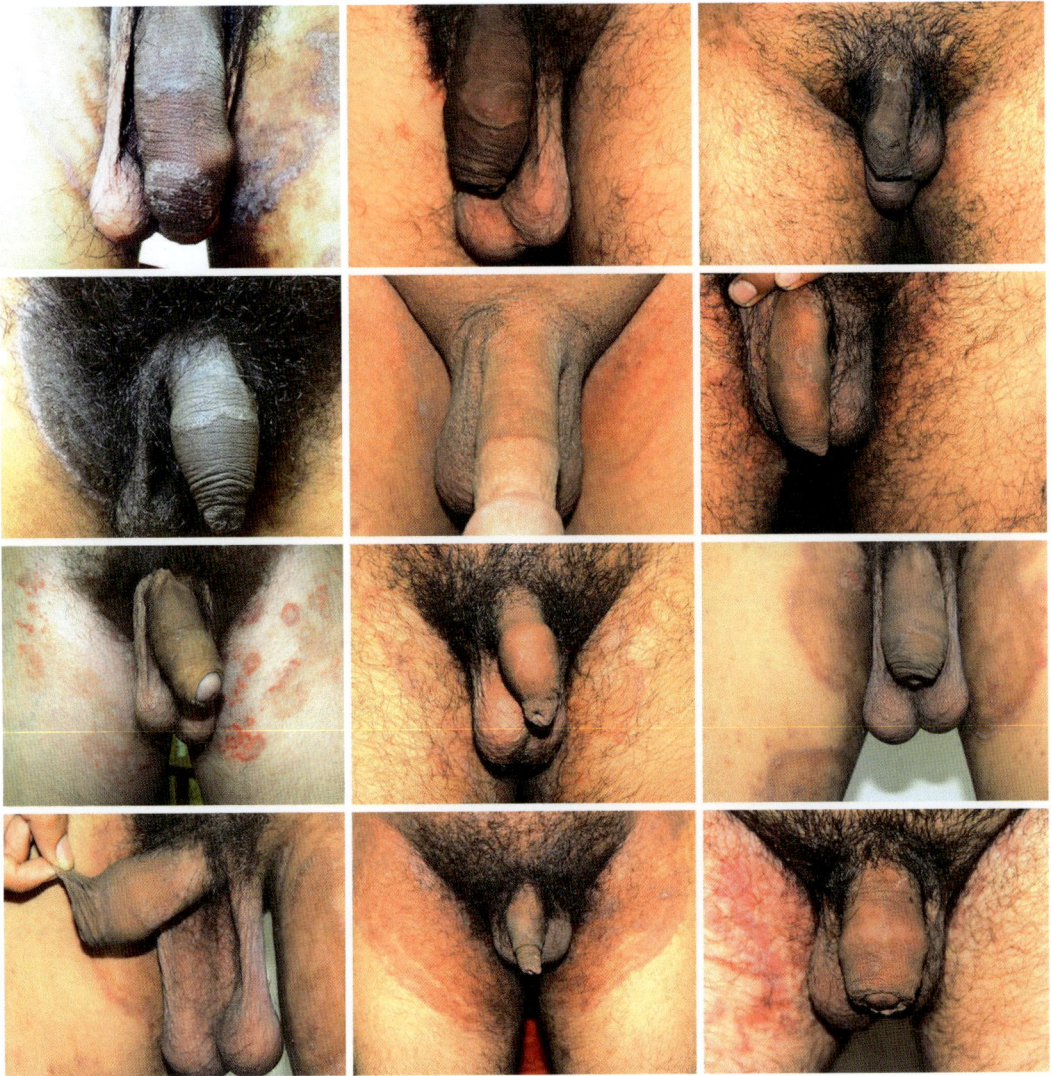

Fig. 14.8 Male genital dermatophytosis as result of topical steroid abuse

on the base of the penis that are hidden by pubic hair as well as on the perineum and scrotum. This makes it mandatory to examine the dorsal/anterior aspect of penis and scrotum, respectively. The patient should be preferably in a reclining position so that the perineal lesions, often extensions of tinea cruris, do not get missed. Not explaining this to the patient often results in inadequate treatment because of the skipped areas. The untreated genitoperineal lesions become a nidus of a chronic infection unresponsive to conventional treatment.

More number of *tinea faciei* are being seen. Most of the patients have infection of other body areas like tinea corporis or tinea cruris. Many of these lesions are probably true examples of tinea incognito because it is not always easy to appreciate the active borders of these lesions (Fig. 14.9). However the pinna of the affected side is often involved as has been reported in tinea capitis in children as "ear sign" [14].

There are said to be more number of cases of adult tinea capitis and these have been found to be extensions from the face or the neck.

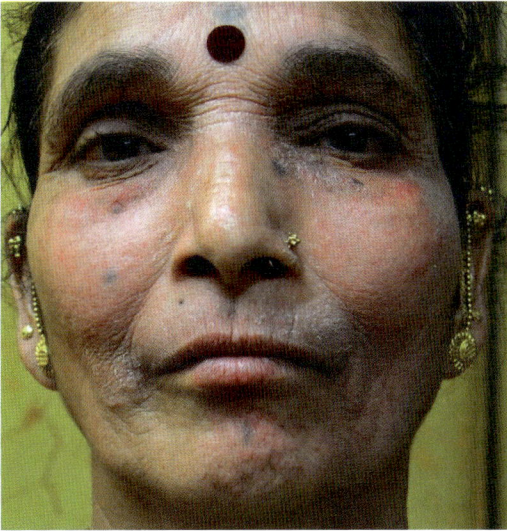

Fig. 14.9 Tinea faciei, often a "true tinea incognito" and clinically confusing

We are seeing more numbers of *erythrodermic variants of tinea corporis* where there is widespread involvement of body surface with variable erythema with profuse scaling (Fig. 14.10). Most of these patients are immunocompetent.

Many of the presentations enumerated above have accompanying stigmata of topical steroid abuse inside as well as in the vicinity of the lesions. The most frequently seen side effects in steroid-modified tinea are striae, hypopigmentation, and atrophy (Fig. 14.11). Among these three it is the striae that show the starkest appearance. Never before have we seen so many cases and such stark presentations of striae induced by topical steroids. They sometimes appear as early as 3–4 weeks of application of fixed drug combinations containing antifungals, antibacterials, and potent steroid molecules like clobetasol propionate. Once formed a minority of them get inflamed, edematous, and even ulcerated with superadded bacterial infections. And it is indeed sad to see patients continuing to apply the same preparations to such striae too leading to a vicious cycle.

This chapter is written not only to describe the morphological diversity of tinea corporis et cruris against the backdrop of steroid abuse but also to alert physicians from all fields to the perils associated with the use of irrational

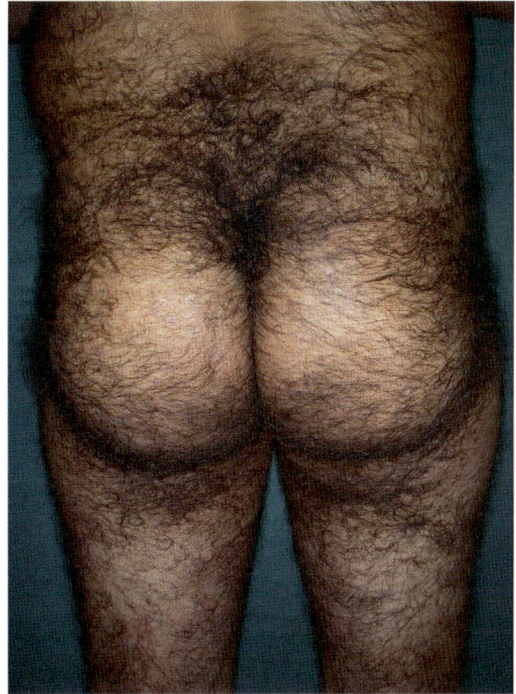

Fig. 14.10 Erythrodermic variant of tinea corporis with erythema and profuse scaling

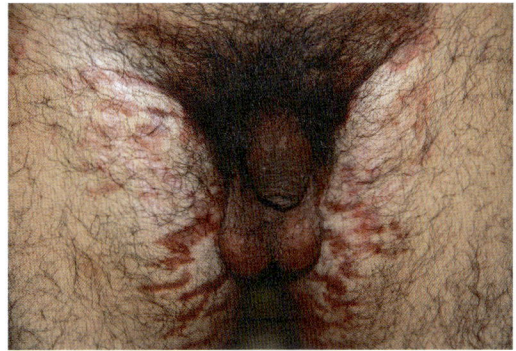

Fig. 14.11 Prominent striae and hypopigmentation

combinations containing antifungal and antibacterial agents with topical steroids, a practice that is common in developing nations. Indian dermatologic literature is replete with scholarly articles on topical steroid abuse not limited to their abuse in dermatophytosis [15–18]. Drug control authorities should take a serious note of this, ban such combinations, and also ensure that the sale of topical steroids is strictly regulated.

References

1. Verma SB. Sales, status, prescriptions and regulatory problems with topical steroids in India. Indian J Dermatol Venereol Leprol. 2014;80:201–3.
2. Verma SB. Topical steroid misuse in India is harmful and out of control. BMJ. 2015;351:h6079.
3. Dogra S, Uprety S. The menace of chronic and recurrent dermatophytosis in India: is the problem deeper than we perceive? Indian Dermatol Online J. 2016;7:73–6.
4. Lim SP, Smith AG. "Tinea pseudoimbricata": tinea corporis in a renal transplant recipient mimicking the concentric rings of tinea imbricata. Clin Exp Dermatol. 2003;28(3):332–3.
5. Verma S, Hay RJ. Topical steroid-induced tinea pseudoimbricata: a striking form of tinea incognito. Int J Dermatol. 2015;54(5):e192–3.
6. Hay RJ, Ashbee HR. Mycology. In: Burns T, Breathnach S, Cox N, Griffiths C, editors. Rook's textbook of dermatology, vol. II. 8th ed. Wiley-Blackwell: West Sussex; 2010. p. 36.1–36.93.
7. Verma SB. A closer look at the term 'Tinea incognito'- a factual as well as grammatical inaccuracy. Indian J Dermatol. 2017;62(2):219.
8. Szepietowski JC. Tinea of the penis: a rare location of the dermatophyte infection. Nouv Dermatol. 1998;17:571–3.
9. Romano C, Ghilardi A, Papini M. Nine male cases of tinea genitalis. Mycoses. 2005;48:202–4.
10. Prohic A, Krupalija-Fazlic M, Sadikovic TJ. Incidence and etiological agents of genital dermatophytosis in males. Med Glas (Zenica). 2015;12:52–6.
11. Vora NS, Mukhopadhyay AK. Incidence of dermatophytosis of penis and scrotum. Indian J Dermatol Venerol Leprol. 1994;60:89–91.
12. Gupta R, Banerjee U. Tinea of the penis. Indian J Dermatol Venereol Leprol. 1992;58:99–101.
13. Verma SB, Vasani R. Male genital dermatophytosis—clinical features and the effects of the misuse of topical steroids and steroid combinations—an alarming problem in India. Mycoses. 2016;59(10):606–14.
14. Agarwal US, Mathur D, Mathur D, Besarwal RK, Agarwal P. Ear sign. Indian Dermatol Online J. 2014;5(1):105–6. doi:10.4103/2229-5178.126064.
15. Rathi SK, D'Souza P. Rational and ethical use of topical corticosteroids based on safety and efficacy. Indian J Dermatol. 2012;57:251–9.
16. Coondoo A. Topical corticosteroid misuse: the Indian scenario. Indian J Dermatol. 2014;59:451–5.
17. Abraham A, Roga G. Topical steroid-damaged skin. Indian J Dermatol. 2014;59:456–9.
18. Lahiri K, Coondoo A. Topical steroid damaged/dependent face (TSDF): an entity of cutaneous pharmacodependence. Indian J Dermatol. 2016;61:265–72.

Use and Misuse of Topical Corticosteroid in Genital Dermatosis

15

Yogesh S. Marfatia and Devi S. Menon

Abstract

Many a time topical corticosteroids are prescribed for genital dermatosis of diverse etiology without establishing a definite cause because of its potent anti-allergic and anti-inflammatory effect. Due to its microenvironment, drug penetration in genitocrural region is highest in the body and hence, it is more susceptible to the adverse effects of topical corticosteroid. The absorption quotient of the scrotum is found to be 40 times that of the forearm. In females, poor sensory discrimination, overlapping symptomatology and high anatomic variability of the vulval skin may obscure the unwarranted side effects of steroids. The post-menopausal vulva is particularly susceptible to the side effects of topical agents. Topical corticosteroids are useful in conditions like balanoposthitis, plasma cell balanitis/zoon's balanitis, lichen sclerosus et atrophicus, balanitis xerotica obliterans, plasma cell vulvitis and contact dermatitis. Genital pruritus can be due to diverse causes and it is essential to find out the exact cause so that unnecessary use of topical corticosteroid is minimized. Alternatives to steroid should be considered like use of calcineurin inhibitors, tacrolimus and pimecrolimus 1%. In many inflammatory dermatoses, circumcision should be advised as first line measure so that prolonged use of corticosteroid can be avoided.

Keywords

Microenvironment • Genitocrural region • Steroid responsive genital dermatoses • Steroid adverse effect • Steroid alternatives

Learning Points

1. Steroid absorption is more in genitocrural region because of the microenvironment in this area.

Y.S. Marfatia (✉) • D.S. Menon
Department of Skin-VD, Medical College Baroda,
Vadodara, Gujarat, India
e-mail: ym11256@gmail.com

© Springer Nature Singapore Pte Ltd. 2018
K. Lahiri (ed.), *A Treatise on Topical Corticosteroids in Dermatology*,
DOI 10.1007/978-981-10-4609-4_15

2. Prescribe topical corticosteroids for steroid responsive genital dermatosis only, avoiding super potent steroids if not indicated. It should be given for a short period while tapering gradually.
3. Think of other causes if response to steroid is not satisfactory after 2–3 weeks.
4. Beware of ADR of topical steroid in groin region like atrophy, tinea incognito, candidial superinfection, striae.
5. Consider steroid alternatives like calcineurin inhibitors, general measures, circumcision, patient education and counselling.

15.1 Introduction

Topical corticosteroids offers treatment, though not curative for many dermatoses of diverse origin.

Because of prompt response to corticosteroid therapy, it is considered as a panacea and its misuse without prescription or medical advice is phenomenal [1].

Genitocrural area, because of its microenvironment, is more susceptible to adverse effects of topical corticosteroids.

15.2 Microenvironment of Genitocrural Region

Body folds provide a unique microenvironment determined by endogenous factors like thinness of skin, concentration of pilosebaceous follicles and exogenous factors like elevated temperature, friction, moisture and partial occlusion provided by skin in these areas [2].

15.2.1 Male

Occlusion provided by foreskin is likely to increase topical steroid absorption. The deep fold that is formed by the junction of the foreskin and the penis proximal to the coronal sulcus is subject to maceration from epithelial debris and glandular secretions, and is a common site of infection and facilitate steroid absorption.

Penetration of drug is correlated inversely with thickness of scrotal skin, therefore drug penetration is highest in scrotal skin. Hence steroid ADR is observed more frequently. In an experiment based on the method of applying C14-labeled hydrocortisone to the skin and measuring 5-day urinary excretion, it was showed that absorption was increased as much as 40-fold on the scrotum, compared with the ventral forearm. That is, if the Absorption Quotient of forearm is taken as 1, that of scrotum is 42 [3, 4].

Occlusion increases the hydration and temperature of scrotal skin, thus enhancing drug penetration by up to ten times [5]. Diseases with impaired barrier function like atopic dermatitis have been associated with increased penetration. Hydration of stratum corneum also enlarges the pathways of diffusion and results in increased permeability. Macerated skin has impaired barrier function which can result in increased percutaneous absorption. Application of potent topical corticosteroid will result in systemic absorption and systemic adverse reactions [6].

In older circumcised men, obesity and the vanishing penis can result in the phenomenon of the 'pseudo-foreskin' where the skin of the penile shaft partially or totally envelopes the glans penis. Such a situation is prone to all the complications and dermatoses found in the uncircumcised state [7]. The relatively fragile skin of the glans penis is susceptible to the influence of exogenous agents, comparable with the vulva, where an increased incidence of contact dermatitis is reported.

15.2.2 Females

Occlusion, friction, exposure to many more physiologic contact irritants like sweat, vaginal secretions, urine, etc. and mechanical trauma trigger contact reaction.

The cells in vulval skin are loosely arranged and it is devoid of stratum corneum with resultant increase in permeability to topically applied steroid up to sevenfold higher than forearm skin. Thus, vulvar skin is highly sensitive to topical agents [8]. Peculiar anatomy and vague symptoms may mask the unwarranted side effects of topically applied steroids [9].

After menopause, vulvar hydration remains unaffected [10]. This may increase susceptibility to water soluble irritants such as propylene glycol, which is one of the content of topical preparations. The postmenopausal vulva is more prone to harmful effect of vigorous cleansing, genital hygiene products and tight clothing or diapers [11]. Sodium lauryl sulphate, parabens, fragrances and other ingredients in the cream base can cause irritation. Ointment base preparations are better but long-term application of ointment occludes skin glands with the risk of development of vulvar sebaceous cysts.

Genital skin is predisposed to adverse effects of topical corticosteroids, particularly if applied for longer periods as in the case of chronic inflammatory genital dermatoses. Absorption of corticosteroid may be as much as fourfold greater with vulvar application than on the forearm [12]. Application of high potency steroid for a period longer than 1 month can result in adrenocortical suppression. High potency steroid should be prescribed only if the symptoms are severe. It is recommended to step down to lower potency steroid once response is obvious. Cutaneous visible adverse effect of topical steroid over vulval skin is not of cosmetic concern and hence, it is more likely that application is continued for a prolonged period as discontinuation leads to recurrence.

15.2.3 Males

15.2.3.1 Balanoposthitis

Balanitis describes inflammation of the glans penis and posthitis means inflammation of the prepuce. It can be of diverse etiology, infective (most common being candidial but occasionally can be herpetic as well) (Figs. 15.1 and 15.2) and non-infective. Balanitis is common in uncircumcised men as a result of poorer hygiene and

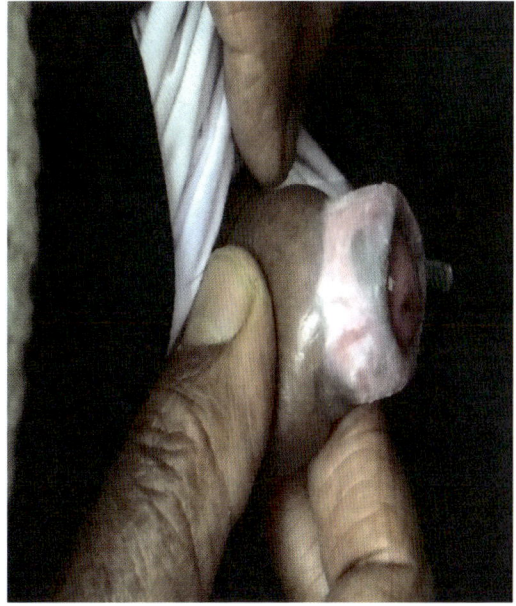

Fig. 15.1 Candidial balanoposthitis in a diabetic patient treated with TS

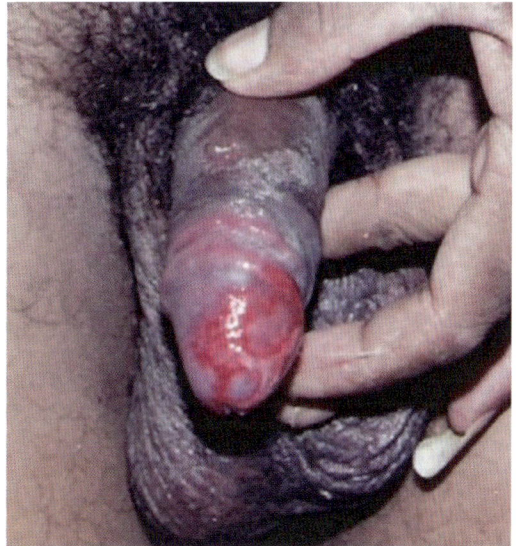

Fig. 15.2 Herpetic balanitis treated with TS

aeration or because of irritation by smegma. Many cases of balanitis seen in practice are a simple intertrigo. Topical corticosteroid alone or in combination with antifungal is a common prescription but simple measures and patient education should be the first priority. Rapid resolution can be achieved by advising the patient to keep his foreskin retracted if possible, having advised him of the risk of paraphimosis. Saline baths are also useful and talcum powders are helpful in drying the area. This advice is simple, but compliance may be challenging. Many patients will present having tried steroid-antifungal creams, often obtained over the counter. Such cases usually come with relapse. The simple measures have a more durable effect [14].

15.2.3.2 Plasma Cell Balanitis/Zoon's Balanitis

It is an idiopathic, benign disorder of uncircumcised male genitalia in middle aged. It is a chronic, reactive, principally irritant, mucositis brought about by dysfunctional prepuce with friction playing a part (dorsal aspect of the glans). It is characterized by a circumscribed, persistent moist plaque with a shiny smooth surface on the glans penis and has minute red specks called 'Cayenne pepper spots'. The keratinized penile shaft and prepuce are spared. Treatment includes moderately potent steroid preparation with or without topical antifungal agents, tacrolimus, CO2 laser and copper vapor LASER. Circumcision is curative.

Ram Chander et al. reported a case of a 70-year-old, married, sexually inactive, uncircumcised male, with biopsy proven plasma cell balanitis with no signs of malignancy. The patient was instructed to apply 0.03% tacrolimus ointment twice daily. Improvement of the lesion was observed after 2 weeks of treatment. The treatment was continued for four more weeks and then tapered over the next 2 weeks. No side effects were observed [15] (Fig. 15.3).

15.2.3.3 Lichen Sclerosus et Atrophicus

Lichen sclerosus et atrophicus (LSA) is inherently itchy condition progressively affecting the prepuce, glans and meatus with propensity for atrophy and penile squamous cell carcinoma. Control of pruritus with antihistamines (sedatives) is the key to offer symptomatic relief and arrest progression. Super potent corticosteroid ointment like clobetasol propionate prescribed in a tapering manner over a period of 10–12 weeks controls pruritus. Role of

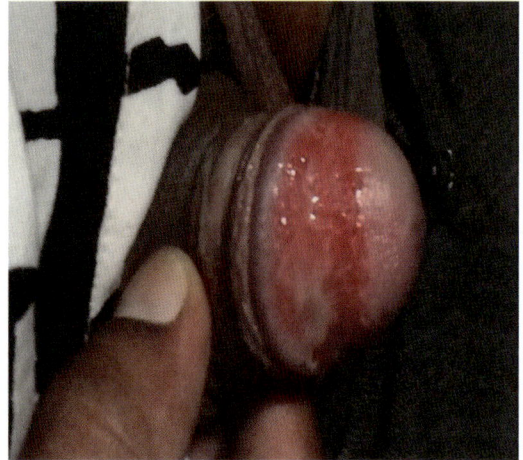

Fig. 15.3 Zoon's balanitis

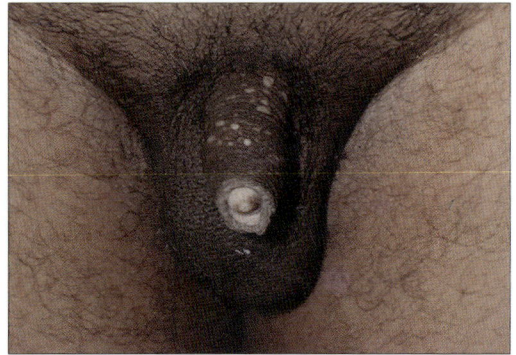

Fig. 15.4 Lichen sclerosus atrophicus with meatal narrowing

emollient cannot be over emphasized. Secondary bacterial and candidial infection should be treated. Other treatment reported to be efficacious include testosterone ointment, oral stanozolol, acitretin, isotretinoin, ACTH, liquid nitrogen cryotherapy, CO2 laser. Surgical interventions like circumcision and plastic repair are indicated in recalcitrant cases [16] (Fig. 15.4).

15.2.3.4 Balanitis Xerotica Obliterans

It is a form of LSA which occurs in uncircumcised men. Whitish smooth atrophic plaques on glans and prepuce are seen with rarely bullae at affected site. External meatus involvement is noticed in 50% cases with consequent stricture formation. SCC may develop in plaques in long standing cases. Steroid creams have been shown to limit the progression of the disease but do not offer a cure in the majority of cases. Studies have shown that applying a potent topical steroid improves BXO in the histologically early and intermediate stages of disease and may inhibit further worsening in the late stages but do not offer a cure in the majority of cases [17].

15.2.3.5 Pseudoepitheliomatous Micaceous and Keratotic Balanitis

It is a rare penile condition which is seen mainly in elderly over 60 years. It is characterized by an initial plaque stage, late tumor stage followed by verrucous carcinoma and transformation to SCC and metastasis. Coronal balanitis with silvery white appearance, mica-like and keratotic horny masses on the glans is seen. The choice of treatment is generally guided by the stage of the disease. Topical measures include 5-FU, podophyllin resin, potent topical steroids and physical measures are cryotherapy, radiotherapy and surgical excision (Fig. 15.5a–c).

15.2.4 Females

15.2.4.1 Plasma Cell Vulvitis

It represents a reaction pattern to an inflammatory condition causing intractable vulvar pruritus. Treatment modalities are topical corticosteroid, lignocaine and misoprostol. Çelik A et al. reported a case of plasma cell vulvitis for which topical clobetasol 17-dipropionate cream 0.05% was applied twice daily. Three weeks after starting the treatment with the topical steroids, 50% of complaints had resolved and the lesions significantly improved. After 3 months, all the symptoms and signs were relieved.

15.2.4.2 Vulvar Lichen Sclerosus Atrophicus

Vulvar lichen sclerosus atrophicus (VLS) is an intensely pruritic chronic inflammatory dermatoses resulting into disfiguring sequelae and having malignant potential. Most commonly occurs on the vulva and around the anus with ivory-white lesions appearing like figure of eight that may be

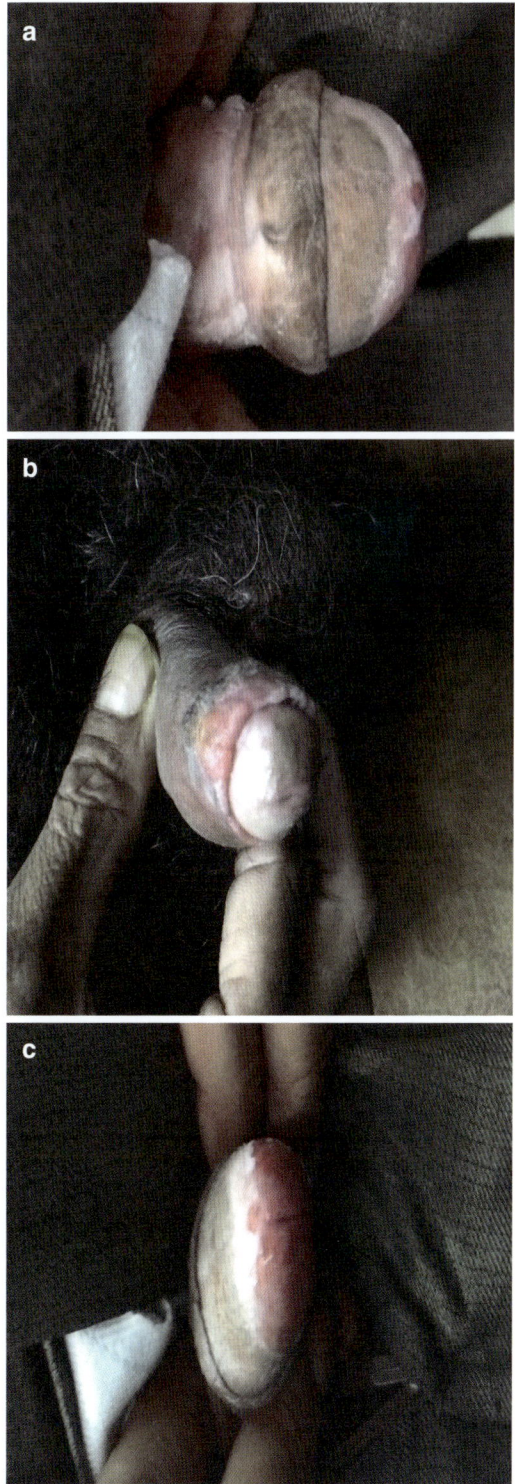

Fig. 15.5 (**a–c**) Pseudoepitheliomatous micaceous and keratotic balanitis

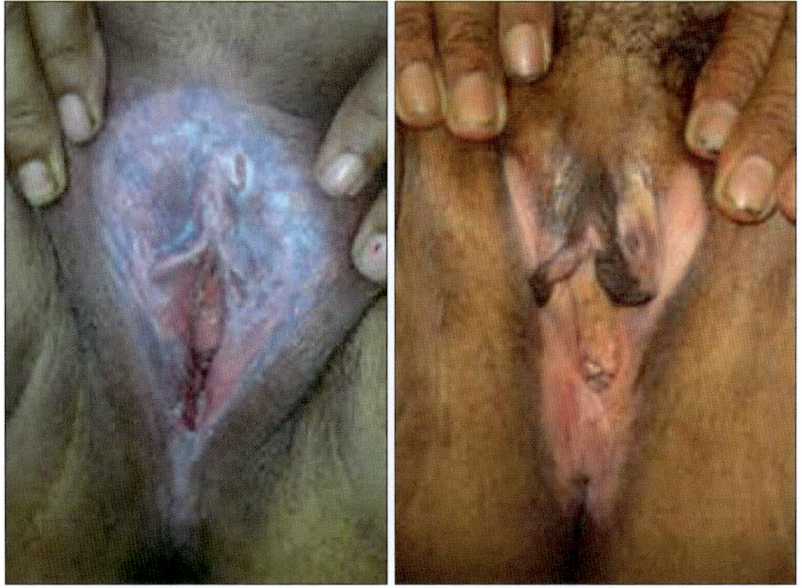

Fig. 15.6 Vulvar lichen sclerosus

shiny. It may be asymptomatic in some cases. Treatment options include potent topical corticosteroids and tacrolimus.

As per the study done by Renaud-Vilmer C et al., prolonged treatment with 0.05% clobetasol propionate ointment resulted in improvement in women older than 70 years and complete regression in younger women with recurrence. Lifelong follow-up is recommended in all cases [18] (Fig. 15.6).

15.2.5 Genital Pruritus

Genital pruritus without apparent skin lesions is empirically treated with topical steroids but common causes should be ruled out. Atopic diathesis is to be considered as an endogenous cause. Exogenous causes include irritation and allergy. Genital allergy can be related to sexual activity, non-sexual causes like topical medication and use of genital hygiene products or even consort contact dermatitis [19].

Psychogenic pruritus should be dealt with accordingly.

As discussed, genital pruritus can be due to diverse causes and it will be prudent to find out the exact cause so that unnecessary use of topical corticosteroid is minimized.

15.3   Side Effects of Topical Steroids (see Table 15.1)

1. Anatomic and physiologic variations of genital skin facilitating more absorption.
2. Occlusive condition increases potential for steroid absorption.
3. Steroid formulations—Absorption is highest with ointment base followed by cream, gel and lotion and hence, ADR more with ointment.
4. Some of the hygiene/personal care products may damage genital mucosa and thereby, increases the chances of absorption.

15.3.1 Factors Affecting Topical Steroid Absorption and Contributing to ADR

Topical steroids are associated with a number of side effects although they are clearly beneficial in the therapy of inflammatory disease [20].

Table 15.1 Genital dermatoses responsive to topical steroids [13]

Diseases very responsive to topical steroids	Diseases less responsive to topical corticosteroids	Diseases where steroids are not first line agents[a]
Atopic dermatitis	Vitiligo	Genital pruritus
Seborrhoeic dermatitis	Pseudoepitheliomatous keratotic and micaceous balanitis	Balanoposthitis
Lichen simplex chronicus	Zoon's balanitis	
Pruritus ani	Plasma cell vulvitis	
Late phase of allergic contact dermatitis		
Late phase of irritant contact dermatitis		
Psoriasis		
Lichen sclerosus/Balanitis xerotica obliterans		

[a]Etiology based treatment is to be preferred

Topical corticosteroid is atrophogenic and atrophic changes can start within 2 weeks of treatment. At microscopic level, there is reduction in cell size and number of cell layers in epidermis. There is decrease in stratum corneum thickness. Epidermal cell differentiation can also be suppressed.

Due to application of TS for a long period, there is increased *transepidermal water loss* and decrease in lipid content affecting barrier function [21].

Dermal atrophy results in thin and brittle skin with striae, local vasodilatation coupled with reduced synthesis of collagen and mucopolysaccharides results in *telangiectasia and purpura*.

15.4 Atrophy Due to Steroid

Prolonged topical steroid use may result in atrophic changes in vulvar skin. Potency, duration and frequency of application are risk factors which contribute to the atrophogenic potential of topical steroids [22, 23].

A case having vulval dermatitis treated with prolonged steroid application developed extensive atrophy in the perineum resulting in secondary 'webbing' and partial obstruction of genital hiatus as well as superimposed dyspareunia was reported [21].

Steroids need to be used cautiously to decrease long-term complications. Starting with higher potency steroids for the shortest duration (up to 2 weeks) followed by tapering coupled with thorough patient education may minimize the unwanted side effects [24].

15.5 Contact Hypersensitivity to TS

Contact hypersensitivity to TS may cause persistence or worsening of skin diseases. It is rare, but its risk increases with prolonged exposure. Nonfluorinated TS (e.g., hydrocortisone hydrocortisone-17-butyrate, and budesonide) results in a higher prevalence of contact allergy in comparison with fluorinated compounds [2].

In addition to topical corticosteroids, vehicles as well as preservatives can also cause contact hypersensitivity [25].

Systemic side effects of TG such as pituitary–adrenal axis suppression are rare but should be considered when treating children because of the potential for growth retardation. Furthermore, children have a higher ratio of total body surface area to body weight (about 2.5- to 3-fold that of adults). The degree of adrenal suppression increases with the potency and concentration of the TG, application area, occlusion and degree of inflamed skin. Other systemic side effects include Cushing's syndrome, the aggravation of diabetes mellitus, and increasing or causing hypertension and osteonecrosis.

15.6 Topical Calcineurin Inhibitors as an Alternative to Steroid in Vulval Dermatoses

Potent topical corticosteroids are frequently needed to treat various forms of vulvar dermatoses, which are often characterized by an abnormal proliferation or activation of T lymphocytes. Atrophogenecity is the limitation of using topical steroid for a prolonged period, so an alternative to topical corticosteroids is to be considered.

Topical immunomodulators like pimecrolimus 1% and tacrolimus block the release of inflammatory cytokines and promote cutaneous innate host defences. Both these topical calcineurin inhibitors are used in the treatment of anogenital lichen sclerosus, genital lichen planus, vulvar lichen simplex chronicus and related pruritic vulvar dermatoses (chronic vulvar pruritus and allergic contact dermatitis of the vulva), although topical pimecrolimus may exhibit a better long-term tolerability profile. They are a useful second-line therapeutic option for patients who are intolerant of or resistant to topical corticosteroids [26]. The plus point is the lack of atrophogenecity and they do not show tachyphylaxis unlike topical steroid.

15.7 Circumcision as an Alternative to Topical Steroid Therapy

Circumcision is reported to protect against many inflammatory dermatoses like phimosis, paraphimosis, balanoposthitis, plasma cell balanitis, circinate balanitis, balanitis xerotica obliterans, psoriasis, seborrhoeic dermatitis, lichen planus and lichen sclerosus.

A retrospective case control study by Eleanor Mallon et al. reported protective effect of circumcision against penile inflammatory dermatoses.

Zoon's balanitis and lichen sclerosus developed almost exclusively in uncircumcised cases. The presence of the foreskin may promote inflammation by a Koebner phenomenon or the presence of infectious agents [27].

In such chronic inflammatory dermatoses, circumcision should be advised as first line measure so that prolonged use of corticosteroid can be avoided.

Conclusion

- The micro-environment of the genital area predisposes to enhanced topical corticosteroid absorption as well as increased adverse reactions.
- Steroid prescription should be restricted to steroid responsive genital dermatoses only and for a short period while tapering gradually.
- Avoid super potent steroids.
- Instruct patient about mode of application, frequency, duration and not to use prescribed steroid for any other indication and in any other person.
- Alternative therapies to topical steroid like calcineurin inhibitors (tacrolimus, pimecrolimus 1%) should be considered.
- General measures should be encouraged.
- Circumcision can be recommended for chronic and recurring genital dermatoses.
- Cases presenting with genital pruritus without any skin lesions must be interrogated to find out possible cause/triggers and should be managed accordingly.
- Patient education regarding avoidance of self medication, OTC preparations and on adverse events due to topical steroid abuse.

References

1. Maibach H, Surber C, editors. Topical corticosteroids. Basel: S. Knrger AG; 1992.
2. Hengge UR, Ruzicka T, Schwartz RA, Cork MJ. Adverse effects of topical glucocorticosteroids. J Am Acad Dermatol. 2006;54:1–15.
3. Feldmann RJ, Maibach HI. Regional variation in percutaneous penetration of 14C cortisol in man. J Invest Dermatol. 1967;48:181–3.

4. Howard I, Maibach MD. Issues in measuring percutaneous absorption of topical corticosteroids. Int J Dermatol. 1992;31(s1):21–5.

5. Brisson P. Percutaneous absorption. Can Med Assoc J. 1974;110:1182–5.

6. Dhar S, Seth J, Parikh D. Systemic side-effects of topical corticosteroids. Indian J Dermatol. 2014;59: 460–4.

7. Singh S, Bunker C. Male genital dermatoses in old age. Age Ageing. 2008;37(5):500–4.

8. Connor CJ, Eppsteiner EE. Vulvar contact dermatitis. Proc Obstet Gynecol. 2014;4(2):1–14.

9. The vulva: Anatomy, physiology, and pathology. Edited by Miranda A. Farage and Howard I. Maibach, New York, New York, Informa Health Care, 2006.

10. Summers PR, Hunn J, et al. Unique dermatologic aspects of the postmenopausal vulva. Clin Obstet Gynecol. 2007;50(3):745–51.

11. Farage MA. Vulvar susceptibility to contact irritants and allergens: a review. Arch Gynecol Obstet. 2005;272:167–72.

12. Farage M, Maibach H. Lifetime changes in the vulva and vagina. Arch Gynecol Obstet. 2006;273:195–202. [Epub October 6, 2005

13. Mehta AB, Nadkarni NJ, Patil SP, Godse KV, Gautam M, Agarwal S. Topical corticosteroids in dermatology. Indian J Dermatol Venereol Leprol. 2016;82:371–8.

14. Pandya I, Shinojia M, Vadukul D, Marfatia YS. Approach to balanitis/balanoposthitis: current guidelines. Indian J Sex Transm Dis. 2014;35:155–7.

15. Chander R, Garg T, Kakkar S, Mittal S. Treatment of balanitis of Zoon's with tacrolimus 0.03% ointment. Indian J Sex Transm Dis. 2009;30(1):56–7.

16. Shah R, Ghiya R, Iyer A, Marfatia YS. Lichen sclerosus: a case report with review of literature. Indian J Sex Transm Dis. 2007;28:40–2.

17. Scheinfeld NS, James WD, et al. Balanitis xerotica obliterans treatment & management. New York: Medscape; 2016.

18. Renaud-Vilmer C, Cavelier-Balloy B, Porcher R, Dubertret L. Vulvar lichen sclerosus effect of long-term topical application of a potent steroid on the course of the disease. Arch Dermatol. 2004;140(6):709–12.

19. Marfatia YS, Patel D, Menon DS, Naswa S. Genital contact allergy: a diagnosis missed. Indian J Sex Transm Dis. 2016;37:1–6.

20. Wiedersberg S, Leopold CS, et al. Bioavailability and bioequivalence of topical glucocorticoids. Eur J Pharm Biopharm. 2008;68(3):453–66. Epub 2007 Aug 8.

21. Sheu H-M, Lee JY-Y, Chai C-Y, Kuo K-W. Depletion of stratum corneum intercellular lipid lamellae and barrier function abnormalities after long-term topical corticosteroids. Br J Dermatol. 1997;136:884–90.

22. Johnson E, Groben P, Eanes A, Iyer P, Ugoeke J, Zolnoun D. Vulvar skin atrophy induced by topical glucocorticoids. J Midwifery Womens Health. 2012; 57(3):296–9.

23. Schoepe S, Schacke H, May E, Asadullah K. Glucocorticoid therapy-induced skin atrophy. Exp Dermatol. 2006;15(6):406–20.

24. ACOG Practice Bulletin No. 93: diagnosis and management of vulvar skin disorders. Obstet Gynecol. 2008;111(5):1243–53.

25. Coondoo A, Phiske M, Verma S, Lahiri K. Side-effects of topical steroids: a long overdue revisit. Indian Dermatol Online J. 2014;5(4):416–25.

26. Goldstein AT, et al. Topical calcineurin inhibitors for the treatment of vulvar dermatoses. Eur J Obstet Gynecol Reprod Biol. 2009;146(1):22–9.

27. Mallon E, Hawkins D, Dinneen M, Francis N, Fearfield L, Newson R, Bunker C. Circumcision and genital dermatoses. Arch Dermatol. 2000;136(3):350–4.

Red Skin Syndrome

16

Mototsugu Fukaya

Abstract

Red skin syndrome (RSS) is a condition that can develop after stopping long-term continuous use of topical steroids. In RSS, erythema or exudative erythema extends from the original location of the rash where topical steroids had been applied to sites where steroids were never used. The disorder may take weeks to several years to resolve and some patients experience repeated seasonal exacerbation long term.

Keywords

Topical steroid addiction (TSA) • Topical steroid withdrawal (TSW) • 11-Beta-HSD2

Learning Points

1. RSS cases have often been misdiagnosed as a flare of the underlying dermatological disorder.
2. RSS can be diagnosed through observation of the rash over time.
3. There is a possibility that the long-term continuous use of topical steroids affects the cortisol production by keratinocytes, thereby causing RSS.

The name RSS was coined by Dr. Rapaport in 2006 [1] to describe a previously unrecognised condition. RSS goes by many names in the literature, and even Rapaport has also used alternative terms such as red scrotum syndrome [2] and red burning skin syndrome [3]. The International Topical Steroid Addiction Network (ITSAN), a patient-led group working to spread awareness about RSS mostly through their website, uses the terms topical steroid addiction (TSA) and topical steroid withdrawal (TSW) in addition to RSS. In Japan, RSS was reported by Dr. Enomoto in 1991 as 'steroid withdrawal syndrome by topical corticosteroid' [4]. The condition has also been called 'steroid dermopathy' or simply 'rebound'.

RSS presents in different ways with a range of diverse clinical features. It occurs after the

M. Fukaya
Tsurumai Kouen Clinic, Nagoya, Japan
e-mail: moto@earth.ocn.ne.jp

© Springer Nature Singapore Pte Ltd. 2018
K. Lahiri (ed.), *A Treatise on Topical Corticosteroids in Dermatology*,
DOI 10.1007/978-981-10-4609-4_16

cessation of chronic continuous use of topical steroids. Symptoms are more severe than the original skin condition (i.e. before treatment with topical steroids). The skin symptoms often appear similar to an exacerbation of the original skin condition that triggered the use of topical steroids in the first place. Therefore, RSS cases have often been misdiagnosed as a flare of the underlying dermatological disorder. RSS can only be diagnosed through observation of the rash over time. However, several features are characteristic, such as the distribution of the rash and its progression.

The first part of this chapter will describe clinical manifestations seen in RSS cases. The second will discuss causes of RSS and the final section will outline treatment of RSS.

16.1 Clinical Manifestation of RSS

RSS often develops in patients with a history of atopic dermatitis (AD). When a patient with AD ceases chronic continuous use of topical steroids, several scenarios may follow [5], including:

1. Simple AD recurrence.
2. Possible RSS. This is difficult to distinguish from recurrent AD symptoms (see Fig. 16.1 for an example).
3. Definite RSS.

Looking at the rash in the series of photographs 1, 2, 3 and 4 in Fig. 16.1, the dermatological diagnosis would clearly be AD. There is no obvious reason to consider the diagnosis of RSS. Photo 1 shows the patient shortly before discontinuing topical steroids where the rash was poorly controlled. Photo 2 was taken 2 months after ceasing topical steroids; photo 3, 7 months after cessation; and photo 4, 12 months after cessation. The patient did not make any lifestyle or environmental changes in those 12 months—all he did was stop the use of topical steroids. If his diagnosis was contact dermatitis secondary to the topical steroids used, then recovery should have been swift. His skin would not have gotten worse as it did—the severity of his symptoms actually peaked during the 2nd month before improving over the next few months. So, if you consider the rash at just one point in time, the diagnosis would almost certainly be AD. However, taking into account the history of topical steroid use and then cessation and the subsequent progression of the rash, the diagnosis of RSS is obvious.

It is easy to make a diagnosis of RSS when the patient's symptoms are severe, as in the case shown in Fig. 16.2. Photograph 1 was taken just before the patient discontinued topical steroids. Here, the patient's skin condition appears too severe to be a typical case of AD. In photo 2, taken 2 months after cessation of topical steroids,

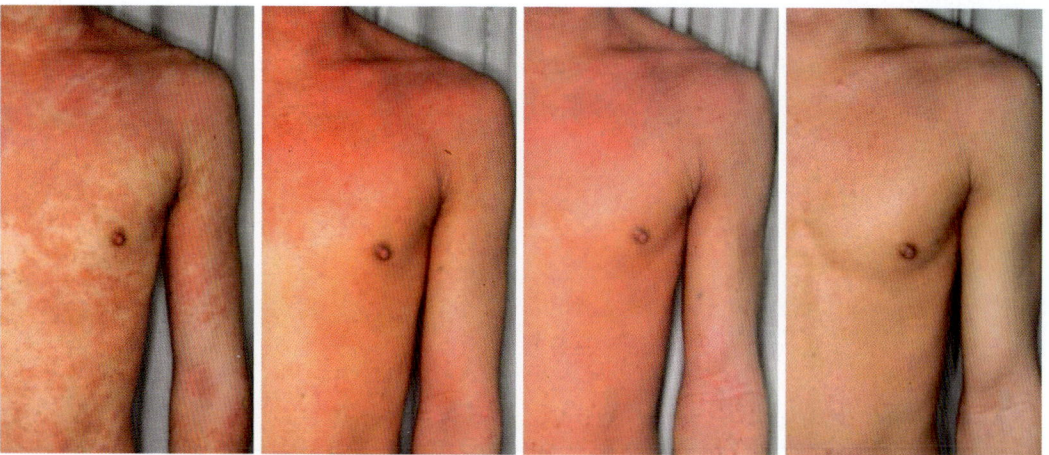

Fig. 16.1 Prior to discontinuation/2 months later/7 months later/12 months later

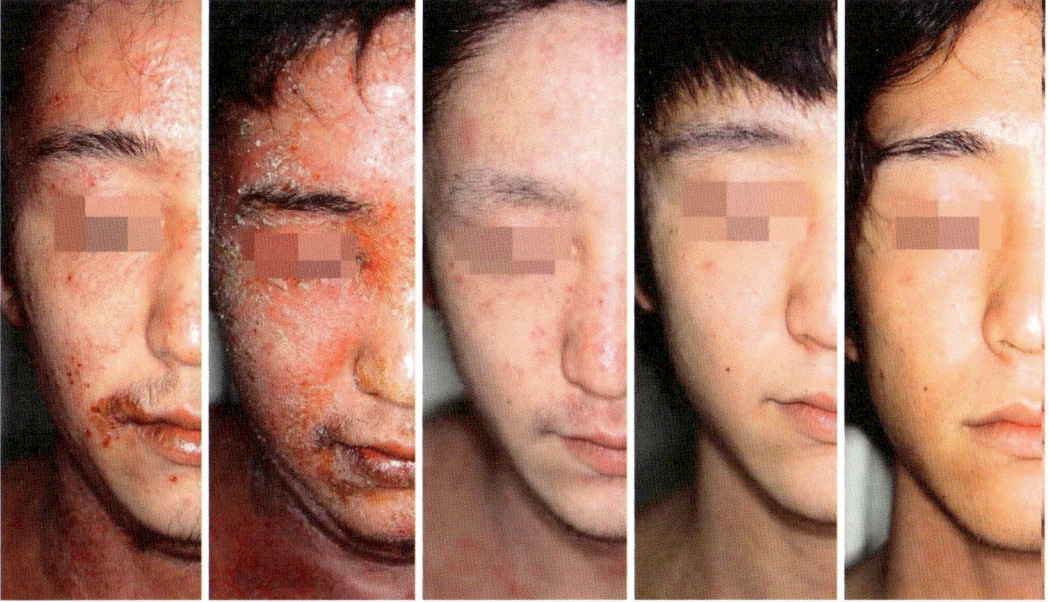

Fig. 16.2 Prior to discontinuation/2 weeks later/3 months later/7 months later/13 months later

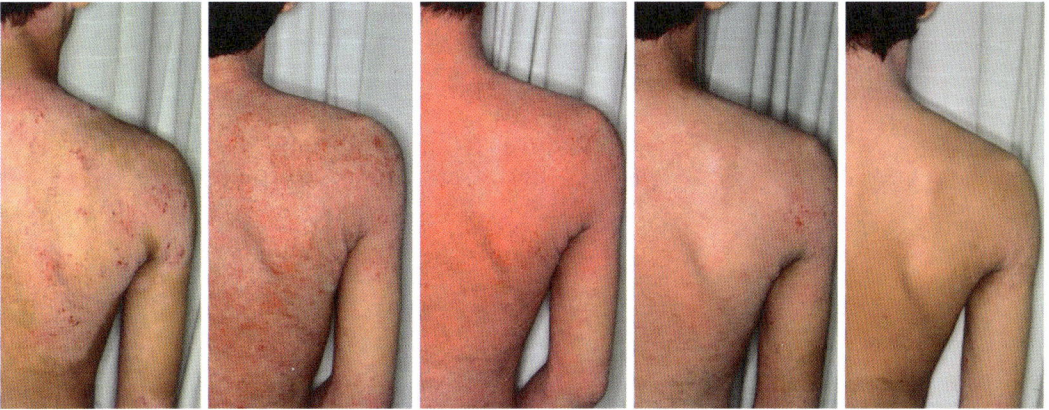

Fig. 16.3 Prior to discontinuation/3 months later/7 months later/11 months later/19 months later

we see exudative erythema, incrustation, exfoliation, pigmentation and scars secondary to scratching. The patient developed a fever of around 40° which lasted 7–10 days and was thus suspected of having adrenal insufficiency. However, his blood cortisol levels were actually raised (not reduced).

In some cases RSS progresses slowly after discontinuation of topical steroids. In these cases both the doctor and patient may become disheartened and doubtful whether management is appropriate. In Fig. 16.3 we see a case where symptoms peaked 7 months after ceasing topical steroids before gradually resolving.

After ceasing topical steroids, a patient with RSS will develop extremely sensitive skin, and dermatitis will appear following exposure to even slight irritation. False positives are common in patch tests done around this time. Temporary exacerbations may result from seasonal changes such as changes in temperature and/or humidity or shedding of hair by pets. Unexpected flares can occur, for example, when a patient moves to a new location. Patients can thus experience a second or third rebound.

Therefore to determine whether a patient is heading towards recovery, the doctor needs to observe the patient for at least 12 months, ideally comparing skin status throughout the seasons over several years. For example, the patient in Fig. 16.3 can be assured of their improvement by comparing photos taken at 7 and 19 months after cessation of topical steroids.

16.2   Causes of RSS

Rapaport focussed on the vasodilation action of nitric oxide (NO) and suggested NO was a cause of RSS [6]. Cork proposed a theory that topical steroids increase protease, which breaks down corneodesmosome, which is in turn known to bind corneocytes to each other, and this is what breaks down the epidermal barrier leading to rebound symptoms [7].

In recent years it has been found that keratinocytes produce cortisol to autoregulate epidermal thickness and differentiation by paracrine and autocrine mechanisms [8]. The author believes that the long-term continuous use of topical steroids affects the cortisol production by keratinocytes, thereby causing RSS [9, 10].

Figure 16.4 shows the epidermal changes seen on the inside forearm of a healthy individual who had applied 0.05% clobetasol propionate twice daily to the area for 2 weeks before stopping. The images shown are of the skin before topical steroid use, day 2 of use, day 15 (i.e. 1 day after ceasing topical steroids) and day 30 (i.e. 16 days after stopping the topical steroid). Immunostaining for anti-PCNA antibodies, anti-cortisol antibodies, anti-11-beta-HSD1 antibodies and anti-11-beta-HSD2 antibodies is demonstrated. Atrophy to epidermis is evident on day 15, and on day 30 this atrophy was seen to be resolving. The intracytoplasmic cortisol in the keratinocytes peaked on day 15, showing the topical steroid use caused an increase in the cortisol production by the epidermis. This response has already been demonstrated in dermal fibroblasts [11]. It appears that the concentration of cortisol in the skin varies almost immediately in response to blood levels of cortisol (which are determined by the adrenal cortex).

Intracytoplasmic cortisol and 11-beta-HSD2 both increase in keratinocytes. 11-Beta-HSD1 is an enzyme that converts cortisone, an inactive steroid, into cortisol, whilst 11-beta-HSD2 converts cortisol into cortisone. Therefore, increased levels of 11-beta-HSD2 indicate cortisol within the keratinocytes is being inactivated.

Figure 16.5 demonstrates a patient's epidermis with immunostaining during RSS and during recovery 2 years later.

The amount of 11-beta-HSD2 near the basal level is increased during RSS. In the recovered epidermis, 11-beta-HSD2 levels had reduced. The epidermal thickness has normalised, as has the granular layer, and the parakeratosis has disappeared. The evidence from this case suggests increased 11-beta-HSD2 in the epidermal basal layer is a cause of RSS. This means cortisol is inactivated to cortisone in the keratinocytes leading to increased proliferation of basal cells and immature keratinisation. This is explained in the diagram in Fig. 16.6.

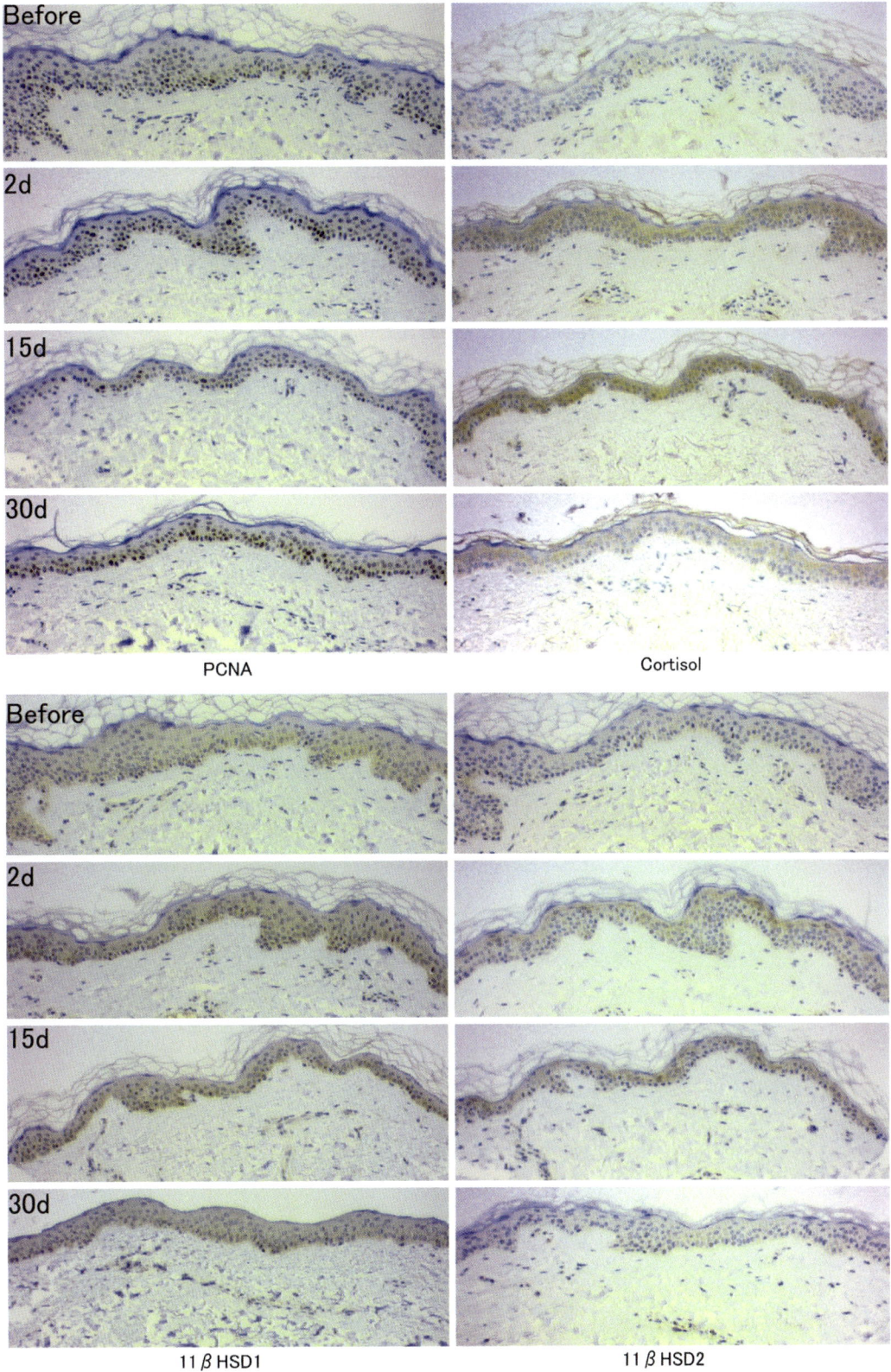

PCNA

Cortisol

11 β HSD1

11 β HSD2

Fig. 16.4 The epidermal changes seen on the inside forearm of a healthy individual who had applied 0.05% clobetasol propionate twice daily to the area for 2 weeks before stopping

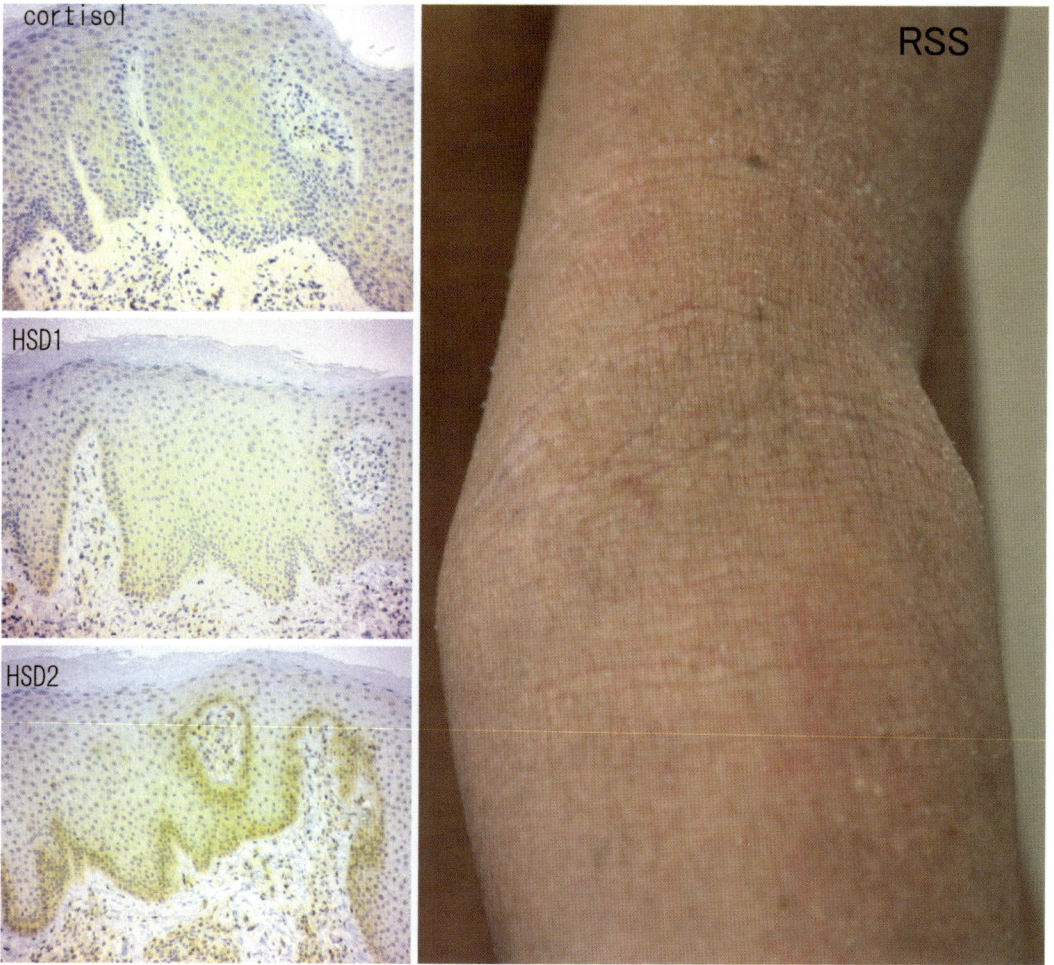

Fig. 16.5 A patient's epidermis with immunostaining during RSS and during recovery 2 years later

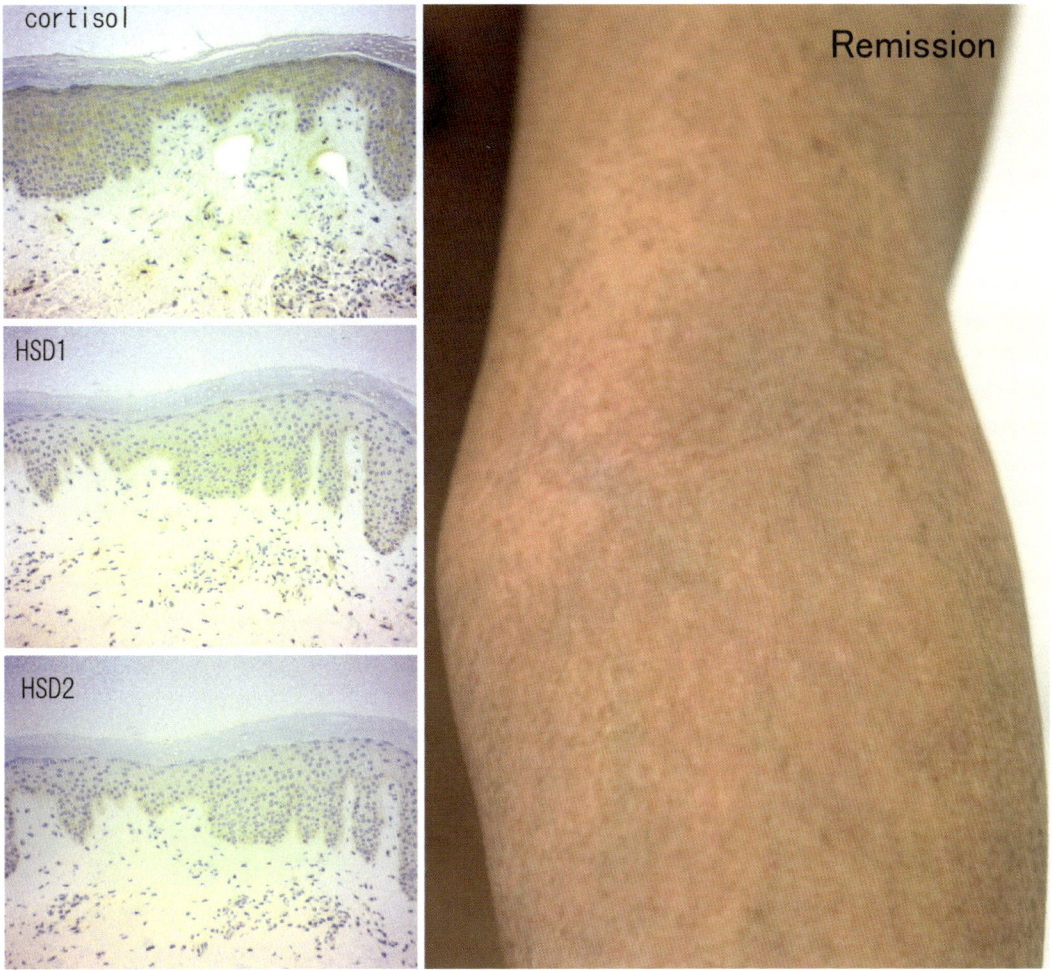

Fig. 16.5 (continued)

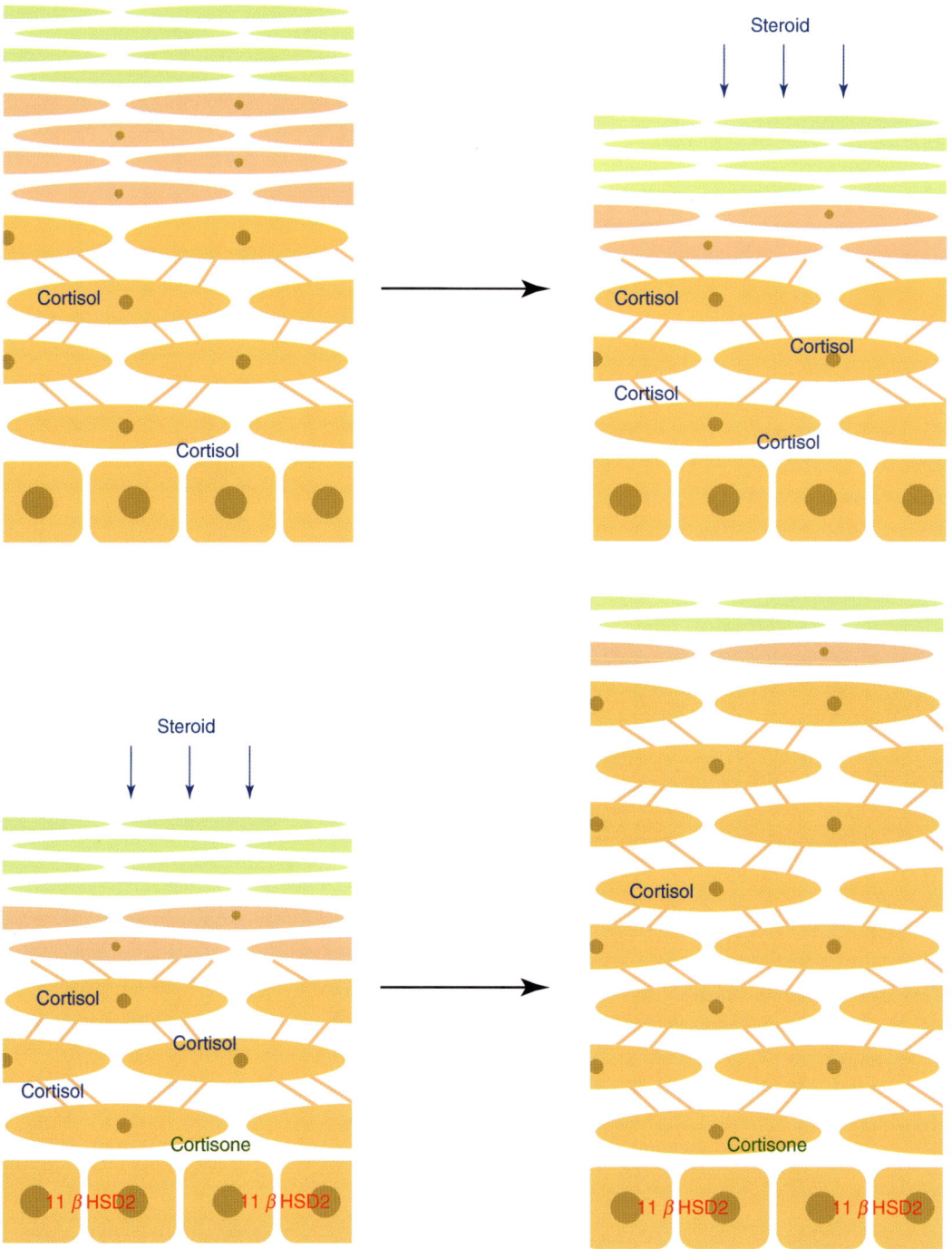

Fig. 16.6 The first picture shows normal epidermis before application of topical steroids. The second shows increased cortisol levels and a thinner epidermis as a result of topical steroid application. The third picture shows the epidermis's progression to topical steroid addiction with increased levels of 11-beta-HSD2 and the conversion of cortisol to the inactive cortisone. The fourth picture shows the epidermis of RSS with abnormal thickening and cortisol still being inactivated to cortisone

16.3 RSS Management

RSS improves spontaneously over time [12]. Therefore, controlled studies are required to determine whether any medical interventions contribute to patient recovery or whether improvements seen around the time of the therapy are coincidental. No controlled studies of treatment for RSS have been published to date.

As RSS is due to the continuous application of topical steroids, the first treatment must logically be the cessation of topical steroids. However, as the diagnosis of RSS can only be made after observation of progression of symptoms following the discontinuation of topical steroids, it can be difficult to determine whether stopping topical steroids should be recommended to an individual patient.

Once the decision to stop topical steroids has been made, the next question is whether to cease treatment immediately (cold turkey) or to gradually taper the amount used. Rapaport and some doctors recommend the cold turkey approach. Other doctors advise gradually reducing the amount of topical steroids applied, and some recommend steroid injections or oral steroids to minimise intense rebound symptoms as required or desired.

When topical steroids are discontinued, steps need to be taken to reduce the risk of infections such as Kaposi varicelliform eruption and septicaemia. Bleach baths may be useful for this purpose [13]. RSS is uncommon in infants (as long-term continuous use of topical steroids is required for the condition to develop); however, occasionally it does occur. In these cases, hypoalbuminaemia and failure to thrive can be problematic and the baby should be monitored closely by a paediatrician familiar with RSS.

Expert opinion suggests moisturising agents are best avoiding when stopping topical steroids. There are some doctors who also advise limiting water intake also. Whilst this may sound irresponsible, it is based on the evidence that skin dryness leads to increased epidermal steroid production [14]. Extremely premature infants that are kept in incubators with low humidity experience a reduction in water loss from their epidermis more rapidly than those exposed to higher humidity, suggesting the low humidity assists with their skin barrier development [15].

It is possible that water restrictions can also contribute to epidermal recovery by increasing blood aldosterone levels (mineralocorticoid receptors in the epidermis bind to cortisol and work similarly to glucocorticoid receptor alpha) [16].

Moisturising has been shown to prevent AD in multiple studies [17, 18]. Thus, it may sound contradictory to advise against moisturising during RSS. However, normal skin is different to the skin seen in a patient with RSS where there has been exposure to long-term continuous use of topical steroids.

Ultraviolet therapy and tar agents are effective in RSS, although the results are not dramatic. Both therapies probably increase the amount of cortisol produced by the skin. Ultraviolet rays have been shown to increase epidermal cortisol concentration [19] and tar agents are metabolised by CYP11A1, which is a cortisol-producing enzyme.

Some doctors recommend glycyrrhizin agents in RSS patients and find these effective. As glycyrrhizin blocks 11-beta-HSD2 [20], this appears to be a logical approach. It has been reported that hyaluronic acid, which has a molecular weight of close to 100,000 daltons, helps to resist epidermal atrophy caused by topical steroid use [21].

Topical PPAR alpha agonist can control RSS symptoms (rebound) in mice [22], and clinical success has been reported in some patients too [23].

Calcineurin inhibitors and immunosuppressive drugs [3] have rarely been reported as being used to manage RSS symptoms. Dermatologists who are unfamiliar with RSS may prescribe these medications for a period before again recommending topical steroids. Doctors and patients who recognise RSS and appreciate it as a side effect of topical steroids may be reluctant to use stronger drugs with the potential for even more serious adverse effects.

Future studies are needed to determine which of these drugs (and the newer biological agents) are helpful in managing RSS symptoms.

References

1. Rapaport MJ, Rapaport V. The red skin syndromes: corticosteroid addiction and withdrawal. Expert Rev Dermatol. 2006;1(4):547–61.
2. Rapaport MJ. Red scrotum syndrome. Cutis. 1998;61(3):128B.
3. Rapaport MJ, Lebwohl M. Corticosteroid addiction and withdrawal in the atopic: the red burning skin syndrome. Clin Dermatol. 2003;21(3):201–14.
4. Enomoto T, Arase S, Shigemi F, Takeda K. Steroid withdrawal syndrome by topical corticosteroid. J Jpn Cosm Sci Soc (Jpn). 1991;15(1):17–24.
5. Fukaya M. Color atlas of steroid withdrawal from topical corticosteroid in patients with atopic dermatitis. Tokyo: Ishiyaku Publishers; 2000.
6. Rapaport MJ, Rapaport VH. Serum nitric oxide levels in "red" patients: separating corticosteroid-addicted patients from those with chronic eczema. Arch Dermatol. 2004;140(8):1013–4.
7. Cork MJ, Robinson DA, Vasilopoulos Y, Ferguson A, Moustafa M, MacGowan A, et al. New perspectives on epidermal barrier dysfunction in atopic dermatitis: gene-environment interactions. J Allergy Clin Immunol. 2006;118(1):3–21.
8. Slominski A, Zbytek B, Nikolakis G, Manna PR, Skobowiat C, Zmijewski M, et al. Steroidogenesis in the skin: implications for local immune functions. J Steroid Biochem Mol Biol. 2013;137: 107–23.
9. Fukaya M. Histological and immunohistological findings using anti-cortisol antibody in atopic dermatitis with topical steroid addiction. Dermatol Ther (Heidelb). 2016;6(1):39–46.
10. Fukaya M. Cortisol homeostasis in the epidermis is influenced by topical corticosteroids in patients with atopic dermatitis. Indian J Dermatol. 2017. (In press).
11. Tiganescu A, Walker EA, Hardy RS, Mayes AE, Stewart PM. Localization, age- and site-dependent expression, and regulation of 11β-hydroxysteroid dehydrogenase type 1 in skin. J Invest Dermatol. 2011;131(1):30–6.
12. Fukaya M, Sato K, Yamada T, Sato M, Fujisawa S, Minaguchi S, et al. A prospective study of atopic dermatitis managed without topical corticosteroids for a 6-month period. Clin Cosmet Investig Dermatol. 2016;9:151–8.
13. Huang JT, Abrams M, Tlougan B, Rademaker A, Paller AS. Treatment of *Staphylococcus aureus* colonization in atopic dermatitis decreases disease severity. Pediatrics. 2009;123(5):e808–14.
14. Agren J, Sjörs G, Sedin G. Ambient humidity influences the rate of skin barrier maturation in extremely preterm infants. J Pediatr. 2006;148(5):613–7.
15. Takei K, Denda S, Kumamoto J, Denda M. Low environmental humidity induces synthesis and release of cortisol in an epidermal organotypic culture system. Exp Dermatol. 2013;22(10):662–4.
16. Boix J, Sevilla LM, Sáez Z, Carceller E, Pérez P. Epidermal mineralocorticoid receptor plays beneficial and adverse effects in skin and mediates glucocorticoid responses. J Invest Dermatol. 2016;136(12):2417–26.
17. Simpson EL, Chalmers JR, Hanifin JM, Thomas KS, Cork MJ, McLean WH, et al. Emollient enhancement of the skin barrier from birth offers effective atopic dermatitis prevention. J Allergy Clin Immunol. 2014;134(4):818–23.
18. Horimukai K, Morita K, Narita M, Kondo M, Kitazawa H, Nozaki M, et al. Application of moisturizer to neonates prevents development of atopic dermatitis. J Allergy Clin Immunol. 2014;134(4): 824–30.
19. Skobowiat C, Dowdy JC, Sayre RM, Tuckey RC, Slominski A. Cutaneous hypothalamic-pituitary-adrenal axis homolog: regulation by ultraviolet radiation. Am J Physiol Endocrinol Metab. 2011; 301(3):E484–93.
20. Teelucksingh S, Mackie AD, Burt D, McIntyre MA, Brett L, Edwards CR. Potentiation of hydrocortisone activity in skin by glycyrrhetinic acid. Lancet. 1990;335(8697):1060–3.
21. Barnes L, Ino F, Jaunin F, Saurat JH, Kaya G. Inhibition of putative hyalurosome platform in keratinocytes as a mechanism for corticosteroid-induced epidermal atrophy. J Invest Dermatol. 2013;133(4):1017–26.
22. Hatano Y, Elias PM, Crumrine D, Feingold KR, Katagiri K, Fujiwara S. Efficacy of combined peroxisome proliferator-activated receptor-α ligand and glucocorticoid therapy in a murine model of atopic dermatitis. J Invest Dermatol. 2011;131(9):1845–52.
23. Fukaya M, Kimata H. Topical clofibrate improves symptoms in patients with atopic dermatitis and reduces serum TARC levels: a randomized, double-blind, placebo-controlled pilot study. J Drugs Dermatol. 2014;13(3):259–63.

Topical Corticosteroid Abuse: Indian Perspective

Meghana Phiske and Rajeev Sharma

Abstract

Topical steroids (TSs) have been used for decades to treat various dermatological disorders due to their various effects, which have become responsible for the various deleterious side effects. Their free availability in India has made them prone for abuse, increasing the risk of local and systemic side effects. The reasons for TSs abuse varies from wrong prescription, dubious marketing by pharmaceutical companies, free availability as OTC drugs and lack of regulations regarding the manufacturing of irrational combinations. The misuse occurs at various levels such as manufacturing, marketing, prescription, sales and end-use by patients/ laymen. TSs are misused for varied indications like acne, pigmentation, fungal infection, pruritus, and as a cosmetic cream. TSs abuse is more common in the younger generation and dark races. The Indian Association of Dermatologists, Venereologists, and Leprologists (IADVL) has formed a task force against TSs abuse, with main aims like raise public awareness, run media campaigns, form study groups for doctors, highlight the problem in journals, and meet with central and state authorities.

Keywords

Topical steroids • TSs abuse • OTC drugs

M. Phiske
Dr. Meghana's Skin Clinic, JK Chambers,
First Floor, Office no 111, Sector-17, Vashi,
Navi Mumbai 400703, India
e-mail: meghanaphiske@rediffmail.com

R. Sharma (✉)
Bishen Skin Centre,
M-69, Janakpuri, Aligarh 202001, India
e-mail: skinaligarh@gmail.com

Learning Points
1. Proper education, sensitization, regularization o prescriptions and strict legal rules and actions would go a long way in curbing the TSs abuse menace.

© Springer Nature Singapore Pte Ltd. 2018
K. Lahiri (ed.), *A Treatise on Topical Corticosteroids in Dermatology*,
DOI 10.1007/978-981-10-4609-4_17

17.1 Introduction

Abuse is inappropriate or excessive use of a drug. In recent years, there has been a dramatic increase in drug abuse. Topical steroids (TSs) which came into existence more than 50 years ago have been used for decades to treat various dermatological disorders. Various effects of TSs like vasoconstrictive, immunosuppressive, antiproliferative, antipruritic, atrophogenic, melanopenic and sex-hormone-like effects lead to rapid response in many dermatoses including infections. But unfortunately these effects have become responsible for the myriad deleterious effects of TSs [1, 2].

Also their free availability over the counter (OTC) without prescription in India has made them prone for abuse, increasing the risk of local and systemic side effects. Betamethasone valerate is the most favored preparation, being popular due to the misconception that it is fairness and anti-acne cream [3].

17.2 Historical Aspects of Steroids

TSs were first introduced in 1951 by Sulzberger. The TS to be introduced was topical hydrocortisone then known as "compound F" [4]. In 1952 Sulzberger and Witten published an article on the effect of topically applied compound F in selected dermatoses [5]. A large number of modifications of the original compound F (hydrocortisone) were discovered in rapid succession. These included fluorohydrocortisone (1955), triamcinolone acetonide (1958), fluocinolone acetonide (1961), betamethasone (1963), clobetasol propionate (1974), clobetasone butyrate (1978), fluticasone (1990), Halobetasone (1990), mometasone (1991) and a host of other molecules. These molecules were of varying potencies as determined by their vasoconstrictive properties [6].

17.3 Reason for Misuse of Steroids

The reasons for rampant TS abuse vary from wrong prescription, dubious marketing by pharmaceutical companies, free availability as OTC drugs (many cosmetic and Ayurvedic products contain unlabeled depigmenting agent and steroids; TSs are available in various irrational combinations) and lack of regulations regarding the manufacturing of irrational combinations [2, 5].

The misuse occurs at various levels such as manufacturing, marketing, prescription, sales and end use by patients and laymen [6].

17.4 Stages at Which Misuse Occurs [6]

1. Manufacturing misuse: Many pharmaceutical companies often market products which they think would be innovative and attractive to the prescriber, to increase their sales. But in the long run such products do more harm than good. Examples include modified Kligman's formula containing mometasone for melasma, superpotent steroids with enhanced penetration and superpotent steroids for use on scalp.

2. Marketing misuse: TSs are often introduced to non-dermatologists without revealing the true aspects of its appropriate usage and information regarding side effects. Unfortunately such marketing practices may not be strictly illegal, leading to abuse of TSs. Though it is illegal for a practitioner of alternative medicine to prescribe allopathic drugs, there is no legal restriction on promotion and sale of TSs by pharmaceutical companies to such practitioners. Hence TS prescriptions coming from alternative medicine are common in India.

3. Prescription misuse: Prescriptions of TSs by dermatologists may be incomplete with respect to quantity to be used, frequency, site and duration. Prescriptions of non-dermatologists ignore the important aspects like potency, site, duration and indication. Also patients with TS prescriptions tend to repeatedly buy the same drug from chemists against medical advice.

4. Sales misuse: TSs in India most are available at very cheap prices since they come under Drug Control Price Order (DPCO) being sold as over-the-counter (OTC) products unlike the

international market. This causes multiple problems:

a. Layman can buy any TSs from chemists for any ailment.
b. Salespersons at chemist counters are considered equal to doctors by many laypersons who encourage buying of TSs to increase their sales. This results in flooding of society with TSs sold and misused freely without a dermatologist's prescription.

5. Misuse by laypersons: Laypersons suffering from various dermatoses tend to apply steroids which are recommended by their friends, neighbors and relatives. Their diseases may also be aggravated on application of steroids. But they do not consult dermatologists initially or even later and continue to use steroids for long time increasing the risk of development of side effects. Another situation where steroids are commonly misused is as fairness cream. Mometasone, hydroquinone and tretinoin containing skin-lightening agent's usage has become very popular especially in India resulting in their aggressive marketing and prescription not just by dermatologists but all physicians resulting in their widespread abuse [2].

17.5 Indications for Misuse

TSs are misused for varied indications, such as acne, pigmentation, fungal infection, pruritus and as a cosmetic or skin cream for any type of rash [5].

17.6 Commonly Abused Steroids

Betamethasone valerate (0.1%), fluocinolone acetonide (0.1%) and betamethasone dipropionate (0.05%) were the main types of steroid abused [7]. The greatest increase in sales in May 2015 was of Panderm Plus Cream, which contains clobetasol, ornidazole, ofloxacin and terbinafine. A modified and vitiated version of the original triple combination of Kligman's formula, intended for use in melasma, contains potent topical corticosteroids such as mometasone in addition to hydroquinone and tretinoin, with a brand called Skinlite

topping the sales in 2015. With total sales of Rs. 2.74 bn in May 2015, these combinations are available over the counter, even though mometasone can cause severe cutaneous adverse effects. Some combination products are marketed and used as whitening creams but can cause long-term and often permanent side effects [8].

17.7 Population Commonly Abusing Topical Steroids

TS abuse is more common in the younger generation who, in the pursuit of looking good and fair, try to procure TSs OTC and use it indiscriminately [2]. In dark-colored races also, TSs have acquired the reputation of being cheap fairness, anti-acne and anti-blemish agents [9].

17.8 Figures on Sales of Topical Steroids

In the Indian market, 1066 brands of TSs are sold. Sale of TSs at the end of December 2013 was 1400 crores, showing an annual growth of 16%. This accounted for 82% of the topical dermatology market, reflecting clearly their popularity. The top-selling combinations contain beclomethasone, neomycin and clotrimazole (sale of Rs. 152 crores in 2013), followed by combination products containing clobetasol, ofloxacin, ornidazole and terbinafine (sale at Rs. 110 crores). According to IMS Health data, most prescriptions for TSs and combinations come from dermatologist followed by general practitioners, obstetrician and gynecologists, pediatricians and physicians [10].

17.9 Magnitude of Steroid Abuse Problem in India

In India all drug combinations are considered new drugs for the first 4 years and therefore need approval from the Drug Controller General of India after safety and efficacy data have been presented. After approval, state licensing authorities allow manufacture and sale throughout the country [8].

By law, steroids, like clobetasol, clobetasone, fluticasone and mometasone, can be sold in India only with a registered medical practitioner's prescription. All steroids are included in schedule H of the Drugs and Cosmetics Rules 1945, but a footnote confusingly excludes topical preparations and eye ointments from the list. This means that the status of these drugs is interpreted as "over the counter" which needs urgent revision. Moreover, existing laws are poorly implemented. Many of India's 800,000 pharmacists sell steroid creams without a prescription, ignoring the box warnings [8].

The situation in India is complicated by these factors:

1. The number of dermatologist in India is currently approximately 7500, of which more than 80% of them practice in urban areas. The population is 1.21 billion out of which about 70% live in villages. So the number of dermatologists is few for the Indian population living in rural areas. Because of this, nonphysicians who are not trained treat dermatoses by prescribing TSs [10]. The top prescribers of topical steroids in India, after dermatologists, are general practitioners, gynecologists, pediatricians and consulting physicians [8].
2. Another major concern regarding selling of prescription drugs as non-prescription drugs is the lack of awareness about medication among the general public, particularly in a developing country like India [6].
3. Inadequate regulation of unscrupulous pharmacists by authorities who act as quasi-dermatologists dispensing reasonably priced superpotent topical steroids either alone or in combination to an unsuspecting populace.
4. "Law related to drugs and cosmetics" indicates that TSs are schedule H drugs; that means they have to be sold strictly only after prescription of a registered medical practitioner. Only clobetasol propionate, clobetasone 17-butyrate, fluticasone propionate and mometasone furoate are included in this list. TS combinations are also not included in the list. From the analysis of the affidavit filed in the Supreme Court in November 2013 in a drug pricing case by the All India Drug

Action Network and others vs Union of India and others, 99.8% of topical steroids have escaped inclusion in the Drug Price Control Order [8, 10].

17.10 General Side Effects of TSs

General side effects noted with topical corticosteroids include telangiectasia, cutaneous atrophy, striae, hyper-/hypopigmentation, tinea incognito, perioral dermatitis, infantile gluteal granuloma and pyoderma [11].

These are likely to occur when superpotent TSs are used on the face, in body folds and on areas with a thin skin (e.g., genitalia). Children are especially liable to these side effects due to their relatively thin skin.

Hypopigmentation is due to impaired melanocyte function and is especially seen with triamcinolone due to its tendency to aggregate owing to its large molecular size. Atrophic changes can affect both epidermis and dermis. The process starts microscopically within 3–14 days of steroid application. Initially epidermis becomes thin due to reduction in epidermal cell size, which reflects a decreased metabolic activity. After prolonged exposure there is reduction in cell layers, that is, the stratum granulosum disappears and the stratum corneum becomes thin. Synthesis of stratum corneum lipids and keratohyalin granules and formation of corneodesmosomes are suppressed.

Dermal atrophy is caused by decreased fibroblast growth and reduced synthesis of collagen. Intertriginous areas are particularly susceptible due to thinner skin, increased moisture, elevated temperature and partial occlusion provided by the skin in these sites. The atrophy is reversible on stoppage of TS, but the normalization may take months [12].

17.11 Side Effects on Face

Another major aspect of TCs abuse is its cosmetic use in dark skinned, particularly in combination with bleaching creams, to make the skin fair [13]. TS-damaged facies is a newly described entity associated with TS abuse.

17.12 Effects of Steroid Abuse on the Face [1, 7, 12–16]

1. Steroid addiction.
2. Red burning skin syndrome.
3. Status cosmeticus.
4. Acneiform eruption.
5. Hypertrichosis.
6. Demodicidosis.
7. Facial plethora.
8. Perioral dermatitis.
9. Steroid rosacea (synonyms – light-sensitive seborrheid, rosacea-like dermatitis, steroid dermatitis resembling rosacea, steroid-induced rosacea, steroidal dermatitis resembling rosacea). It is a dermatitis resembling rosacea following repeated or chronic unsupervised application of TSs. Not only the abuse but even excessive, regular use of topical fluorinated steroids on face is associated with this eruption. It presents as an erythematous papule that dries and evolves into diffuse erythema, pustules and nodules. It requires 6 months for development, but it is also potency dependent.
10. "Topical steroid-dependent face" (TSDF). This follows unsupervised application of TSs on the face even after resolution of the primary dermatosis for which the TS was intended. It presents with severe rebound erythema, burning and scaling on the face on any attempted cessation of the application. Also included in this definition are flares of photosensitivity, papules and pustules.

17.13 Less-Known Cutaneous Side Effects

Hypertrichosis, cutaneous dyschromias, delay in wound healing and flare of skin infections are less common [12].

17.14 Ocular Complication

Ocular complications include steroid-induced open-angle glaucoma with reversible increased intraocular tension, irreversible glaucomatous cupping of the optic disk and visual field defects [17].

17.15 Systemic Side Effects

Systemic side effects of TCs are known to occur when superpotent or potent TSs are used for a long time on areas with thin skin, e.g., the face and on raw/inflamed surfaces [12].

The side effects include:

1. Ocular-Cataract (posterior cortical), open-angle glaucoma.
2. Ocular-Cataract disease, mineralocorticoid effects especially with hydrocortisone and 9-α-fluoroprednisolone.
3. Metabolic glucose intolerance.
4. Reduced bone mineral density.
5. Osteopathy.
6. Decreased growth rate.
7. Electrolyte balance.
8. Edema.
9. Hypocalcemia.
10. Hypertension.
11. Suppression of the HPA axis.
12. Factors causing HPA suppression are as mentioned below [[12]:]
    a. Applying TSs over large areas.
    b. Using higher concentrations of TSs.
    c. Using TSs under occlusion.
    d. Increased application of moderately potent TSs.
    e. Increased steroid penetration (especially in atopics).
    f. Modest use of more potent derivatives.
    g. This can cause iatrogenic Cushing disease, corticosteroid-related Addison crises, growth retardation and death. The HPA axis recovers spontaneously in a fortnight.

17.16 Awareness Campaign in India

The first major article about TS abuse from India was published in the *Indian Journal of Dermatology* in 2006. In the same year, a thread named "Topical steroid misuse menace" was initiated in the ACAD IADVL group of IADVL and a delegation of IADVL led by Dr. Suresh Joshipura, the then President of IADVL and Dr. Koushik Lahiri, the then Hon. General Secretary of IADVL, submitted a memorandum on this issue to the Union Minister of Health and to the Ministry of Chemicals and Fertilizers.

Since the first report on abuse, many more articles have been published from India. Patients presenting with steroid abuse are being discussed in ACAD IADVL and dermatologists have been actively posting photographs and discussing this issue in a Facebook group devoted to this issue named "No steroid cream on face without a doctor's prescription." The issue is also discussed in lay print and electronic medium. The social media is also being utilized for a similar purpose [6].

17.17 Task Force (ITATSA) Concept and Its Journey So Far

The Indian Association of Dermatologists, Venereologists and Leprologists (IADVL) has formed a task force against TS abuse, with main aims like raise public awareness, run media campaigns, form study groups for doctors, highlight the problem in journals and meet with central and state authorities. The task force has started to collect relevant data and has asked the drug controller to bring topical steroids under schedule H, disallowing their unrestricted sale and has demanded explanation as to why the authorities authorize irrational combinations [8].

A brief timeline for the journey so far is as follows:

a. On 5 November 2006, just 7 days after IADVL ACAD group was created by the then Honorary General Secretary Dr. Koushik Lahiri, he started a mail thread on the issue of topical steroid abuse. It evoked great discussion between members. This was the *first* time this issue was discussed on a national platform.
b. The same year Dr. Koushik Lahiri and Dr. Arijit Coondoo moved a proposal in the General Body meeting of the association at Chennai in 2007 (STOP OTC sale of Topical Corticosteroid without prescription) and got it passed.

c. The term TSDF was coined by Dr. Koushik Lahiri on 20th March 2008 on IADVL ACAD group.
d. Between April and June 2008, as the principle investigator Dr. Koushik Lahiri initiated a countrywide multicenter study to analyze and assess the scenario, another first in IADVL history, Dr. Abir Saraswat agreed to prepare the manuscript as first author. That group of erudite and committed investigators from all corners of India, namely, Drs. Koushik Lahiri, Abir Saraswat, Shyam B Verma, Arijit Coondoo, CR Srinivas, Asit Mittal, Rajeev Sharma, Saumya Panda, Anil Abraham, Shyamanta Barua, Manas Chatterjee and Murlidhar Rajagopalan, formed the initial nidus for ITATSA.
e. This highly rated and quoted historic article was finally published in 2011 in IJDVL.
f. In 2012, Dr. Koushik Lahiri then started the Facebook page (No steroid on Face without Dermatologists Prescription). It created history by number of hits from all over the world.
g. 23 May 2014: The petition at change.org was started.
h. 30 May: IADVL, Varanasi came forward to support the movement; news were published in Dainik Jagran.
i. 31 May: 500 signatures.
j. 1 June: Writer Taslima Nasreen joins the crusade and tweets supporting the cause.
k. 3 June: IADVL, WB comes forward to support.
l. 4 June: Crossed 1000 signature mark.
m. 4 June: IADVL, Karnataka Branch comes forward to support.
n. 5 June: IADVL, NE branch comes forward to support.

IADVL Taskforce Against Topical Steroid Abuse (ITATSA):

a. 29 June 2014: IADVL, national body officially endorses the movement and forms a dedicated task force ITATSA (Dr. Koushik Lahiri as the Chair and Dr. Abir Saraswat as the Convener).
b. 30 June: Yahoo Groups was formed.
c. 30 July: INSTEAD joins hand.
d. 16 August: ITATSA endorsed by IADVL CC.

e. 23 September: ITATSA approached DCGI.

f. 10 October: An appeal from IADVL to our industry partners to support our crusade against topical steroid misuse.

g. 28 October: Celebrity activity proposed by Dr. Venkatram Mysore.

h. 12 February 2015: ITATSA endorsed by GB

i. 13 February: IADVL celebrity activity, treat your skin right program unveiled.

j. 18 February: OPPI came forward in support.

k. 3 March: ITATSA WhatsApp group created.

l. 24 April 2015: Meeting with the following was held:
  • Secretary, Department of Pharmaceuticals, Dr. VK Subburaj
  • Joint Drug Controller General of India, Dr. S Eswara Reddy
  • Director General of Health Services, Dr. Jagdish Prasad

m. 27 April 2015: Meeting with DCGI Dr. GN Singh.

n. May 2015: DCGI issues circular.

o. November 2015: Follow-up meeting with DCGI Dr. GN Singh.

p. December 2015: DCGI issues another circular.

q. February 2016: New team with Dr. Kiran Nabar as Chairperson and Dr. Rajetha Damisetty as Convener was formed. Though Dr. Kiran Nabar later resigned.

r. 1 April 2016: Follow-up meeting with DCGI.

s. 14tApril 2016: Dr. Rajeev Sharma was inducted as the Chairperson.

t. 12 August 2016: Gazette published including all the topical steroids under schedule H and deleting the footnote excluding topicals from the list.

u. 14 January 2017: Dr. Shyam Verma took over as the Chairperson of ITATSA, Dr. Rajetha Damisetty continued as the Convener.

17.18 Studies on Topical Steroid Abuse

1. Early reports of TS dependence or addiction were published in 1973 by Burry and in 1976 by Kligman and Frosch [6].

2. A landmark study in India by Saraswat et al. revealed that most TS abusers belonged to the 20- to 30-year age group. Betamethasone valerate alone or in combination was most commonly abused. TSs use as a fairness/general purpose/aftershave was in 29% and for acne was in 24%.Steroid combinations were used by 59.6% of patients. The rural/suburban populace and younger population used potent and superpotent TSs. Non-prescription TS use was in 59.3% and out of these, 90.3% were for potent/superpotent steroids. Among 40.7% physician prescriptions, 44.3% were from non-dermatologists. Adverse effects were seen in 90.5% TS users. In acne or acne exacerbation, topical steroid-dependent faces were common side effects. In 93%, TSs were used unnecessarily, in excess, were of the wrong potency, or were instituted without a diagnosis [1].

3. A study conducted in Bastar, Chhattisgarh, by Dey revealed that lightening of skin color was the main reason for using TSs followed by melasma and suntan. The commonest side effects were acne (37.99%), plethoric face with telangiectasia (18.99%), puffy face and acneiform eruptions with papulopustular lesions [11].

4. Another study by Jha et al. revealed that the majority (42.9%) of 410 patients studied self-prescribed TSs; 20% recommended by their friends, family members or neighbors; 18.2% recommended by a non-dermatologist practitioner; 10.2% recommended by a dermatologist; and 8.5% recommended by beauty parlors. Steroid-induced acne was the commonest adverse effect of topical steroids (42.9%) followed by hypopigmentation in 14.1%. The commonest abused TS was betamethasone valerate which was dispensed in 92 patients (22.4%) as fairness cream/anti-acne cream, Kligman formula in 43 patients (10.4%) for melasma/other hyperpigmented lesion and TS-containing antifungal/antibiotic cream in 41 patients (10%) for tinea faciei/other facial dermatoses [3].

17.19 Treatment

TS addiction and side effects can be treated and results in significant improvement in the quality of life. Treatment of facial adverse effects of TSs requires complete cessation of usage. In case of addiction, progressively less potent TSs are introduced over a period of weeks to months and the dose is gradually tapered off. Stinging, pruritus and photosensitivity are treated using emollients, topical calcineurin inhibitors, and sunscreens. Systemic agents include antihistamines, nonsteroidal anti-inflammatory drugs, tetracyclines and isotretinoin [2].

17.20 Measures to Reduce the Problem of Steroid Misuse

Measures that need to be taken at different levels to prevent steroid abuse include:

1. Sensitization and education of general practitioners and pharmacists – General practitioners and pharmacists are often the first point of contact for most of the patients. Training and sensitizing them regarding possible complications of these drugs and the extent of problem in the society would help to reduce the incidence of TS-related side effects [5]. Continuing medical education for residents in the dermatology department is also greatly needed. Also dissemination of information in this regard to the masses by means of mass media is of paramount importance.
2. Legal action – Legislation/stronger implementation of existing laws is required to limit public access and advertising of potent TCs. A law should be enacted enforcing immediate ban on the non-prescription sale of TCs. The authorities should also be requested to ensure that such laws are strictly enforced both in "letter and spirit" [6].
3. Audit of prescriptions – To reduce TS-related side effects especially with prolonged use, the rational use of TSs should include careful consideration of the patient's age, total area of application, quantity to be applied, efficacy of the selected steroid and frequency of application. Hence, one step to achieve rational prescribing is periodic auditing of prescriptions [18].
4. Proper prescriptions – There should be more emphasis on rational and complete prescription of TSs. The prescription of very potent steroids should be limited. The prescription pattern may be influenced by availability in the hospital pharmacy and choice of dermatologist. The medical community should prescribe with a social perspective in mind and should not follow practices which would be detrimental to the society.
5. Education about dispensing TSs – To achieve maximum effectiveness, patients must be encouraged to apply TSs appropriately. Dermatologists must inform the patients about the TSs to be applied on different parts of the body. The use of FTU, which provides guidelines regarding the amount of ointment needed based on specific anatomic areas, should be practiced widely to reduce variations in the use of TSs and to encourage adherence to therapy [18].
6. Revision of hospital formulary – There is a need to revise hospital formulary where low-potency TSs should be included along with potent ones so that the latter can be avoided in conditions where they are unnecessary. The hospital authorities should make low-potency steroids available in the hospital pharmacy keeping in mind the adverse effects of potent steroids.
7. Evaluation of drug utilization pattern – There is a need to do periodic evaluation of drug utilization pattern to enable suitable modification in the prescription of drugs to reduce the side effects and improve benefit [18].
8. Sensitization of policy makers – The potential hazards of TS abuse need to be explained and discussed with policy makers in order to sensitize them to the grave problem of steroid abuse [10].
9. Inclusion of TSs under schedule H – The Indian government should bring TSs, except for those with low potency, under schedule H to ensure their production and sale are regulated [8].

Conclusion

Pathetic misuse of TSs is becoming endemic at an increasing rate in the Indian rural setup. In India, free availability without a prescription from a registered physician has allowed many of these drugs to become household names, where they are hardly regarded as drugs anymore [2].

Misuse of TSs especially over the face and also as a cream for any skin problem is increasing at an alarming rate. Proper education, sensitization, regularization of prescriptions, and strict legal rules and actions would go a long way in curbing the TS abuse menace.

References

1. Saraswat A, Lahiri K, Chatterjee M, Barua S, Coondoo A, Mittal A, et al. Topical corticosteroid abuse on the face: a prospective, multicenter study of dermatology outpatients. Indian J Dermatol Venereol Leprol. 2011;77:160–6.
2. Sinha A, Kar S, Yadav N, Madke B. Prevalence of topical steroid misuse among rural masses. Indian J Dermatol. 2016;61(1):119.
3. Jha AK, Sinha R, Prasad S. Misuse of topical corticosteroids on the face: a cross-sectional study among dermatology outpatients. Indian Dermatol Online J. 2016;7:259–63.
4. Hengge UR, Ruzicka T, Schwartz RA, Cork MJ. Adverse effects of topical glucocorticosteroids. J Am Acad Dermatol. 2006;54:1–18.
5. Nagesh TS, Akhilesh A. Topical steroid awareness and abuse: a prospective study among dermatology outpatients. Indian J Dermatol. 2016;61(6):618–21.
6. Coondoo A. Topical corticosteroid misuse: the Indian scenario. Indian J Dermatol. 2014;59(5):451–5.
7. Rathi S. Abuse of topical steroid as cosmetic cream: a social background of steroid dermatitis. Indian J Dermatol. 2016;51:154–5.
8. Verma SB. Topical corticosteroid misuse in India is harmful and out of control. BMJ. 2015;351:H6079.
9. Mahe A, Ly F, Aymard G, Dangou JM. Skin diseases associated with the cosmetic use of bleaching products in women from Dakar, Senegal. Br J Dermatol. 2003;148:493–500.
10. Verma SB. Sales, status, prescriptions and regulatory problems with topical steroids in India. Indian J Dermatol Venereol Leprol. 2014;80(3):201.
11. Dey VK. Misuse of topical corticosteroids: a clinical study of adverse effects. Indian Dermatol Online J. 2014;5:436–40.
12. Coondoo A, Phiske M, Verma S, Lahiri K. Side-effects of topical steroids: a long overdue revisit. Indian Dermatol Online J. 2014;5:416–25.
13. Chohan SN, Suhail M, Salman S, Bajwa UM, Saeed M, Kausar S, Suhail T. Facial abuse of topical steroids and fairness creams: a clinical study of 200 patients. J Pak Assoc Dermatol. 2014;24(3):204–11.
14. Mehta AB, Nadkarni NJ, Patil SP, Godse KV, Gautam M, Agarwal S. Topical corticosteroids in dermatology. Indian J Dermatol Venereol Leprol. 2017;82:371–8.
15. Ljubojeviae S, Basta-JuzbaSiae A, Lipozeneiae J. Steroid dermatitis resembling rosacea: aetiopathogenesis and treatment. J Eur Acad Dermatol Venereol. 2002;16:121–6.
16. Sneddon I. Adverse effect of topical fluorinated corticosteroids in rosacea. Br Med J. 1969;1:671–3.
17. Mandapati JS, Metta AK. Intraocular pressure variation in patients on long-term corticosteroids. Indian Dermatol Online J. 2011;2:67–9.
18. Rathod SS, Motghare VM, Deshmukh VS, Deshpande RP, Bhamare CG, Patil JR. Prescribing practices of topical corticosteroids in the outpatient dermatology Department of a Rural Tertiary Care Teaching Hospital. Indian J Dermatol. 2013;58(5):342–5.

Topical Corticosteroid Abuse in Nepal: Scenario

18

Anil Kumar Jha, Subekcha Karki, and Sagar Mani Jha

Abstract

Nepal is a developing country, and at present, there are no proper health insurance plans readily accessible to all citizens. Anyone who has health issues hesitates to visit a doctor. Rather than treating any problem at its initial stage and preventing complications, patients do the pre-doctor trial method. One of the major problems this tendency has led to is the increase in steroid abuse and steroid-induced dermatosis. So the underlying problem to be addressed to minimise this problem is *ignorance and illiteracy*. The pain is not just that the patient wastes their money on such preparation; the real pain is when these preparations increase the problem and add new ones too.

Keywords

Steroid abuse • Steroid-induced dermatosis • Over-the-counter medications (OTC medications)

A.K. Jha (✉)
DI Skin Health and Referral Centre, Maharajgunj, Kathmandu, Nepal
e-mail: dranilkjha@hotmail.com; docanilabe@yahoo.co.in

Nepal Medical College, Attarkhel, Jorpati, Kathmandu, Nepal

S. Karki
DI Skin Health and Referral Centre, Maharajgunj, Kathmandu, Nepal
e-mail: doctorakarki@gmail.com

S.M. Jha
DI Skin Health and Referral Centre, Maharajgunj, Kathmandu, Nepal

Shree Birendra Army Hospital, Kathmandu, Nepal
e-mail: sagarmanijha@gmail.com

Learning Points

1. Masking effects of topical steroids.
2. Raise awareness among patients, general public and also doctors and health care givers about the steroid induced dermatosis.

18.1 Introduction

Corticosteroids have anti-inflammatory, immunosuppressive, anti-proliferative and vasoconstrictive effects. It is the most frequently

© Springer Nature Singapore Pte Ltd. 2018
K. Lahiri (ed.), *A Treatise on Topical Corticosteroids in Dermatology*,
DOI 10.1007/978-981-10-4609-4_18

prescribed dermatologic drug products (Fig. 18.1). Steroids are effective at reducing the symptoms of inflammation, but do not address the underlying cause of the disease [1].

Common conditions where topical steroids are prescribed (alone or in combination with other medications) [1] are as follows:

Psoriasis
Atopic dermatitis
Seborrheic dermatitis
Intertrigo
Nummular eczema
Lichen simplex chronicus
Lichen planus
Allergic contact dermatitis
Papular urticaria
Common adverse effects of topical steroids [1–3]:
Skin atrophy

Acneiform reactions, steroid-induced acne/rosacea/perioral dermatitis
Hypertrichosis
Pigmentary changes
Development of infections
Steroid-induced dermatosis

18.2 Current Scenario

This chapter is an overview of the current scenario that we dermatologists practising in different parts of Nepal deal with in our day-to-day practice.

Nepal is a developing country, and at present, there are no proper health insurance plans readily accessible to all citizens. Anyone who has health issues hesitates to visit a doctor. Rather than treating any problem at its initial stage and

---

GENERIC NAME
Class 1–Superpotent
  Betamethasone dipropionate 0.05% optimized vehicle
  Clobetasol propionate 0.05%

  Diflorasone diacetate 0.05%
  Fluocinonide 0.1% optimized vehicle
  Flurandrenolide, 4 mg/cm²
  Halobetasol propionate 0.05%
Class 2–Potent
  Amcinonide 0.1%
  Betamethasone dipropionate 0.05%

  Desoximetasone 0.25%
  Desoximetasone 0.5%
  Diflorasone diacetate 0.05%

  Fluocinonide 0.05%
  Halcinonide 0.1%
  Mometasone furoate 0.1%
Class 3–Potent, upper mid-strength
  Amcinonide 0.1%
  Betamethasone dipropionate 0.05%
  Betamethasone valerate 0.1%
  Diflorasone diacetate 0.05%

Fluocinonide 0.05%
Fluticasone propionate 0.005%
Class 4–Mid-strength
  Betamethasone valerate 0.12%
  Clocortolone pivalate 0.1%
  Desoximetasone 0.05%
  Fluocinolone acetonide 0.025%
  Flurardrenolide 0.05%
  Hydrocortisone probutate 0.1%
  Hydrocortisone valerate 0.2%
  Mometasone furoate 0.1%
  Prednicarbate 0.1%
  Triamcinolone acetoride 0.1%
Class 5–Lower mid-strength
  Betamethasone dipropionate 0.05%
  Betamethasone valerate 0.1%
  Fluocinolone acetonide 0.025%
  Flurandrenolide 0.05%
  Fluticasone propionate 0.05%
  Hydrocortisone butyrate 0.1%
  Hydrocortisone valerate 0.2%
  Prednicarbate 0.1%
  Triamcinolone acetonide 0.1%
Class 6–Mild strength
  Alclometasone dipropionate 0.05%
  Desonide 0.05%

  Fluocinolone acetonide 0.01%

Class 7–Least potent
  Topicals with dexamethasone, flumethasone, hydrocortisone
  Methylprednisolone, predrisolone

Fig. 18.1 List of topical corticosteroids according to their potency [1]

preventing complications, patients do the pre-doctor trial method. One of the major problems this tendency has led to is the increase in steroid abuse and steroid-induced dermatosis.

Many topical preparations are sold in pharmacy as an over-the-counter medication (OTC), i.e. these can be given to patients without doctor prescription. There are no definite guidelines for OTC and prescription medication. Hence, when there are several problems, especially in relation to dermatology such as itching, urticaria and pigmentation, etc., people take the advice of the person in pharmacy and without any proper examination start OTC. Currently one of the most frequently selling OTC products is topical steroids. In the lack of proper law and also absence of licenced pharmacists, topical steroids are sold like common household products (it would not be wrong to say that it is sold like toothpaste).

18.3 Patient Perspective

Also from the patients' side since they do not know about the strength, effects, side effects and contraindications of topical steroids, they use it. As we all know, topical steroids reduce inflammation: the patient feels relieved after its use, no matter what the real problem is, and instead of consulting the experts, they continue using it.

So be it, knowingly or unknowingly topical steroids are being abused by the person in pharmacy as well as the patients themselves. Several times there are also unlabelled, non-licenced creams and other topical preparations which are sold in the market, beauty parlour, cosmetic shops and advertising agencies claiming to be herbal, special formulations or authentic skin creams with no medications. Several times even the topical cosmetic creams sometimes repack steroids or mix steroids with cosmetic creams and label them as being pure cosmetics.

But no matter who is abusing it or why the trend is increasing, ultimately the patient suffers! When the indications are not correct, usually *steroids mask the real problem*; they give temporary relief, and the patient gets habituated to its use. There is development of steroid dependency; whenever the patient uses steroid, there is relief from the problem, but once they try to stop it, either the problem comes back again or it even gets worse with other new problems.

Hereby, we shall discuss few such common scenarios: *steroid-induced dermatosis due to steroid abuse*.

18.4 Scenario

18.4.1 Case 1

A 23-year-old unmarried female who is living and working in Kathmandu as a sales girl in a supermarket noticed hyperpigmentation over her B/L cheeks and nose area; she asked her friend who had clearer skin and was told she was using some cream given to her at the pharmacy. Without giving it a second thought, she went to the pharmacy and asked if they had cream for her problem and was given mometasone furoate.

18.4.1.1 Problem
The person at the pharmacy was not a trained or licenced pharmacist; he was like any other shopkeeper, selling and making profit. There was no diagnosis, treatment was incorrect and no guidelines for its use were given.

18.4.1.2 Result
After few weeks since there was lightening of the pigmentation, she started using mometasone like a night cream. She was unaware of the harm that it would do in the long run. She also got complements from her friend that her skin was getting better. Weeks to months to years, then she developed 'steroid dependency'.

She visited my clinic with multiple acnes; hyperpigmentation over the forehead, nose, and B/L cheek; and sun sensitivity which also got worse if she stops using mometasone.

Steroid-induced dermatosis is one of the most common causes of dermatology consultation in Nepal. But patients are unaware.

18.4.2 Case 2

A 20-year-old male student working in a tea shop had itching around the groin area; he went to a nearby pharmacy and got some cream which after 2 days of application relieved his itching. After a few days, there was itching again, and he continued the remaining cream. This went on for few months, and in the meantime, he was also using the cream over other body parts which were itching. On the sixth month, he realised the itching was becoming more severe, and even after applying the cream, there was only temporary relief and the itching was back again. He also noted that there were many patches of white to red in colour over different body parts.

18.4.2.1 Problem

This 'it's just an itch' kind of thought either from the patient's side or unauthorised people selling medicines either from shops, parlours, door-to-door salesperson or pharmacy has made simple fungal infection, i.e. tinea infection into tinea incognito, i.e. in simple terms one that was treated with wrong medications and has flared up.

18.4.2.2 Result

The boy spent almost 100–200 every month on those creams, once he was able to see the lesions himself and the look of it scared him. Six months after having the problem, he visited the clinic with tinea incognito with steroid-induced striae over the thigh areas. The challenge was not only to treat him but also to convince him he was using all wrong kinds of medicines under different brand names.

These few cases are only examples of how topical steroid has been misused in our country (Figs. 18.2, 18.3 and 18.4). Topical steroids are given as OTC (over the counter) for any kind of

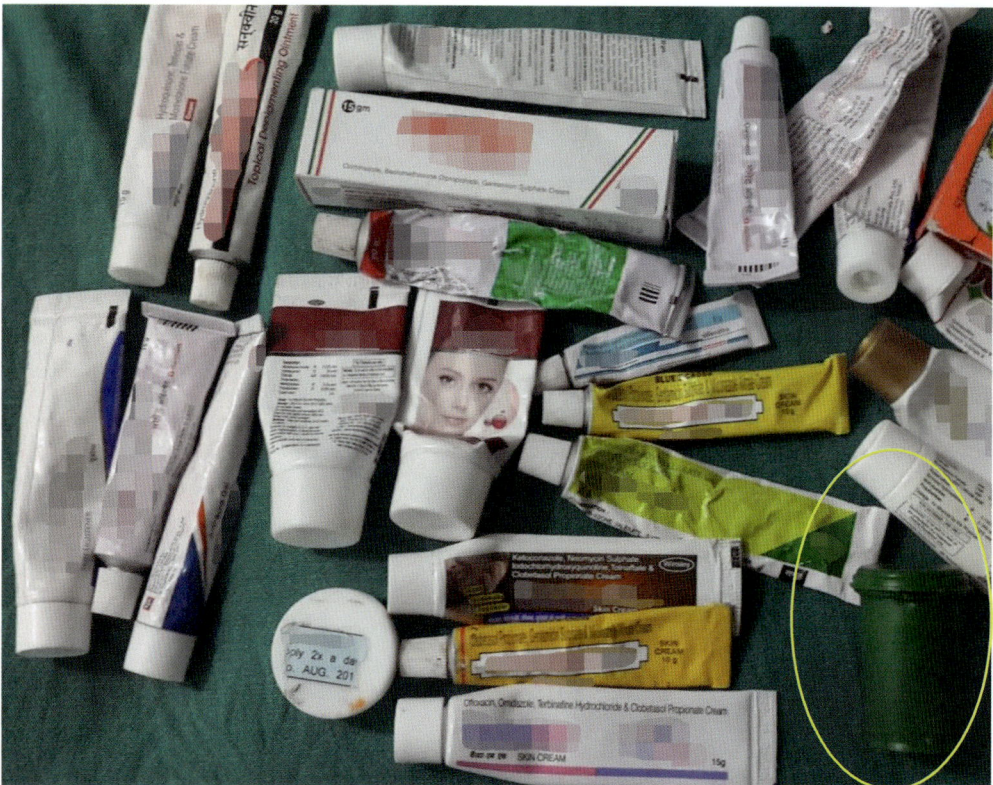

Fig. 18.2 Within a period of 3 months while preparing for the article, we started collecting such topical medications which patients had been abusing unknowingly and had brought along with for evaluation

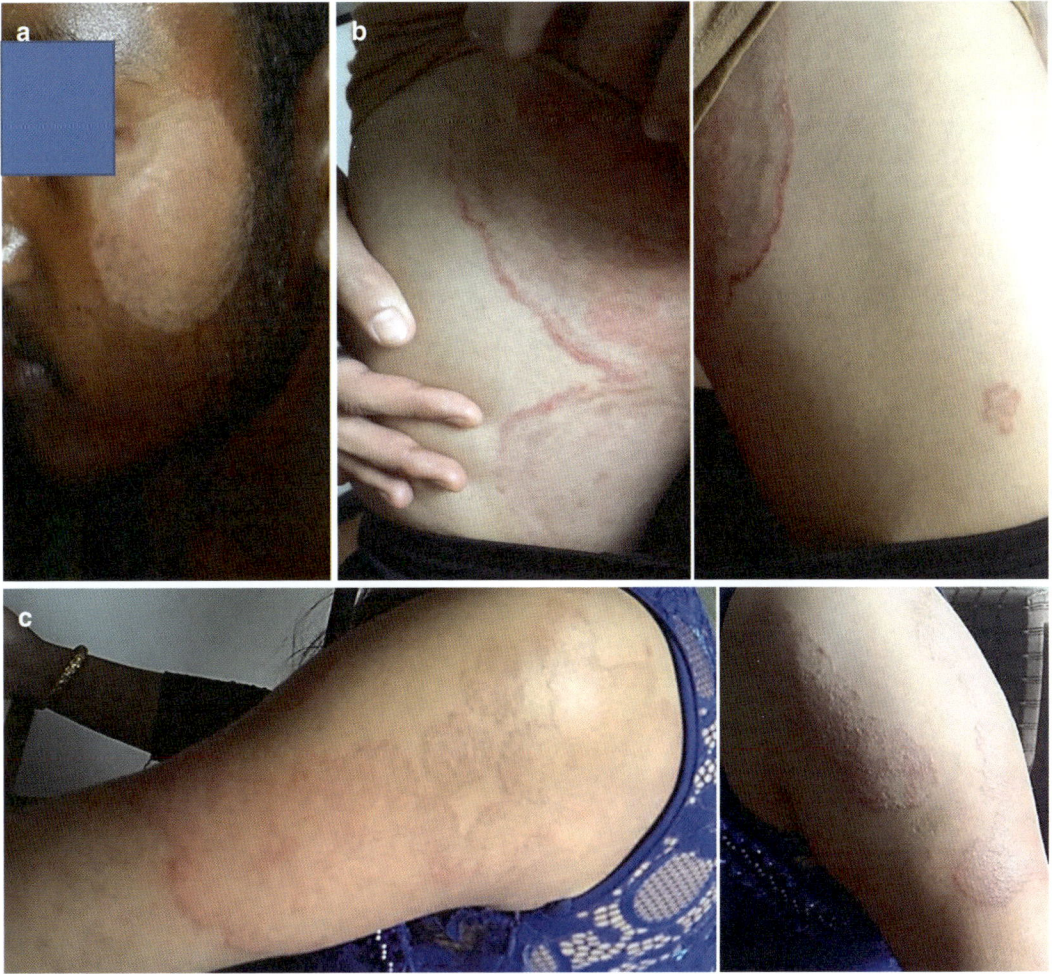

Fig. 18.3 Tinea incognito: (**a**) tinea fasciei, (**b**) tinea cruris and (**c**) tinea corporis. (Photo courtesy: Dr. Subekcha Karki, MD)

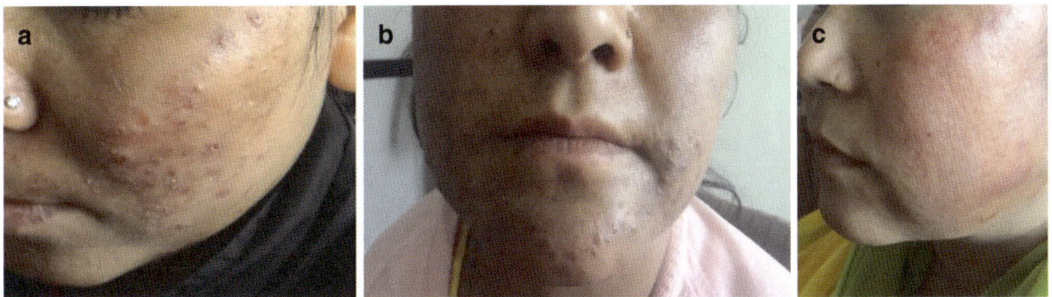

Fig. 18.4 Steroid-induced facial dermatosis: (**a**) acneiform eruption, (**b**) hyperpigmentation, (**c**) rosacea and (**d**) telangiectasia

problem, be it melasma, freckles, allergies, fungal infection, bacterial infection, etc.

List of common steroids abused for a period ranging from 5 months to 3 years among the patients visiting DI Skin Health and Referral Center (DISHARC) OPD consultation (list from the most common to the least common):

Mometasone furoate in combination with hydroquinone + tretinoin

Mometasone furoate + hydroquinone 4%

Clotrimazole + *beclomethasone*

Clotrimazole + *beclomethasone* + gentamicin

Clobetasol propionate + gentamicin + miconazole cream base

Clobetasol propionate + neomycin + tolnaftate + iodochlorhydroxyquinolone + ketoconazole

Ofloxacin + ornidazole + terbinafine + *clobetasol propionate*

Clobetasol propionate + neomycin + clotrimoxazole

Unlabelled in small plastic containers

A 3-month data analysis of OPD cases at DI Skin Health and Referral Center (DISHARC) with various steroid abuse-related dermatoses:

- Over a period of 3 months, we did a data analysis at DI Skin Health and Referral Center (DISHARC). There were 36 new cases of steroid misuse causing steroid-induced dermatosis and tinea incognito.
- There were 15 male and 24 female patients.
- There were 27 cases of tinea incognito and 12 steroid-induced facial dermatoses.

A 3-month data analysis of OPD cases at Shree Birendra Army Hospital, Kathmandu, Nepal, Department of Dermatology with various forms of topical steroid abuse

Conclusion

Both data are from two different health centres situated in Kathmandu City which is also the capital of the country. This reflects the scenario where people who have access to specialist abuse topical medications. Hence, it would not be wrong to say that the problem is severe in rural areas (Figs. 18.5, 18.6, 18.7, 18.8 and 18.9).

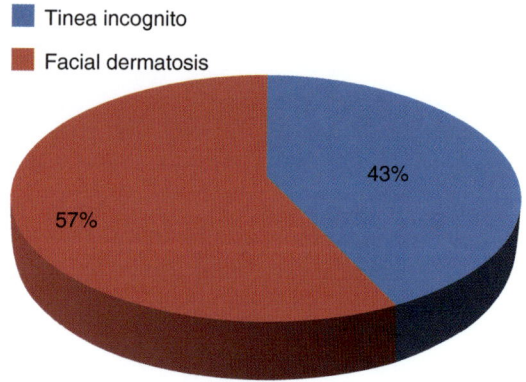

Fig. 18.5 Disease distribution

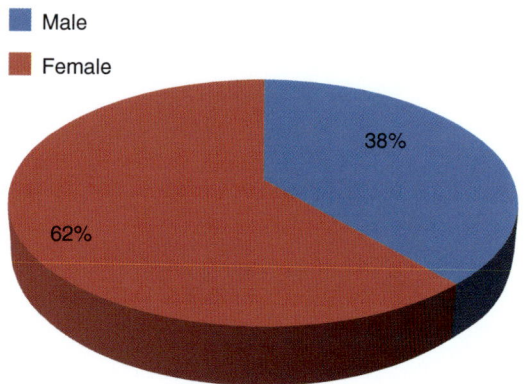

Fig. 18.6 Sex distribution

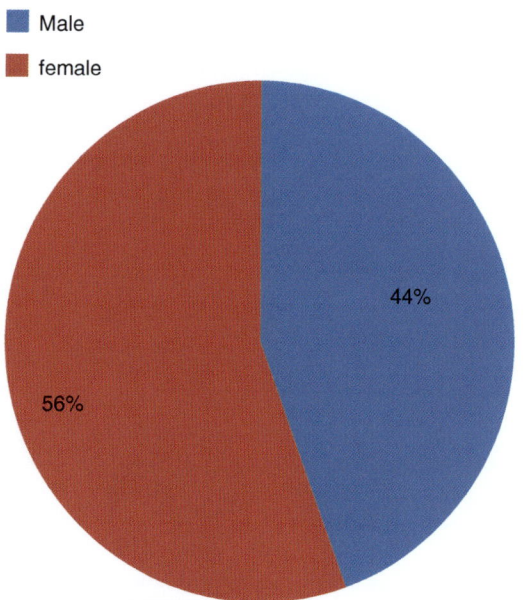

Fig. 18.7 T. incognito

Fig. 18.8 Facial dermatosis due to steroid abuse

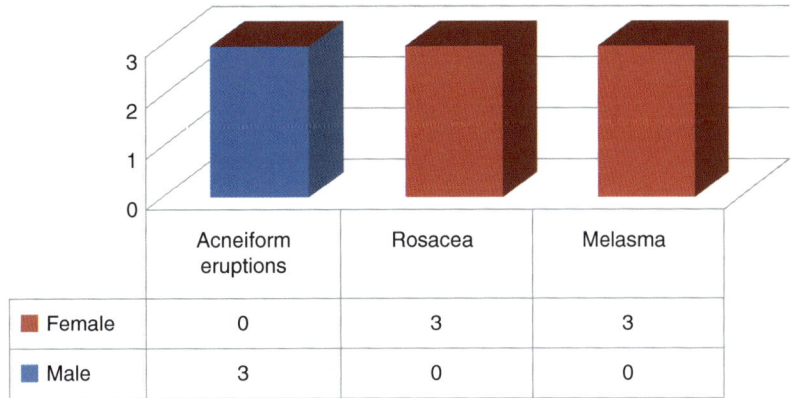

	Acneiform eruptions	Rosacea	Melasma
Female	0	3	3
Male	3	0	0

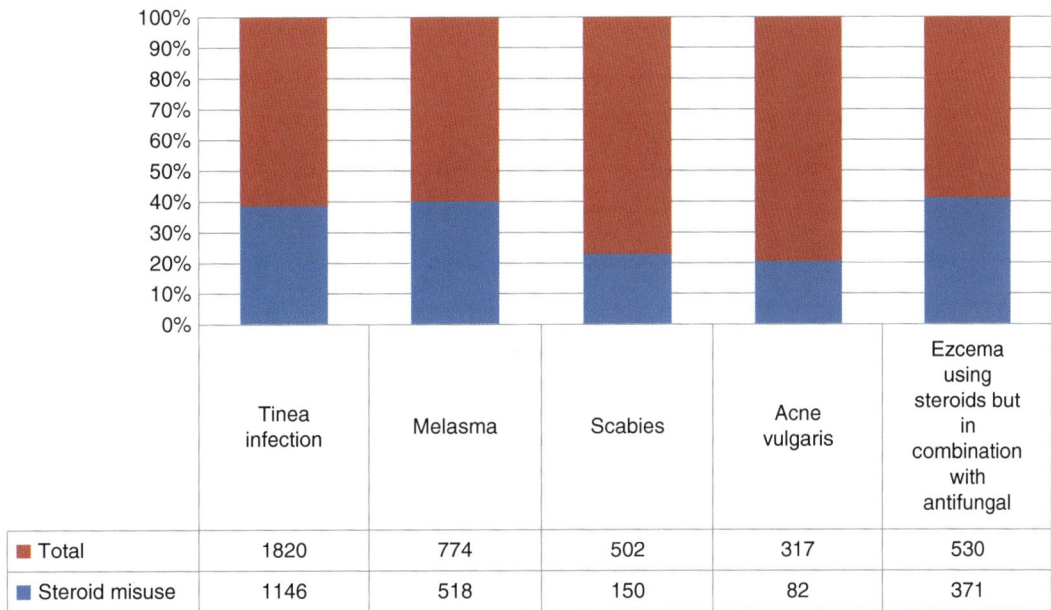

	Tinea infection	Melasma	Scabies	Acne vulgaris	Ezcema using steroids but in combination with antifungal
Total	1820	774	502	317	530
Steroid misuse	1146	518	150	82	371

Fig. 18.9 Percentage of cases with steroid abuse prior to specialist consultation

The data show a significant amount of patient with topical steroid abuse and also various dermatoses due to its abuse. The condition among rural are as where people do not have any access or the lack of specialist is suffering from steroid-induced dermatosis. The steroid abuse is usually carried out without the knowledge of the patient themselves. The creams they avail from various places are considered to be harmless and hence used continually which result to various complications.

So the underlying problem to be addressed is how to minimise IGNORANCE AND ILLITERACY.

The current need is to:

- Monitor and set laws for selling of unlabelled products.
- Make people aware through mass media about the reality.
- Regulate for not selling such preparations without prescriptions.

The pain is not just that the patient wastes their money on such preparation; the real pain is when these preparations increase the problem and add new ones too. It is very disappointing to see people trust these people who themselves are unaware about what the problem is, what they are giving is, what consequences it carries and how morbid the patients become.

Acknowledgement Registration offices of DI Skin Health and Referral Center, Maharajganj, Kathmandu, Nepal, Department of Dermatology and Shree Birendra Army Hospital, Kathmandu, Nepal.

References

1. Wolff K, Goldsmith L, Katz S, Gilchrest B, Paller AS, Leffell D. Topical steroids. In: Fitzpatrik's dermatology in general medicine, Ch-216. 7th ed. p. 2102.
2. James WD, Berger T, Elston D. Andrews' diseases of the skin. In: Clinical dermatology. Philadelphia, PA: Saunders; 2011. p. 968.
3. Bolognia JL, Jorizzo JL, Schaffer JV. Dermatology. 4th ed. Brasil: Elsevier; 2015.

Topical Corticosteroid Abuse: Bangladesh Perspective

19

M.U. Kabir Chowdhury

Abstract

Topical corticosteroid abuse is a major dermatological problem in Bangladesh. Rampant over the counter sale of potent steroid containing creams is the main reason. These creams are being misused by the ignorant citizens as fairness products or as antifungal creams. The quacks, general physicians, non dermatological physicians and even homeopaths prescribe potent steroids without realising the impending danger from these products. A stringent law and strict application of such law is needed to stop this menace.

Keywords

Corticosteroids • Steroid creams • Steroid abuse

Learning Points

1. Topical steroid abuse is a shameful reality in Bangladesh today.
2. Potent steroid containing creams are available OTC.
3. The side effects of indiscriminate usage can lead to catastrophic consequences.
4. Strict law and application of such law is needed.

M.U. Kabir Chowdhury
Principal, Shamorita Medical College Hospital, Dhaka, Bangladesh

Professor of Dermatology, Holy Family Medical College, Dhaka, Bangladesh

Director, Kabir National Skin Centre, Dhaka, Bangladesh

Ex Visiting Professor, Faculty of medicine, University of Ottawa, Ottawa, Canada
e-mail: mukabir@gmail.com

History of glucocorticoid use is not very long but only started in 1920. Anabolic steroid use starts in the early twentieth century. Testosterone is the prime hormone which guides the body to have strength and energy. Testosterone propionate injection was first introduced in human in the late 1930s only.

Use of topical steroid was successfully introduced in 1952 with good results.

All topical steroids have got anti-inflammatory activities with vasoconstrictive abilities. Longtime use of topical steroid causes numerous side effects and damages of the skin.

Topical corticosteroids are in use for various dermatological ailments with good success, though long and continued use of topical steroid may cause skin atrophy with telangiectasia. Sometimes it causes tachyphylaxis, which means particular topical steroid is not effective anymore. However side effects depend on the potency and type of corticosteroids.

© Springer Nature Singapore Pte Ltd. 2018
K. Lahiri (ed.), *A Treatise on Topical Corticosteroids in Dermatology*,
DOI 10.1007/978-981-10-4609-4_19

197

Use of topical corticosteroids depends on the types and duration of dermatological disorders. Also types of preparation like ointments, emulsions, liquids, and gels are used according to the type of the particular lesion, site, and disease entity.

Commonly used steroids are adrenocortical hormones in dermatological disorder due to potent anti-inflammatory activities.

According to potency, local corticosteroids are generally classified into five grades:

Strongest
- Clobetasol propionate
- Diflorasone diacetate

Very strong
- Amcinonide
- Diflucortolone valerate
- Difluprednate
- Fluocinonide
- Mometasone furancarboxylate

Strong
- Beclomethasone propionate
- Betamethasone valerate
- Fluocinolone acetonide
- Prednisolone acetate

Medium or mild
- Alclometasone propionate
- Clobetasone butyrate
- Dexamethasone
- Flumethasone pivalate
- Hydrocortisone butyrate
- Triamcinolone acetonide

Weak
- Hydrocortisone acetate
- Methylprednisolone acetate
- Prednisolone

The effect and potency of a topical corticosteroid depend on the formulation and the base of the application. Potency is also increased when a formulation is used under occlusive dressing or in flexor areas. In general, ointments are more potent than creams or lotions.

Topical steroids have wide use in dermatology in many dermatoses and dermatitis. Major use of topical steroids are in pruritus, psoriasis vulgaris, asteatotic eczema, nummular dermatitis, seborrheic dermatitis, lichen planus, lichen simplex, lichen simplex chronicus, atopic dermatitis, discoid lupus, lichen sclerosus et atrophicus, and alopecia areata.

Longtime uses of topical steroid may cause tachyphylaxis; to prevent such problem, we usually ask patient to apply such drugs with thin film and low quantity. Some patients are advised to stop the topical steroid after a week and re-start on alternate days. This process helps to prevent tachyphylaxis.

All types of topical steroids that are in use almost always have magical results, but side effects also are very noticeable. It depends on potency and type of topical steroid.

Local side effects or adverse effects of topically applied steroids are as follows:

- Steroidal acne (Fig. 19.1)
- Capillary telangiectasia (Fig. 19.2)
- Delayed wound repair

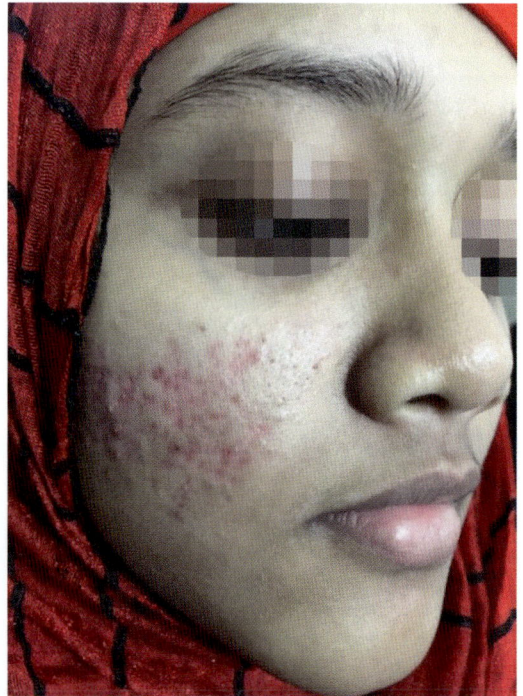

Fig. 19.1 Steroid acne

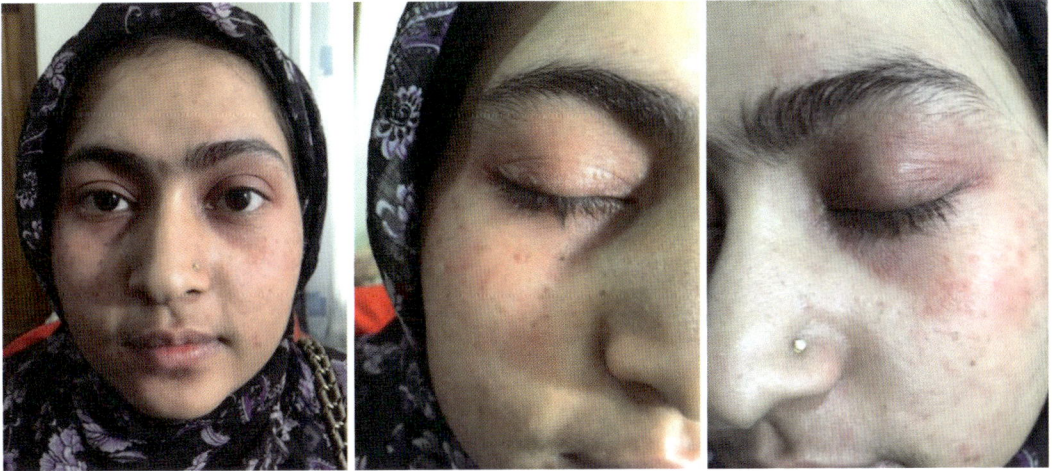

Fig. 19.2 Severe erythema with skin atrophy in telangiectasia

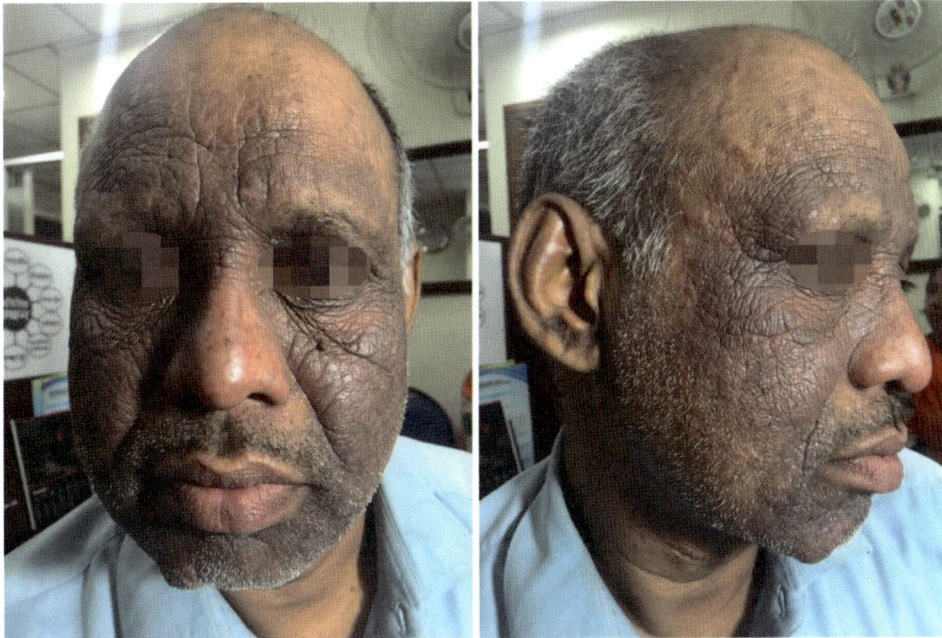

Fig. 19.3 Steroid abuse with whitening agent caused photodermatitis with solar prurigo

- Hypertrichosis due to excessive use of steroid
- Photodermatosis due to sun sensitivity (Fig. 19.3, Fig. 19.4)
- Pigmentation disorder
- Rosacea-like dermatitis
- Skin atrophy (Fig. 19.2)
- Steroid acne milium/colloid milium
- Steroid elastosis
- Steroid purpura/flush
- Steroid skin injury
- Steroidal contact dermatitis
- Striae atrophicans
- Susceptibility to bacterial, fungal, and viral infections
- Xeroderma/ichthyosiform cutaneous symptoms

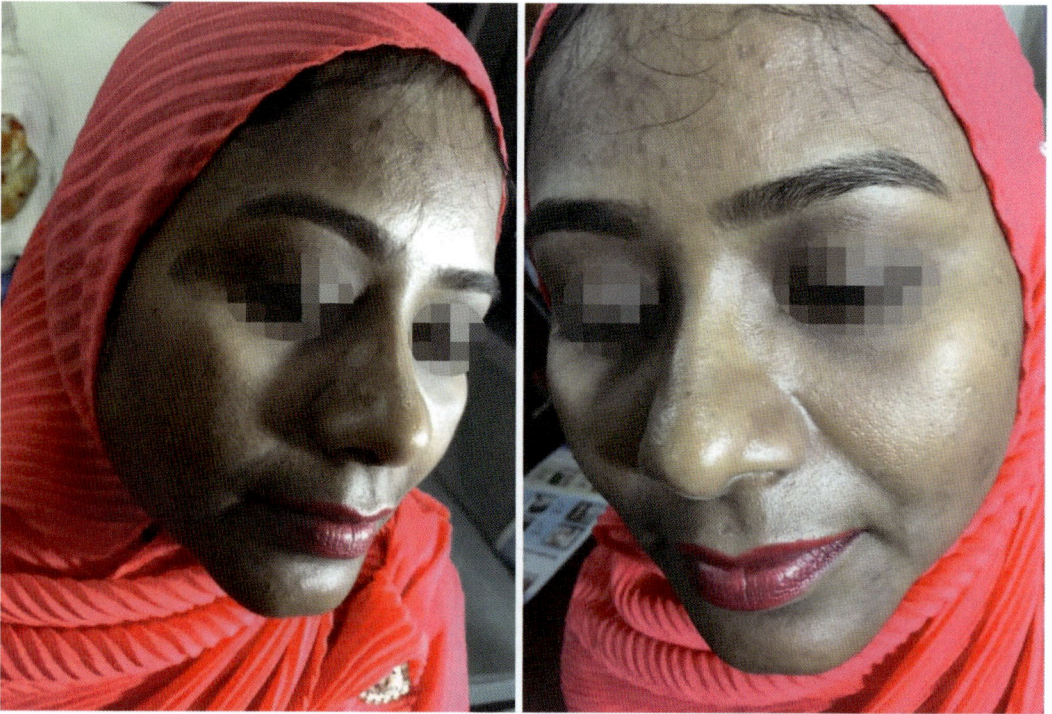

Fig. 19.4 Severe photosensitivity after over use of steroid with combination of whitening agent

Also glaucoma or cataract may develop due to topical use of eye ointments or drops.

Systemic side effects of potent topical steroids are also noticed due to percutaneous absorption which is common in infant and young children.

Topical corticosteroids are widely used and also misused and even abused. In our country these medications are sometimes unsupervised and even used without prescription, just like OTC medicine. These sorts of condition cause unnoticed bad effects, side effects, and adverse effects which are undesirable. These sorts of problems are commonly seen in the use of corticosteroid on the facial skin.

Use of steroid over the face is mainly done by females, which is common in Bangladesh. The commonest misused drug in Bangladesh is betamethasone valerate. The most common side effect observed is acneiform eruptions followed by steroid dependency and steroidal dermatitis resembling rosacea or red face.

This type of misuse is done by quacks and patients themselves mostly due to unknown knowledge of consequence or ignorance.

Repeated use of topical corticosteroids in various skin problems in Bangladesh is common, which is detrimental for facial skin. For magic symptomatic relief in many skin diseases, our patients use steroid topically without knowing its side effects.

In Bangladesh, so many dark complexion women and even men use steroid as a fairness cream solely or with the combination of known fairness cream.

In close observation for 30 years, I have noticed most of the abusers are young people who come from poor socioeconomic families and uneducated background. They usually get this information from the neighbors, relatives, friends, colleagues, and even from advertisement in electronic media.

Other than steroid so many persons in Bangladesh use different types of whitening and lightening fairness cream which is common in dark complexion girls or women. Those creams sometimes contain hydroquinone and inorganic mercury and even mixed with steroid also.

Bleaching effects of these creams usually have severe side effects. Sometimes these products are phototoxic and cause photodermatitis resulting in hyper- or hypopigmentation of skin surface.

These sorts of mixed formulation have multidimensional mechanisms of action which lightened dark skin in pursuit of fair complexion. So many persons, boys and girls, adults and adolescents, and even elderly women, are victims of these circumstances. They need no prescription as topical steroids are sold in local pharmacies even cosmetics or grocery shops in Bangladesh.

As discussed, the side effects of topical steroids with or without other agents cause more serious side effects instead of fairness. These sorts of creams may cause contact dermatitis and exogenous ochronosis with irreversible whitening of the skin, and also severe hyperpigmentation is not uncommon which usually happened due to phototoxicity.

So many students and young female garment workers are victims of the circumstances of skin lightening creams. Misguided by advertisements of steroid containing lightening cream, they are attracted to use those creams and continue to use them until it causes serious burning and hyper- and hypopigmentation of their facial skin. These gullible individuals are erroneously advised to use these creams by their relatives, friends and neighbors. Abuse of topical steroid is a big problem in Bangladesh.

Sometimes users became habituated or addicted with the use of steroid, so it is difficult for them to leave it suddenly.

The following creams are available in Bangladesh as a fairness or beauty cream: (1) Stillman's Bleach® cream, (2) Golden Pearl®, (3) GM Cream, and (4) Shirley Cream, and so many fairness cream named or unnamed are widely used in Bangladesh.

Unnoticed, unwarranted, and unauthorized use of fairness cosmetics are creating problem in Bangladesh which need special attention from the Drug Control Authority of the country. Only then can we save the young generation from side effects of abusing steroid, fairness cream, and other complicated skin preparations.

Considering the benefit of topical corticosteroids of early symptomatic relief, this drug is prescribed for patients of almost all type of dermatoses except fungal and bacterial infections. Even sometimes it is wrongly used for the treatment of the diseases in fungal infection causing worsening of the condition. Adverse conditions have to be managed by skin specialist in Bangladesh. Abuse of topical corticosteroid in Bangladesh is common due to easy availability of the drugs. Sometimes topical corticosteroids are abused for the treatment of acne which reduces inflammation though it comes back with double magnitude after withdrawal of the medication. Abuse of topical steroid is a burning issue in Bangladesh.

The situation of abuse of steroid is alarming in this country because the young generation is using this sort of steroid cream for cosmetic purpose, though it is not recommended by the dermatologist.

Improper and wrong use of topical steroid causes many problems in this society. Sometimes potent steroids are used in the body folds, face, and other parts of the body which causes flare of fungal infections and thinning of the skin. In my practice I have overcome these types of problem which is increasing day by day. Use of steroid in fungal infection causes diagnostic dilemma for the dermatologist in those patients. Abuse of steroid is an emerging problem in Bangladesh.

It is well known that steroid reduces inflammation resulting in wonderful outcome, but it relapses after withdrawal of the drug with high magnitude.

In dermatological practice, titration dose of steroid is used to overcome withdrawal relapse and tachyphylaxis.

Abuse of corticosteroid is already a big problem which needs countrywide awareness through social, electronic, and paper media.

In Bangladesh, we need extensive awareness among the doctors, patients, and general population. All of us must know the magnitude of abuse causing impairment of daily quality of life index of the abuser of topical steroids.

More than three decades in practice in Bangladesh as a dermatologist, I found so many patients of steroid overuse, misuse, and abuse. We as dermatologists use topical steroid in so many indications of skin problems. However, systemic use of steroid is limited in the practice of dermatology. But I have seen that due to ignorance of unregistered medical practitioners, both urban and rural areas use steroid in undiagnosed cases of skin diseases. Even in every month, I do see more than 100 patients who attended to my OPD with serious side effects of topical steroids on the face which is difficult to handle. Most of them developed tachyphylaxis with telangiectasia and atrophy. In those cases sometimes, I have to use topical steroid again to withdraw gradually or tapering doses. Mometasone furoate is the best topical application that is applied to withdraw from topical steroid abuse. Sometimes it takes weeks or months to come out from steroid addiction. Other than the face, there are lots of complications of topical steroid including striae and thinning of skin. Steroidal striae are sometimes very serious and became untreatable due to severe thinning of the skin. In those cases they cannot use anymore topical steroid which aggravates the existing lesions. In atopic dermatitis children, use of topical steroid may cause systemic side effects due to absorption through the skin. In any patient of topical steroid use, we should take extra care for prevention of steroidal side effects. Using titration or tapering doses of steroid is the best way to prevent of steroidal side effects. Proper use of steroid needs extensive research awareness for medical practitioners. It will help to do counseling for the patient population of the country. My recommendation for Bangladesh is "any type of steroid must not be easy available or as an otc product."

Not only is the topical steroid abuse a problem but also systemic corticosteroid abuse is well known in Bangladesh. A Reuter report says, "Young females in Bangladesh that are involved in prostitution take steroids to get weight and bulk up. Ninety percent (90%) prostitutes at the 15 legal whorehouses from Bangladesh apply the corticosteroid Oradexon. Ninety percent equal to 900 young prostitutes that use this corticosteroid regularly. Steroid is also used in Bangladesh for fattening of Cattle."

All concerned government and nongovernment organizations should fight together to control abuse of steroid in Bangladesh within no time.

Bibliography

Al-Dhalimi MA, Aljawahiri N. Misuse of topical corticosteroids: a clinical study from an Iraqi hospital. East Mediterr Health J. 2006;12:847–52.

Al-Saleh I, Shinwari N, Al-Amodi M. Accumulation of mercury in ovaries of mice after the application of skin lightening creams. Biol Trace Elem Res. 2009;131: 43–54.

Aso M, Shimao S. Problems in steroids for topical use. Hifubyo Shinryo. 1988;10:984–91. (in Japanese)

Chen AYY, Zirwas MJ. Steroid-induced rosacea like dermatitis: case report and review of the literature. Cutis. 2009;83:198–204.

Del Rosso JQ. Management of papulopustular rosacea and perioral dermatitis with emphasis on iatrogenic causation or exacerbation of inflammatory facial dermatoses. J Clin Aesthet Dermatol. 2011;4: 20–30.

Ghosh A, Sengupta S, Coondoo A, Jana AK. Topical corticosteroid addiction and phobia. Indian J Dermatol. 2014;59:465–8.

Hameed AF. Steroid dermatitis resembling rosacea: a clinical evaluation of 75 patients. Dermatology. 2013;2013:1–4. doi:10.1155/2013/491376.

Leyden J, Thew M, Kligman AM. Steroid rosacea. Arch Dermatol. 1974;110:619–22.

Mahe A, Ly F, Aymard G, Dangou JM. Skin diseases associated with the cosmetic use of bleaching products in women from Dakar, Senegal. Br J Dermatol. 2003;148:493–500.

Mukhopadhyay AK, Baghel V. A study to evaluate the efficacy and safety of hydrocortisone aceponate 0.127% lipophilic cream in steroid responsive dermatoses in Indian patients. Indian J Dermatol Venereol Leprol. 2010;76:591.

Pitche P, Afoune A, Amage U, et al. Prevalence of skin disorders associated with the use of bleaching cosmetics by Lome women (French). Sante. 1997;7(3):161–4.

Rathi SK, Kumrah L. Topical corticosteroid induced rosacea like dermatitis: a clinical study of 110 cases. Indian J Dermatol Venereol Leprol. 2011;77:42–6.

Sangeeta M. Fair war. A case study on fairness cream. Int J Contemp Bus Stud. 2012;3:46–54.

Saraswat A, Lahiri K, Chatterjee M, et al. Topical corticosteroid abuse on face: a prospective multicenter study of dermatology outpatients. Indian J Dermatol Venereol Leprol. 2011;77:160–6.

Shankar PR, Subish P. Fair skin in South Asia: an obsession. J Pak Assoc Dermatol. 2007;17:100–4.

Shimao S. Problems in topical steroid therapy: Q & A. Hifubyo Shinryo. 1983;5:77–83. (in Japanese)

Sin KW, Tsang HF. Large-scale mercury exposure due to a cream cosmetic: community-wide case series. Hong Kong Med J. 2003;9:329–34.

Sulzberger MB, Witten VH. The effect of topically applied compound F in selected dermatoses. J Invest Dermatol. 1952;19:101–2.

Ullah H, Noreen S, Fozia et al. Comparative study of heavy metals content in cosmetic products of deferent countries marketed in Khyber Pakhtunkhwa, Pakistan. Arabian J Chem. 2013. Available from: http://dx.doi.org/10.1016/j.arab. Accessed 25 Dec 2013.

WHO. Mercury in skin lightening products. 2013. Available from: www.who.int/ipcs/assessment/public_health/mercury_flyer.pdf. Accessed 24 Dec 2013.

Bangladesh's dark brothel steroid secret by Mark Dummett BBC News.

Topical Corticosteroid Use in the Middle East

20

Hassan Galadari

Abstract

The use of topical steroids in the Middle East is quite common as the regulations of dispensing to patients are lax. Even though the uses of these medications are limited in the pediatric population in fear of their possible side effects, their use in adults is mainly in the treatment of pigmentary disorders. Given that such conditions are common, abuse is highly possible. The occurrence of adverse events, such as atrophy, is common in this population group.

Keywords

Middle East • Pigmentary disorders • Steroids • Prescription • Education

Learning Points

1. Topical steroids are an important part of the dermatologists' armamentarium in the treatment of many inflammatory conditions.
2. The use of topical corticosteroids is important in children as they are the gold standard in the treatment of atopic dermatitis, a condition that is common in the Middle East.
3. Abuse of these medications occurs in adults especially for the treatment of conditions such as melasma.
4. Strict regulation should be enforced when prescribing such drugs so as they do not get dispensed without a prescription.
5. Regulation should also be enforced on outlets that promote compounded medications without label as some might contain strong corticosteroids as part of their ingredient.
6. Education is important among the public to ensure informed decision-making in their health care.

H. Galadari, MD, FAAD
College of Medicine and Health Sciences,
United Arab Emirates University,
Al Ain, United Arab Emirates
e-mail: hgaladari@uaeu.ac.ae

© Springer Nature Singapore Pte Ltd. 2018
K. Lahiri (ed.), *A Treatise on Topical Corticosteroids in Dermatology*,
DOI 10.1007/978-981-10-4609-4_20

The use of topical corticosteroids in the Middle East is quite high comparatively to that of the United States and the West. Though there is an apprehension of their use given perceived side effects, such limitation only exists in the pediatric population. The use of the creams, however, is made more readily available due to the lack of regulatory bodies controlling their dispensing. Pharmacies do not require prescriptions in order for them to hand in even Class I steroid creams. The patient may either ask for it by name or the pharmacist would volunteer giving the medication if the patient describes that he or she has eczema or an itchy lesion. That being said, the patient may still have that apprehension if they are aware that the cream they are handed out is actually steroid in nature.

Thus, it is important to break down patients into two distinct groups: pediatric and adult. This is done so, given the fact that their reaction to a steroid-based medication is different as well as the reason why they are using it to begin with.

20.1 Pediatric Population

The general consensus of people from the Middle East is that in children steroid creams are bad. Parents fear that their children may become addicted to the medications and also fear of systemic adverse events, such as striae and weight gain. This apprehension is at times in a manner disproportionate to the actual reason why such medications may be prescribed, and this may cause an impediment to treatment. Some patients' parents would refuse steroid-containing creams to treat their child's atopic dermatitis no matter how severe. This poses a great challenge to the practitioner when it comes to the use of such medications, and that is why other nonsteroidal agents, such as calcineurin inhibitors, are preferred. Even with the black box label associated with tacrolimus and pimecrolimus, their uses are much less maligned by the general population than steroid-containing agents.

To help counter the negative publicity associated with steroids, doctors, including dermatologists, have sought to compounding glycerin-containing

ointments with a Class III or IV steroids. Those may be sold from mainly doctors' offices as well as pharmacies. Some doctors do not mention the ingredients of these agents, and they are not disclosed on the containers that they are sold from. This is done mainly to help appease the population's fear of the use of steroid agents.

As for the agents used in the pediatric population, the main class of steroids are those that are Class III or IV with mometasone being the most widely used. Other agents include hydrocortisone valerate and hydrocortisone butyrate. Rarely, Class I or II, such as clobetasol and betnovate, is prescribed, and those are usually reserved for extremely severe cases.

The population is still not accepting the concept of control and maintenance therapy when it comes to the use of these agents for treating chronic conditions. The medicines would be applied up to a certain time, usually 2 weeks, and then abruptly stopped. This causes, of course, a relapse in the condition. When the medicines are prescribed again, patients refuse using them given that they had had an unsatisfactory prior history of their use. This further adds fuel to the fear of using steroids, as they are generally seen as a temporary and unreliable fix.

20.2 Adult Population

Adults follow two different trains of thought when it comes to the use of topical steroids. In the first instance, which relates to their use in chronic conditions, such as atopic dermatitis, psoriasis, and vitiligo, they are thought of in a similar apprehensive fashion as that seen in the pediatric population. Adults would not readily use such agents and would rather use other alternative treatment modalities than steroids. Fear of adverse events is the key issue to noncompliance, but the other would be the temporary effect of steroids in treating these conditions. Unlike in the West, health literacy is not high in the Middle Eastern population even though living in affluent countries of the Gulf. A survey conducted by Zayed University of the United Arab Emirates showed that less than half (48%) had a reasonable level of knowledge based on an understanding of food labels, despite the majority studying public health and nutrition (78.6%). Among those who had "inadequate" understanding, there was a correlation with family education levels; 91% had a father who had a lower education level than the student, and 71.4% had a mother who had a lower education level. The literacy of this cohort is 100% with the most relying on online forums and social media as sources of health information. That being said, chronic conditions that are receptive to treatment but with no cure are not thought of as such. The population still believes that topical agents should in finality cure their psoriasis, for example. If they do not, then these agents are deemed inferior and may not be used again because of this. In addition, patients are not loyal to one doctor, with second opinions sought by many. Due to this practice, dermatologists end up switching patients from one agent to another, even a generic of the same, without the knowledge that such agents are one and the same.

The second practice pertaining to the adult population is the use of these medications in cosmetic procedures. Pigmentary disorders, such as melasma and postinflammatory hyperpigmentation in the Middle Eastern population, are quite high, due to fact that the majority are of Fitzpatrick skin type IV and V. In addition, intertriginous parts of the body as well as the elbows and knees are naturally darker. Steroids in the forms of creams and ointments are usually prescribed as part of treatment regimen to help "whiten" dark areas [1]. Those are usually combined with a retinoid cream and hydroquinone. Steroids in this form are readily acceptable. The mixture may be found premixed, or patients are prescribed these agents and instructed to mix these agents on the palm prior to applying them on the face. When prescribed in such manner, there is no issue that is related to this. The dilemma occurs when patients begin to self-medicate, and they do so either by acquiring agents directly from the pharmacy given that they do not require a prescription or even from Internet sites. These mixtures are sold as bleaching agents and are used heavily [2]. These agents are those that give steroids their notoriety, and their general misuse is a huge impediment to proper health care. The horror stories associated with steroid use emanate from this population group; people who are not content with their complexion and seek a remedy to "unify" their skin tone. This population is vulnerable to the gaffe in the system where Class I steroids are prescribed without a prescription, leading to atrophy and reported cases of cataracts and blindness [3].

In conclusion, it is important that the use of topical steroids be regulated in the Middle East. No country that belongs to the region requires a prescription for the patient to receive the medication from the pharmacy. In addition, they can also be sold online through social media sites promising fairer skin of a lighter tone. Health literacy does help in this regard, with those knowing the potential dangers undertaking a much more informed approach in their self-care and self-image. People should not fear the use of these agents and should not overuse them with a promise of perceived beauty. Only when this approach is taken will proper use of not just topical steroids but all prescription-based medications be deemed safe for use [4].

References

1. Nnoruka E, Okoye O. Topical steroid abuse: its use as a depigmenting agent. J Natl Med Assoc. 2006;98(6):934–9.
2. Sinha A, Kar S, Yadav N, Madke B. Prevalence of topical steroid misuse among rural masses. Indian J Dermatol. 2016;61(1):119. doi:10.4103/0019-5154.174081.
3. Dey VK. Misuse of topical corticosteroids: a clinical study of adverse effects. Indian Dermatol Online J. 2014;5(4):436–40. doi:10.4103/2229-5178.142486.
4. Nagesh TS, Akhilesh A. Topical steroid awareness and abuse: a prospective study among dermatology outpatients. Indian J Dermatol. 2016;61(6):618–21.

Topical Corticosteroid Abuse: Southeast Asia Perspective

21

Evangeline B. Handog
and Maria Juliet Enriquez-Macarayo

Abstract

Topical corticosteroids (TCS), since its discovery in 1952, have been very useful for many dermatologic conditions, particularly inflammatory dermatoses. TCS abuse and misuse have been published and yet continue to exist. Considering that the indication of TCS use is correct, the duration of use, areas of application, and TCS potency/vehicle are the most important factors that may lead to potential side effects. To avoid TCS abuse, it is important to educate our patients well. Adverse reactions from TCS are similar in all countries. Frequency and degree vary due to different factors such as adherence to government policies, availability of different classes of TCS, and cultural differences and beliefs. Avoidance of abuse is vital and patient education plays a major role in this aspect.

Keywords

Topical corticosteroids • Use and misuse • Southeast Asia • Striae • Telangiectasia • Skin atrophy • Acneiform eruptions • Perioral dermatitis • Fungal infections • Furunculosis • Folliculitis • Perilesional hypopigmentation • Topical steroid dependent face • Cushingoid appearance

Learning Points

1. The benefits a patient derive from Topical Corticosteroids (TCS) are immense, however the misuse and abuse are really alarming as we see complications in our daily practice.
2. There should be awareness of the consequences of improper use of TCS due to patient's misinformation or lack of knowledge.
3. The risk of having TCS complications are almost the same for Southeast Asian patients.

E.B. Handog (✉)
Department of Dermatology,
Asian Hospital and Medical Center,
2205 Civic Drive, Alabang, Muntinlupa City 1780,
Philippines
e-mail: vangee@handog.net

M.J. Enriquez-Macarayo
Department of Dermatology, AUF Medical Center,
Pampanga, Philippines

© Springer Nature Singapore Pte Ltd. 2018
K. Lahiri (ed.), *A Treatise on Topical Corticosteroids in Dermatology*,
DOI 10.1007/978-981-10-4609-4_21

21.1   Introduction

For 65 years, topical corticosteroids (TCS) have evolved from their discovery by Sulzberger and Witten [1] to the development of multiple possible combinations with other molecules. There is no part of the world where TCS are non-existent.

Topical corticosteroid has been an important prescription for most inflammatory conditions. The result of TCS application has been almost dramatic in most cases, such that dermatologists, medical practitioners, and patients adhere to its use. As corticosteroid-responsive dermatoses [2, 3] have grown in the past years, so did the list of known adverse reactions from its use [4–7]. Efficacy and adversity of TCS are entangled in its potency, absorption and adequacy [8]. Guidelines have been set and constantly updated by expert groups on the proper handling and use of TCS. In this day and age, every medical practitioner and even the patients have easy access as to the the pros and cons of using TCS. However, topical steroid abuse does not seem to cease.

21.2   In Southeast Asia

There might not be major differences in practice with regards to TCS use in different parts of the world, including Southeast Asian countries (i.e., Brunei, Cambodia, East Timor, Indonesia, Laos, Malaysia, Myanmar, the Philippines, Singapore, Thailand, and Vietnam). As evident in a study conducted by Chan et al. [9], 91–100% of the respondent dermatologists from Southeast Asia utilize topical corticosteroids in children with mild to moderately severe atopic dermatitis. Judicious use of TCS for atopic dermatitis was likewise discussed in the consensus guidelines set by an Asia-Pacific expert panel [10] and acknowledged by a review led by Giam et al. [11]. What may be different are the following: formulation (branded and generic) availability, accessibility issues, socio-economic factors, country regulations, patient attitude and beliefs.

21.3   Factors Related to TCS Abuse

In our many years in the practice of dermatology, we have observed the following as significant factors in the occurrence of side-effects from TCS use:

Medical practice-wise:
- Misdiagnosis/product misinformation that leads to incorrect use of TCS
- Poor doctor-patient communication: medical history taking not thorough; insufficient instructions and patient education as to the proper use of TCS
- Improperly filled in prescriptions as to the amount and duration of TCS use

Pharmaceutical practice-wise:
- Source of "prescription": medical practitioners must be the only source of TCS prescription; however, with the laxity in restrictions, this is not the case. In many countries, advice as to its use comes from the pharmaceutical field (manufacturers, drugstores), paramedical personnel, media, family, friends, and neighbors.
- Easy accessibility: TCS (i.e., in pure forms, in fixed-dose combinations, in lightening products) may be procured as over-the-counter (OTC) medications in a majority of drugstores; the necessity of a medical prescription is not adhered to at all times whether it is the first purchase or a refill.

Media-wise:
- Internet and social media consults: medical information and management are easily availed, making the patients confident in treating themselves.
- Advertisements promoting several TCS products lead to confidence in procuring the product without proper consultation to a medical practitioner.

Patient/consumer-wise:
- Poor patient-doctor communication: language barrier leading to miscommunication; reluctance in asking questions; medical history not divulged in full.

- Poor patient education: leads to irresponsible usage of TCS; more so, amidst the proper instructions and education, persistence of indiscriminate use of TCS abounds. On the other hand, fear of use is another issue; factor to this is the misconception and misinformation on the viability of TCS use.
- Economics: avoidance of proper medical consultations to reduce expenses, resorting to paramedical or nonmedical consults and self-treatments.

21.4 Abuse from TCS: Clinical Presentations

In Southeast Asia, abuse from TCS comes in many forms, from local to systemic. Considering that the indication of TCS use is correct, the duration of use, areas of application, and TCS potency/vehicle are the most important factors that may lead to potential side effects.

Among the known cutaneous adverse effects [5], most commonly encountered in our region are:

Striae
- May be present on any area of application (Figs. 21.1, 21.2, 21.3, 21.4, and 21.5) but commonly seen on thin areas like the axillae

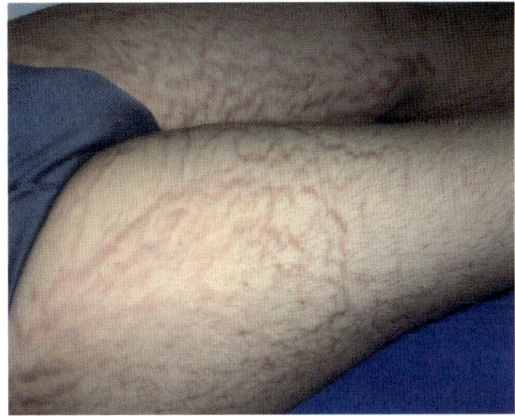

Fig. 21.2 Multiple striae on the thighs of an Indonesian male patient after daily application of clobetasol cream for over a month (Courtesy of Prof. Indropo Agusni, MD-DV, Indonesia)

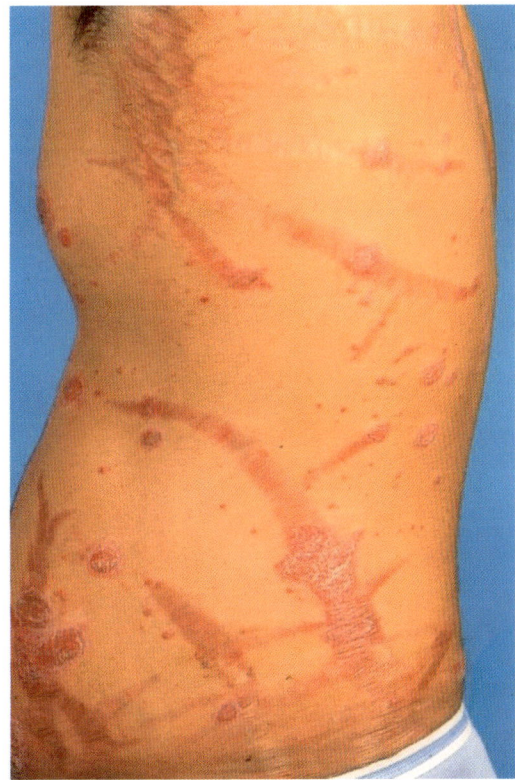

Fig. 21.3 Steroid-induced striae on the abdomen of a psoriatic Singaporean patient (Courtesy of National Skin Centre, Singapore)

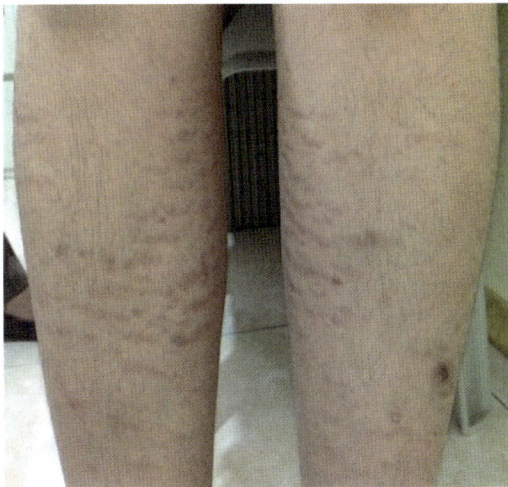

Fig. 21.1 Striae on the legs of a psoriasis teenage Filipino patient from prolonged application of clobetasol (Dermovate) cream (Courtesy of Dr. Ana Lucia Dela Paz, Philippines)

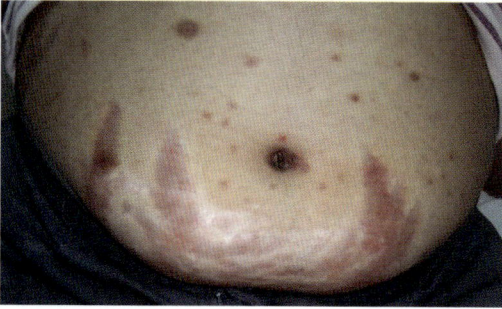

Fig. 21.4 Deep abdominal striae in a psoriatic Indonesian patient after application of many kinds of TCS (Courtesy of Prof. Indropo Agusni, MD-DV, Indonesia)

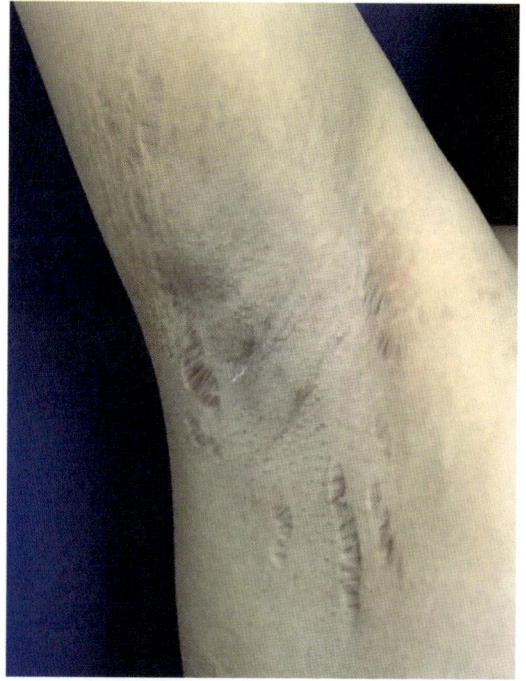

Fig. 21.6 Deep striae of the axillary regions in a 23-year-old Filipina female from a 1-month continuous application of topical clobetasol intended for "whitening" purposes, as prescribed by a medical doctor (Courtesy of Dr. Christene Pearl Arandia, Philippines)

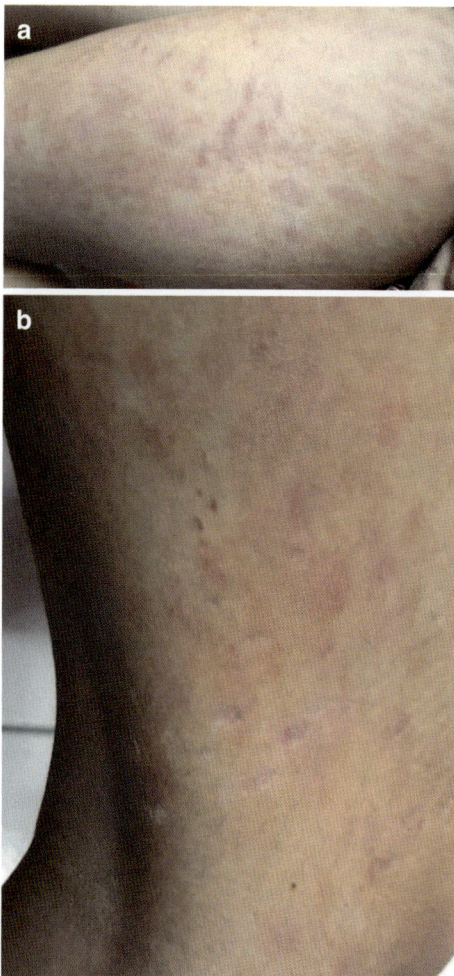

Fig. 21.5 Striae on the inner arms (**a**) and thigh areas (**b**) in a 13-year-old Filipina patient with psoriasis after 2 months of self-administered topical halobetasol propionate in petroleum jelly (Courtesy of the Department of Dermatology, Research Institute for Tropical Medicine, Philippines)

(Figs. 21.6, 21.7, 21.8, and 21.9) and groins (Figs. 21.10 and 21.11)

Telangiectasia
• Mostly on the face (Fig. 21.12) but on other areas of application as well (Fig. 21.13)

Skin atrophy (Figs. 21.11, 21.14, and 21.15)
• Though commonly seen in patients using superpotent TCS, prolonged use and excessive amounts of lower-potency TCS like triamcinolone can lead to atrophy [4, 5] (Fig. 21.16).
• As TCS suppresses proliferation of cells in the epidermis and later in the dermis, collagen synthesis is likewise inhibited [4]. Thinning becomes evident as loose crinkled skin, along with striae of various depths and hypopigmentation.

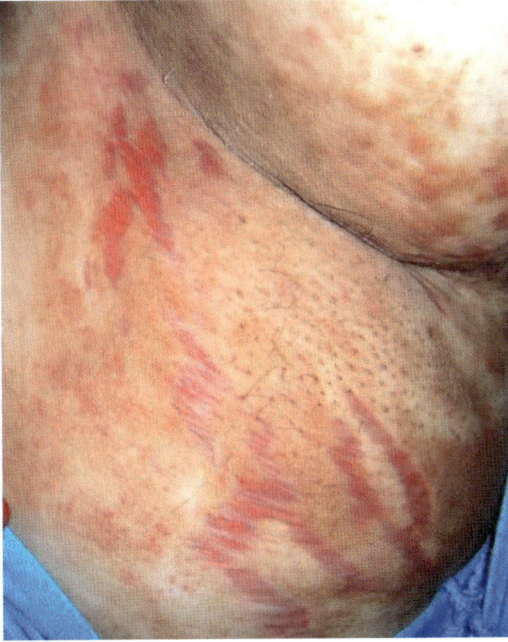

Fig. 21.7 Deep axillary striae in a 45-year-old Filipina female after prolonged application of betamethasone valerate cream 2× daily for 6 months on contact dermatitis lesions from herbal medications (Courtesy of Dr. Noemie Ramos, Philippines)

Acneiform eruptions
- Known to exist as a common side-effect of oral intake of corticosteroid but commonly seen with application of TCS (Figs. 21.17, 21.18, 21.19, 21.20, and 21.21) and even with inhaled steroid forms (Fig. 21.22).
- Though prolonged use of TCS may be a factor, there are some cases when only after a week's use of low-potency TCS like dexamethasone cream, acneiform lesions erupt.
- Appearance is the same for all and although improvement comes with stopping the steroid use, treatment is difficult in many patients and quality of life is much affected.
- The positive anti-inflammatory effect of the steroids may take its toll by leading to the undesirable increase in the cutaneous free fatty acids and pilosebaceous duct bacteria that may lead to comedogenesis [5, 12].

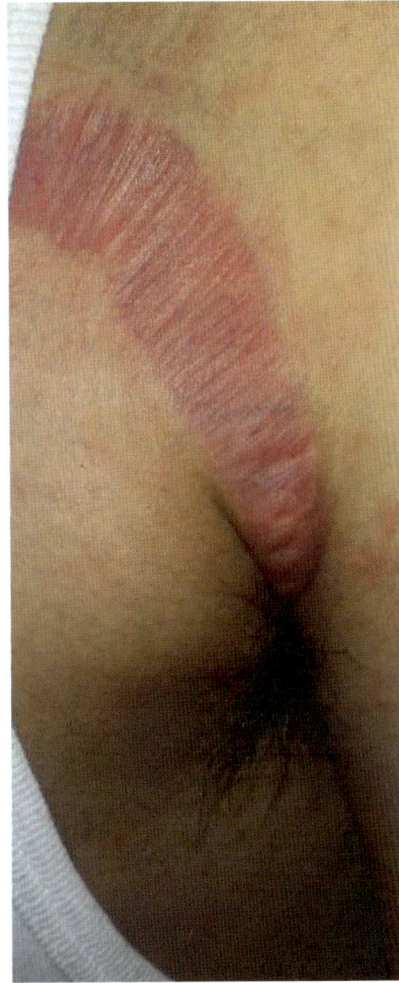

Fig. 21.8 Very deep striae on the axillae from prolonged topical steroid use in a Filipino male (Courtesy of the Department of Dermatology Jose R Reyes Memorial Medical Center, Philippines)

Aggravation of existing acne (Fig. 21.23)
- Occurs when acne cases are mistaken for a dermatitis treatable by TCS and when consumers are misled by misinformation on some OTC drugs (i.e., "BL" cream with clobetasol propionate and ketoconazole as ingredients, with indications as fungal infections and eczema and with price range of USD 30 cents—USD 1)

Perioral dermatitis (Fig. 21.24)
- When this occurs from injudicious use of TCS, even from low- to mid-potent strength,

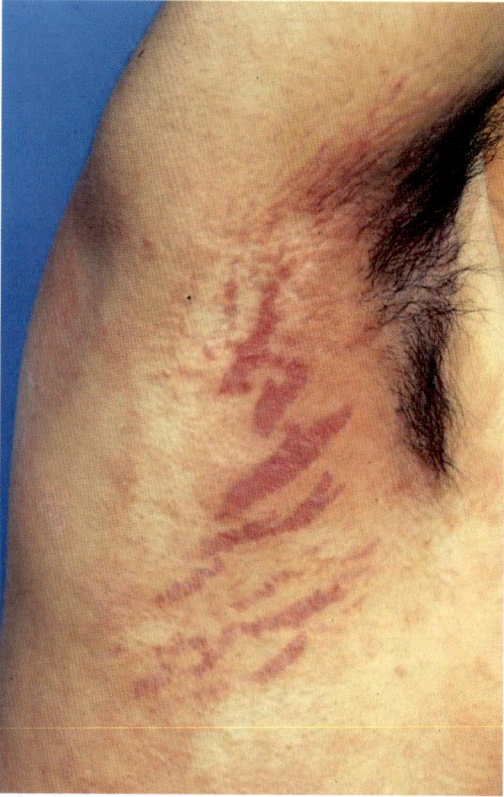

Fig. 21.9 Steroid-induced striae on the axillae in a Singaporean patient (Courtesy of National Skin Centre, Singapore)

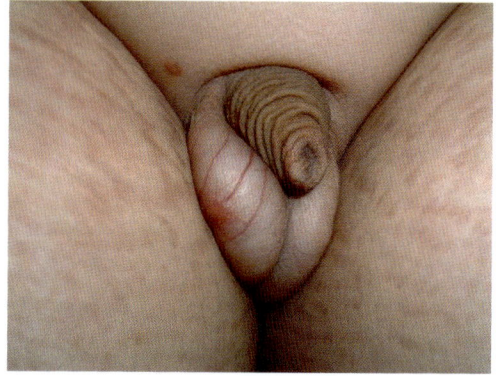

Fig. 21.11 Striae in the inguinal areas and atrophy of the scrotal skin from topical steroid application for diaper rash in a child (Courtesy of Dr. Rataporn Ungpakorn, Institute of Dermatology, Thailand)

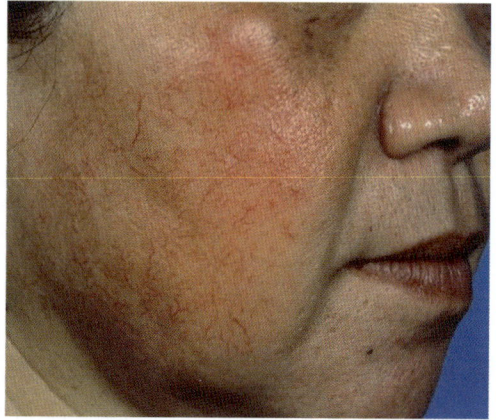

Fig. 21.12 Steroid-induced facial telangiectasia (Courtesy of National Skin Centre, Singapore)

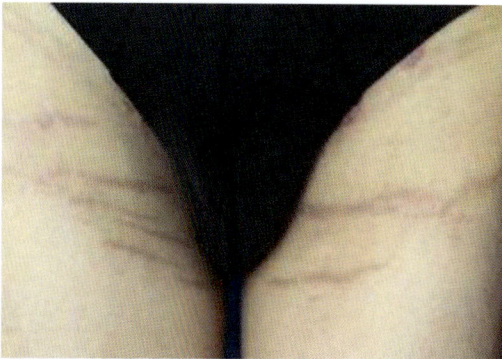

Fig. 21.10 Striae on both inguinal and thigh areas in a 21-year-old Filipino male with psoriasis who self-medicated with halobetasol propionate ointment and clo-betasol propionate ointment for 6 months (Courtesy of the Department of Dermatology, Research Institute for Tropical Medicine, Philippines)

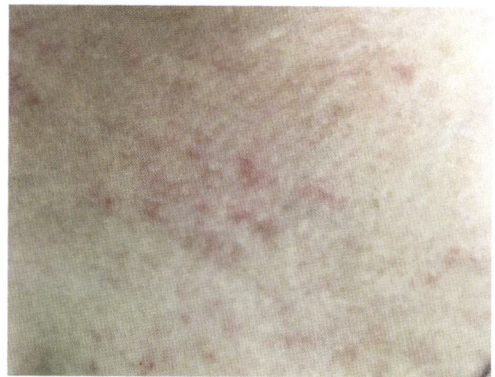

Fig. 21.13 Multiple telangiectatic atrophic lesions on the chest of a 46-year-old Filipina with folliculitis who self-medicated with clobetasol propionate cream 2× daily for 3 months (Courtesy of the Department of Dermatology, Research Institute for Tropical Medicine, Philippines)

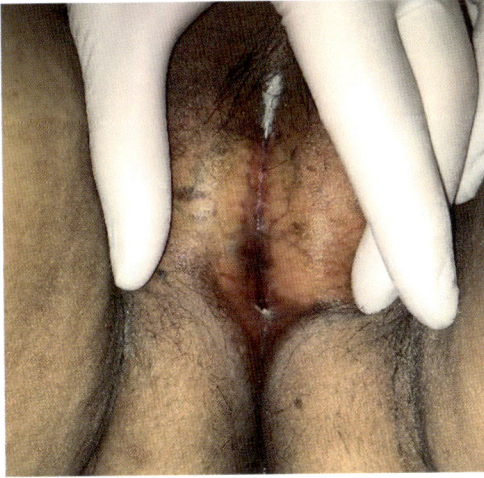

Fig. 21.14 Atrophic skin-colored patches with telangiectasia on the labia majora in a 69-year-old Filipina with mucosal lichen planus, noted with application of prescribed halobetasol propionate and betamethasone dipropionate ointment for 1 year (Note that resorption of labia minora has occurred prior to starting topical corticosteroid) (Courtesy of the Department of Dermatology, Research Institute for Tropical Medicine, Philippines)

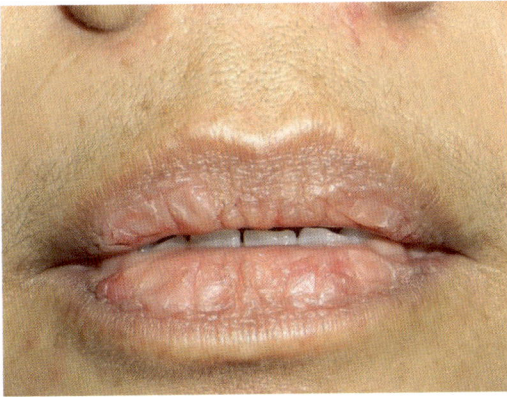

Fig. 21.15 Upper lip atrophy from potent topical steroid in a Thai patient (Courtesy of Dr. Rataporn Ungpakorn, Institute of Dermatology, Thailand)

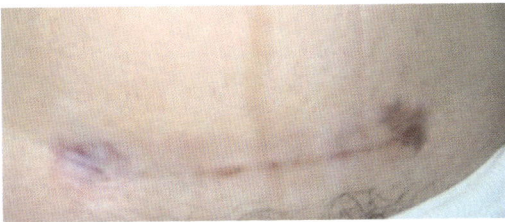

Fig. 21.16 Deep skin atrophy seen on this post-CS scar due to excessive use of triamcinolone creams (Courtesy of Prof. Indropo Agusni, MD-DV, Indonesia)

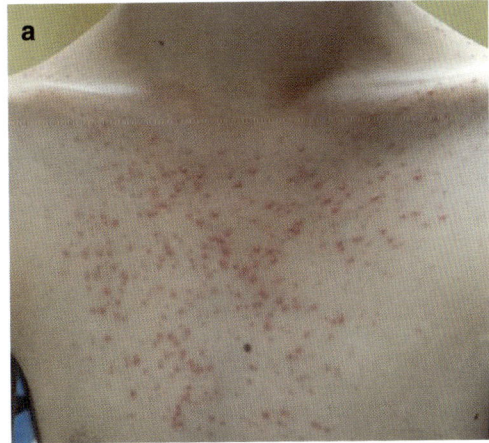

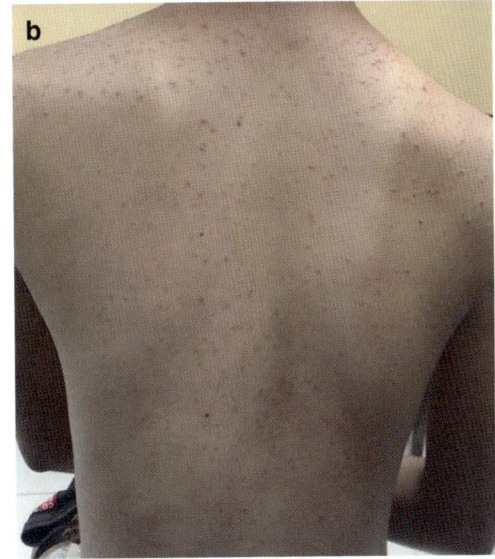

Fig. 21.17 Acneiform dermatitis on the (**a**) chest and (**b**) back in a 16-year-old Filipino male who applied a 2-week-prescribed desonide lotion 2× daily for 16 weeks for his pityriasis rosea (Courtesy of Dr. Roberto Pascual, Philippines)

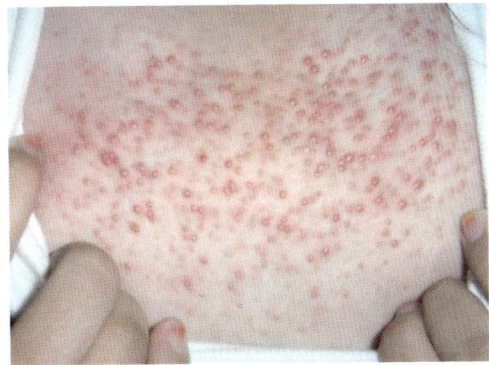

Fig. 21.18 Acneiform dermatitis on the chest of an Indonesian female (Courtesy of Prof. Indropo Agusni, MD-DV, Indonesia)

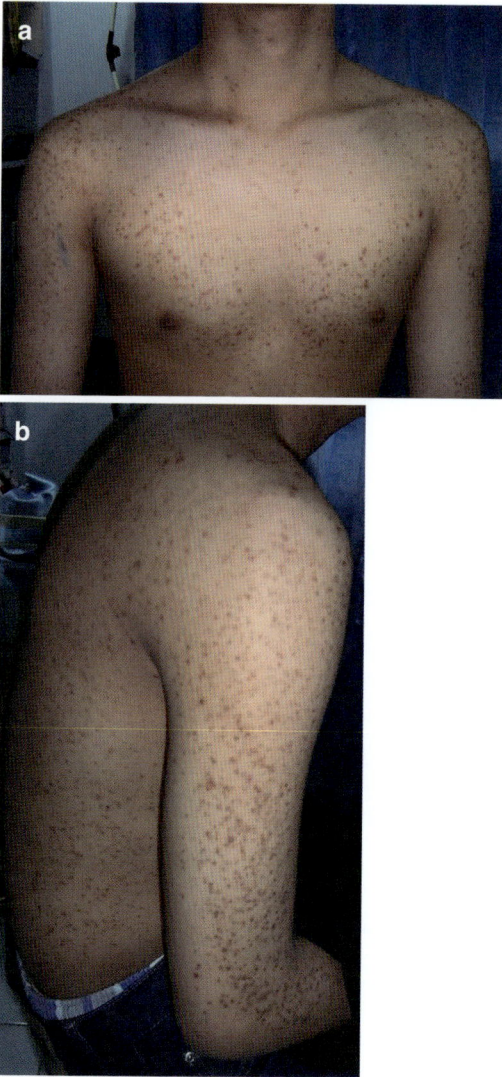

Fig. 21.19 Acneiform dermatitis, truncal (**a**) and extremities (**b**), in an Indonesian male (Courtesy of Prof. Indropo Agusni, MD-DV, Indonesia)

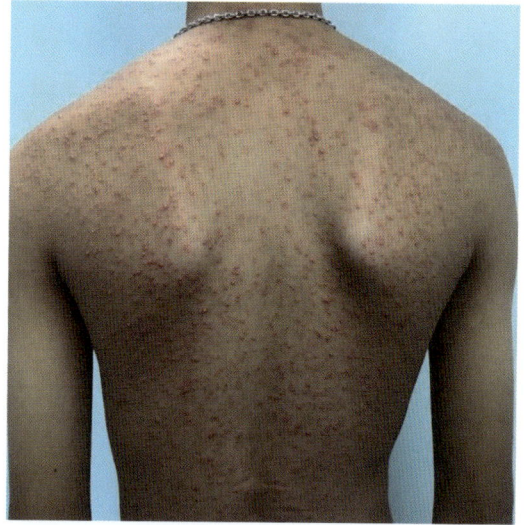

Fig. 21.20 Acne lesions in a Thai male treated with topical steroids for pityriasis versicolor (Courtesy of Dr. Rataporn Ungpakorn, Institute of Dermatology, Thailand)

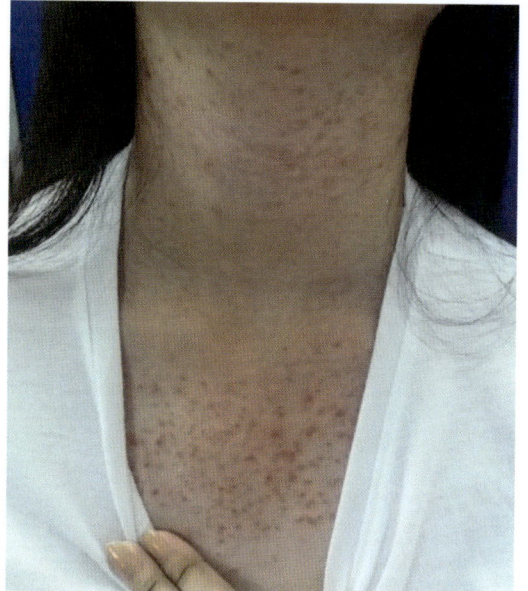

Fig. 21.21 Aggravation of acne lesions and eruption of acneiform papules due to application of BL cream (OTC clobetasol-ketoconazole combination cream) for 3 months in a 20-year-old Filipina patient (Courtesy of the Department of Dermatology, Research Institute for Tropical Medicine, Philippines)

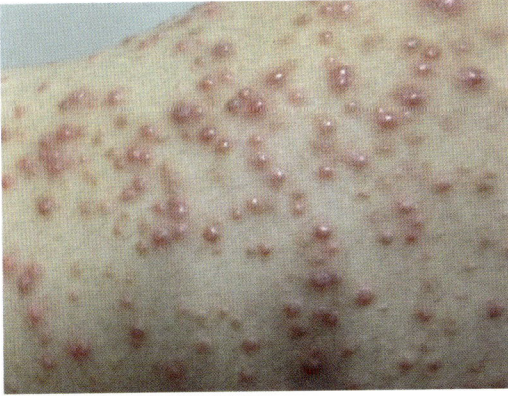

Fig. 21.22 Steroid acne developing in a Filipino patient after prolonged use of asthma inhaler (Courtesy of Dr. Ma. Flordeliz Abad-Casintahan, Philippines)

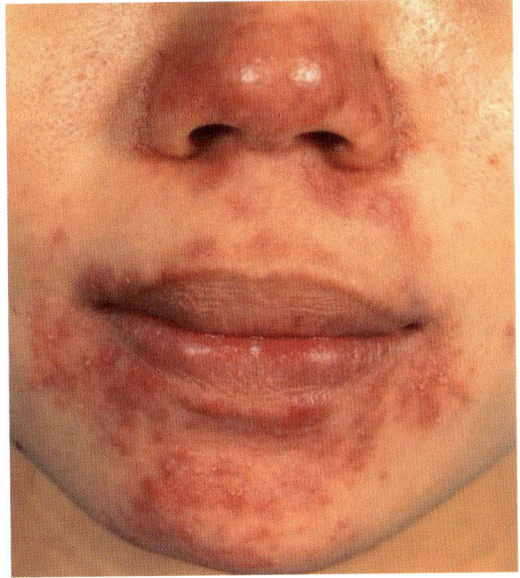

Fig. 21.24 Perioral dermatitis (Courtesy of National Skin Centre, Singapore)

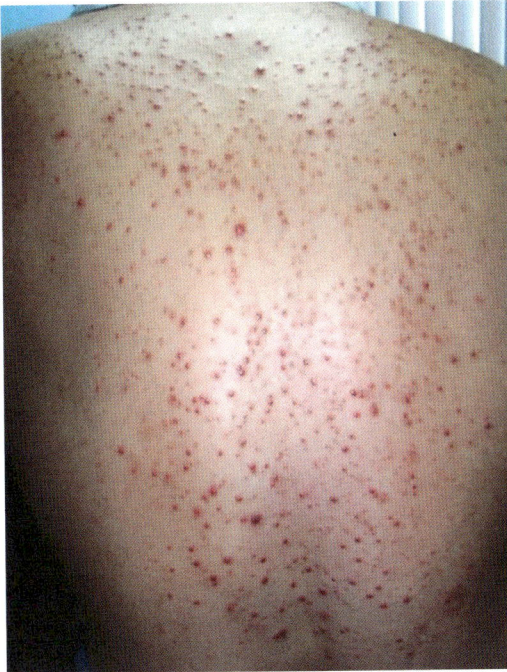

Fig. 21.23 Aggravation of acne lesions on the back in a 35-year-old Filipino male after being prescribed with mometasone furoate lotion once daily for 2 months (Courtesy of Dr. Noemie Ramos, Philippines)

withdrawal from TCS is the immediate solution, but resolution of the condition is at times slow and frustrating.

Fungal infections
- May appear as a consequence of prolonged application of TCS especially in the groin area (Fig. 21.25) or as tinea incognito when TCS are applied on existing fungal infections (Figs. 21.26, 21.27, 21.28, 21.29, and 21.30). Either way, immunosuppression invites overgrowth of dermatophytes and yeasts.

Furunculosis and folliculitis
- Most commonly seen bacterial infections with imprudent use of TCS (Figs. 21.31, 21.32, and 21.33)

Perilesional hypopigmentation
- Often seen in all age groups (Figs. 21.34 and 21.35) but especially among the pediatric patients with atopic dermatitis (Fig. 21.36)
- Seen even with low-potency TCS and intermittent application

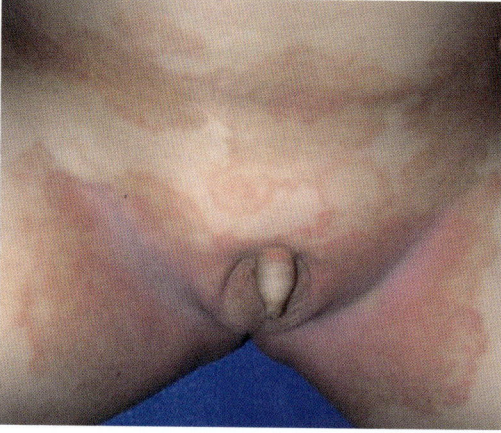

Fig. 21.25 Fungal infection on this child developed after application of several steroids (Courtesy of Prof. Indropo Agusni, MD-DV, Indonesia)

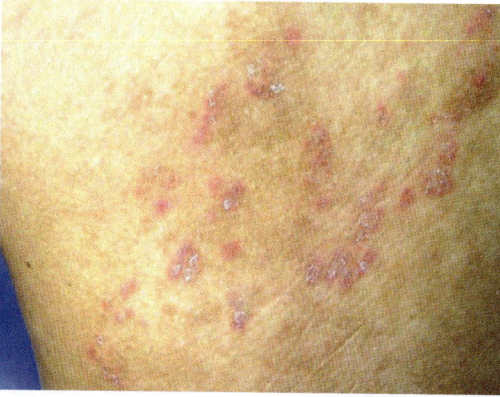

Fig. 21.26 Tinea corporis (KOH + fungal hyphae) on the back of this 50-year-old diabetic Filipino male led to persistence and aggravation after application of mometasone cream 1× daily × 3 weeks (Courtesy of Dr. Noemie Ramos, Philippines)

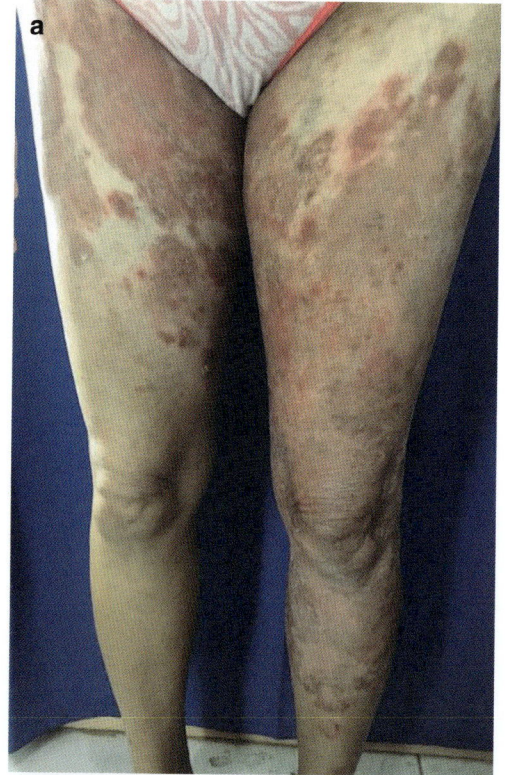

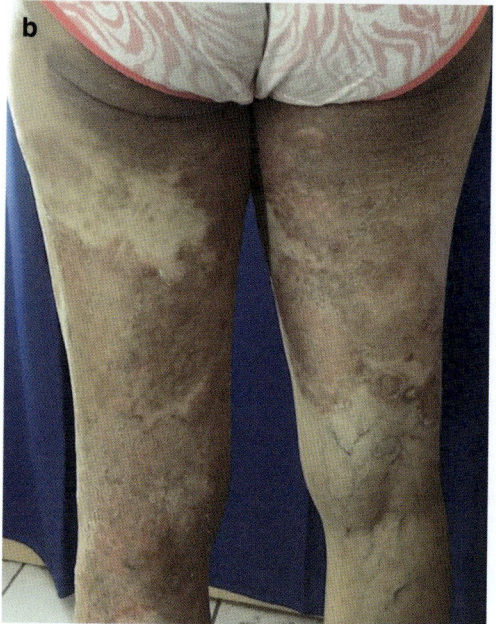

Fig. 21.27 Self-medication of multiple pruritic erythematous scaly plaques on the inguinal areas (**a**) and buttocks (**b**) with BL cream irregularly for 6 months led to increase in severity and extent of this Tinea Incognito in a 52-year-old Filipina (Biopsy showed hyphae and spores in the stratum corneum) (Courtesy of the Department of Dermatology, Research Institute for Tropical Medicine, Philippines)

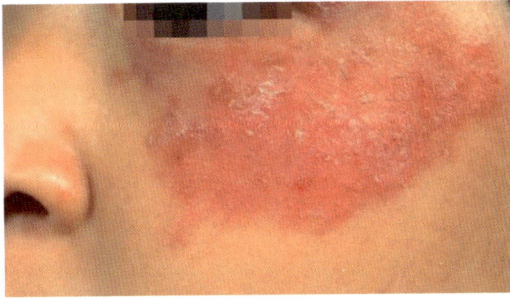

Fig. 21.28 Tinea incognito from TCS (Courtesy of National Skin Centre, Singapore)

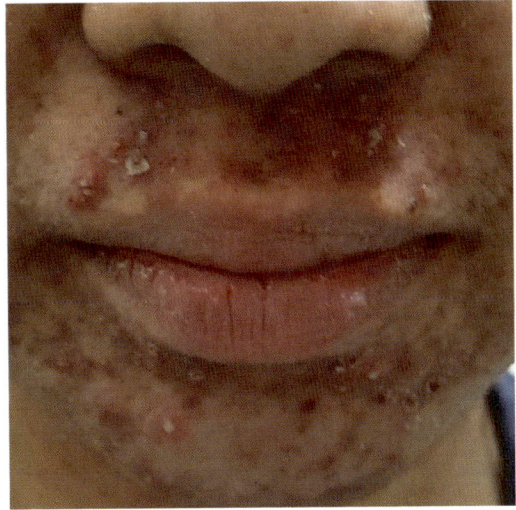

Fig. 21.29 Application of "BL" cream led to the aggravation of tinea corporis on this Filipino patient (Courtesy of Dr. Ana Lucia Dela Paz, Philippines)

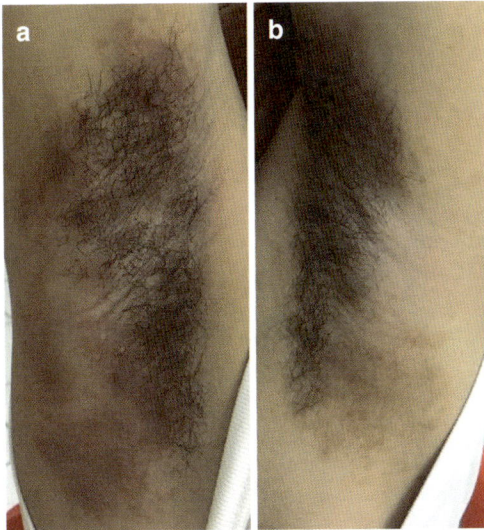

Fig. 21.30 Hyperpigmented patches on both axillae (**a**, **b**) with persistent pruritus treated with "BL cream" for 2 weeks in an 18-year-old Filipino male, later diagnosed as Tinea Incognito (Courtesy of the Department of Dermatology, Research Institute for Tropical Medicine, Philippines)

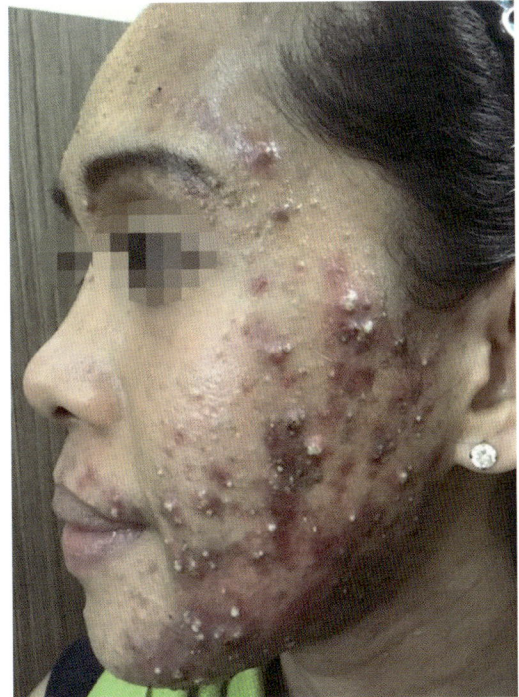

Fig. 21.31 Perioral folliculitis in a 34-year-old Filipino female after 1-month use of topical fluocinonide cream as treatment for her acne (Courtesy of Dr. Johannes Dayrit, Philippines)

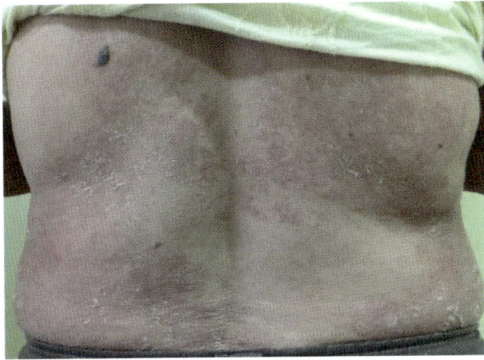

Fig. 21.32 Furunculosis and folliculitis in a Filipina patient after application of topical steroid for her acne lesions (Courtesy of the Department of Dermatology, Jose R. Reyes Memorial Medical Center, Philippines)

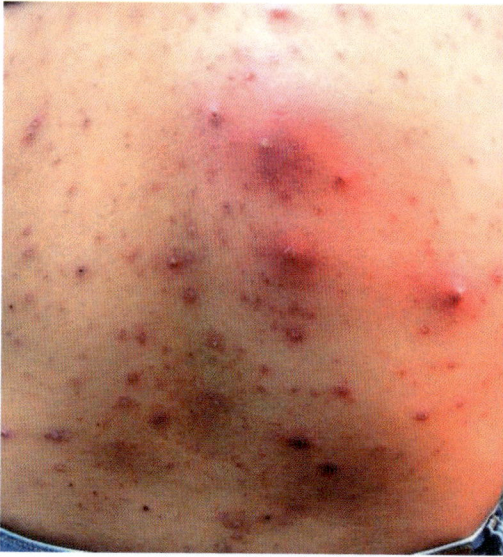

Fig. 21.33 Furunculosis and folliculitis developed in this 28-year-old Filipino male after application of clobetasol cream on his acne lesions for 1 month (Courtesy of Dr. Noemie Ramos, Philippines)

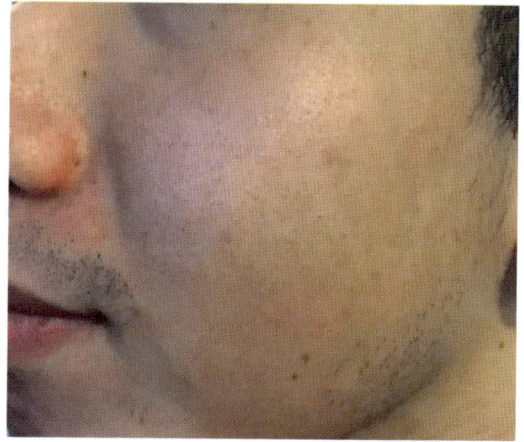

Fig. 21.35 Persistent hypopigmentated patch on the left cheek of a 29-year-old Filipino male who, 7 years ago, self-medicated his acne lesions with mometasone furoate cream 2× daily for 1 month (Courtesy of the Department of Dermatology, Research Institute for Tropical Medicine, Philippines)

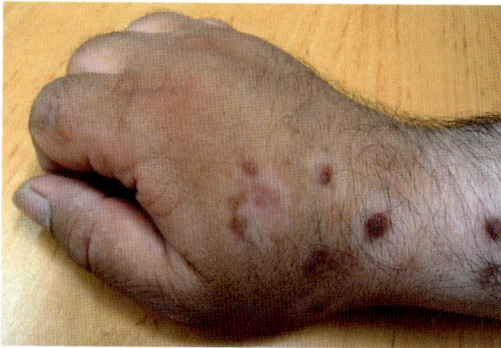

Fig. 21.34 Depigmentation around chronic eczema lesions on the arm of a Thai patient from prolonged application of clobetasone (Courtesy of Dr. Rataporn Ungpakorn, Institute of Dermatology, Thailand)

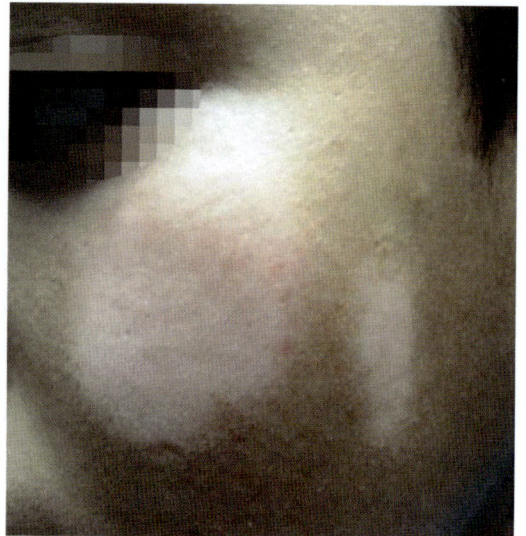

Fig. 21.36 Hypopigmented patches on the left cheek of a 5-year-old Filipino boy after his mother applied clobetasol propionate cream 2× daily for 1 week on face rashes (Courtesy of Dr. Noemie Ramos, Philippines)

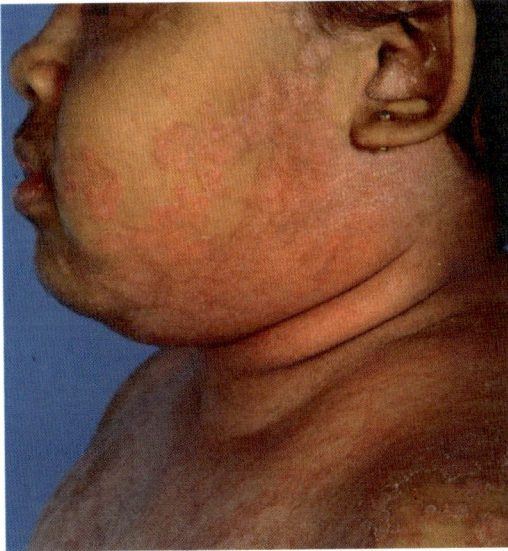

Fig. 21.37 Cushing's syndrome from prolonged use of TCS in a child with psoriasis (Courtesy of National Skin Centre, Singapore)

Decrease in skin pigmentation on areas of TCS application, though considered a complication, has been capitalized by many fairness cream formulations [5] abounding in Asian markets. As part of the whole Asian culture, where the color of one's skin is a concern and at times an obsession, misuse of TCS as part of lightening creams is disturbing [3, 13–23]. Apart from this, a topical steroid-dependent face (TSDF) has been described in scientific articles where facial rebound erythema, burning, and scaling become evident upon stopping the TCS use after prolonged usage [24–26]. Worse, the need to avoid these withdrawal effects leads to further use of even more potent TCS leading to what authors termed as steroid addiction [20, 25, 27–29].

Systemic side effects may be seen such as adrenal suppression and Cushingoid appearance (Fig. 21.37). This appears to be more common among chronic skin conditions (i.e., psoriasis, atopic dermatitis) where there is a need of continuous treatment. Unfortunately, TCS is the most common medication that is being continued by medical practitioners and the patients themselves.

21.5 Pearls to Live By

- Classification of TCS by potency [30] must be known by heart, not only by the medical practitioners but also by the pharmaceutical and paramedical personnel. This will increase awareness of the side effects that may be brought about by the wrong prescription, wrong refill, and wrong advice.
- Highly potent and ointment-based TCS produce more untoward effects on the areas of application, especially the face and thin-skinned areas, if applied too frequently, too long, and too much [31].
- Comparing adults to children, the latter are more susceptible to be inflicted with systemic reactions based on their higher ratio of total body surface area to body weight. Undesirable effects are dependent on the TCS chemical composition, location, method, and duration of application [4].
- Physicians must be able to extract a complete history from their patients with steroid-responsive dermatoses, especially that of existing comorbidities. Awareness of these aspects will lead to a more judicious prescription and instruction to the patient.
- Guidelines for appropriate and reasonable utilization of TCS have been set and periodically updated. It is the responsibility of every physician to be constantly informed.
- The medical profession and the pharmaceutical field must work symbiotically toward actively reporting adverse drug reactions from TCS.
- Adverse reactions from TCS are similar in all countries. Frequency and degree vary due to different factors such as adherence to government policies, availability of different classes of TCS, and cultural differences and beliefs.

References

1. Sulzberger MB, Witten VH. The effect of topically applied compound F in selected dermatoses. J Invest Dermatol. 1952;19(2):101–2.
2. Ference JD, Last AR. Choosing topical corticosteroids. Am Fam Physician. 2009;29(2):135–40.

3. Kannan S, Khan W, Bharadwarj A, Rathore S, Khosia PP. Corticosteroid-induced cutaneous changes: a cross-sectional study. Indian J Pharm. 2015;47(6):696–8.

4. Hengge UR, Ruzicka T, Schwartz RA, Cork MJ. Adverse effects of topical glucocorticosteroids. J Am Acad Dermatol. 2006;54(1):5.

5. Coondoo A, Phiske M, Verma S, Lahiri K. Side-effects of topical steroids: a long overdue revisit. Indian Dermatol Online J. 2014;5(4):416–25.

6. Singh N, Rieder MJ, Tucker MJ. Mechanisms of glucocorticoid-mediated anti-inflammatory and immunosuppressive action. Paediatr Perinat Drug Ther. 2004;6:107–15.

7. Rathi SK, Kumrah L. Topical corticosteroid-induced rosacea-like dermatitis: a clinical study of 110 cases. Indian J Dermatol Venereol Leprol. 2011;77:42–6.

8. Ciccone S, Marini R, Bizzarri C, El Hachem M, Cappa M. Cushing's syndrome in a 6-month-old boy: a rare side-effect due to inadequate use of topical corticosteroids. Acta Derm Venereol. 2016;96:138–9.

9. Chan YC, Tay YK, Sugito TL, Boediardja SA, Chau DD, Nguyen KV, et al. A study on the knowledge, attitudes and practices of Southeast Asian dermatologists in the management of atopic dermatitis. Ann Acad Med Singap. 2006;35(11):794–803.

10. Rubel D, Thirumoorthy T, Soebaryo RW, Weng SCK, Gabriel TM, Villafuerte LL, et al. Asia-Pacific consensus group for atopic dermatitis. Consensus guidelines for the management of atopic dermatitis: an Asia-Pacific perspective. J Dermatol. 2013;40:160–71.

11. Giam YC, Herbert AA, Dizon MV, Bever HV, Tiongco-Recto M, Kim KH, et al. A review on the role of moisturizers for atopic dermatitis. Asia Pac Allergy. 2016;6(2):120–8.

12. Momin S, Peterson A, Del Rosso JQ. Drug-induced acneform eruptions: definitions and causes. Cosmet Dermatol. 2009;22:28–37.

13. Saraswat A, Lahiri K, Chatterjee M, Barua S, Coondoo A, Mittal A, et al. Topical corticosteroid abuse on the face: a prospective, multicenter study of dermatology outpatients. Indian J Dermatol Venereol Leprol. 2011;77:160–6.

14. Ambika H, Vinod CS, Yadalla H, Nithya R, Babu AR. Topical corticosteroids abuse on face: a prospective, study on outpatients of dermatology. Dermatol Online. 2014;5:5–8.

15. Rathod SS, Motghare VM, Deshmukh VS, Deshpande RP, Bhamare CG, Patil JR. Prescribing practices of topical corticosteroids in the outpatient dermatology department of a rural tertiary care teaching hospital. Indian J Dermatol. 2013;58(5):342–5.

16. Jha AK, Sinha R, Prasad S. Misuse of topical corticosteroids on the face: a cross-sectional study among dermatology outpatients. Indian Dermatol Online J. 2016;7(4):259–63.

17. Sinha A, Kar S, Yaday N, Madke B. Prevalence of topical steroid misuse among rural masses. Indian J Deramtol. 2016;61(10):119.

18. Nagesh TS, Akhilesh A. Topical steroid awareness and abuse: a prospective study among dermatology outpatients. Indian J Dermatol. 2016;61:618–21.

19. Bains P. Topical corticosteroids abuse on face: a clinical study of 100 patients. Int J Res Dermatol. 2016;2(3):40–5.

20. Lu H, Xiao T, Lu B, Dong D, Yu D, Wei H, et al. Facial corticosteroid addictive dermatitis in Guiyang city, China. Clin Exp Dermatol. 2010;35:618–21.

21. Dhalimi MA, Aljawahiry N. Misuse of topical corticosteroids: a clinical study in an Iraqi hospital. East Mediterr Health J. 2006;12:847–52.

22. Kumar S, Goyal A, Gupta YK. Abuse of topical corticosteroids in India: concerns and the way forward. J Pharmacol Pharmacother. 2016;7(1):1–5.

23. Inakanti Y, Thimmasarthi VN, Anupama KS, Nagaraj A, Peddireddy S, Rayapati A. Topical corticosteroids: abuse and misuse. Dermatol Online. 2015;6(2):130–4.

24. Rathi SK, D'Souza P. Rational and ethical use of topical corticosteroids based on safety and efficacy. Indian J Dermatol. 2012;57:251–9.

25. Lahiri K, Coondoo A. Topical steroid damaged/dependent face (TSDF): an entity of cutaneous pharmacodependence. Indian J Dermatol. 2016;61(3):265–72.

26. Coondoo A. Topical corticosteroid misuse: the Indian scenario. Indian J Dermatol. 2014;59(5):451–5.

27. Ghosh A, Sengupta S, Coondoo A, Jana AK. Topical corticosteroid addiction and phobia. Indian J Dermatol. 2014;59:465–8.

28. Liu ZH, Du XH. Quality of life in patients with facial steroid dermatitis before and after treatment. J Eur Acad Dermatol Venereol. 2008;22:663–9.

29. Hajar T, Leshem YA, Hanifin JM, Nedorost ST, Lio PA, Paller AS, Block J, Simpson EL (the National Eczema Association Task Force). A systematic review of topical corticosteroid withdrawal ("steroid addiction") in patients with atopic dermatitis and other dermatoses. J Am Acad Dermatol. 2015;72:541–9.

30. Burkhart G, Morrell D, Goldsmith L. Dermatological pharmacology. In: Brunton LL, Chabner BA, Knollmann BC, editors. Goodman and Gilman's the pharmacological basis of therapeutics. 12th ed. New York, NY: McGraw Hill; 2011. p. 1806–8.

31. Kligman AM, Frosch PJ. Steroid addiction. Int J Dermatol. 1979;18:23–31.

Topical Corticosteroid Abuse: A Japanese Perspective

22

Mototsugu Fukaya

Abstract

Abuse of topical steroids has been a problem in Japan since at least the 1990s due in a large part to the nature of the National Health Insurance (NHI) system and the "drug price margin" issue. The Atopic Dermatitis Treatment Guidelines published in 2000, which emphasise the safety of topical steroids, do not discuss potential adverse effects such as red skin syndrome.

Keywords

Drug price margin • Overprescribing • Lawsuit • Media • Guidelines

Learning Points

1. Topical steroid abuse in Japan started in 1980s related with overprescribing by doctors.
2. Japanese authoritative dermatologists got involved in lawsuits and discussion about side effects of topical steroids became taboo.
3. Guidelines are not successfully functioning for preventing side effects of topical steroids such as Red Skin Syndrome.

22.1 Topical Steroids Available Over the Counter in Japan

Mild to potent topical steroids are available over the counter (OTC) in Japan. They are sold in stores where a pharmacist or registered sales clerk is permanently stationed. (Registered sales clerks need to pass an examination to obtain a qualification.) When selling OTC topical steroids, education is provided to the customer, unless the customer advises the pharmacist (or clerk) that such education is not necessary.

22.2 Precautions on the Package Inserts of OTC Topical Steroids

The following is an example of the precautions given to people buying OTC topical steroids in Japan:

M. Fukaya
Tsurumai Kouen Clinic, Nagoya, Japan
e-mail: moto@earth.ocn.ne.jp

© Springer Nature Singapore Pte Ltd. 2018
K. Lahiri (ed.), *A Treatise on Topical Corticosteroids in Dermatology*,
DOI 10.1007/978-981-10-4609-4_22

This medication is used to treat skin disorders, so please do not use it as make-up or after-shave. If you are using high doses or using the product for a long period of time, you may develop acne or skin breakouts (pimples), reddening of the facial skin, facial swelling, dryness or roughness of the skin and increased hairiness. Therefore, please take particular caution when using them on the face. In addition, please do not use this product unnecessarily after symptoms have improved.

How to use topical steroids correctly when self-medicating:

*Please apply the correct quantity to the affected region. Under normal circumstances apply twice daily; however, if symptoms are severe, apply three times daily.

*Once symptoms improve reduce frequency of use.

*Please do not use for more than 1 week.

*If your skin does not improve in 5–6 days, or if your symptoms worsen, the diagnosis may be incorrect. Self-medication is no longer appropriate. Please stop using the topical steroid and discuss your condition with your doctor, pharmacist or registered sales clerk.

*If you have used topical steroids over an extensive area on the trunk that exceeds the area of 2–3 palms, self-medication is no longer appropriate. Please discuss your condition with your doctor, pharmacist or registered sales clerk.

What is an appropriate amount of topical steroid to use?

The "finger-tip" unit is useful in guiding topical steroid use. 0.5 g of topical steroid is approximately the amount of topical steroid squeezed from a tube from the tip of an adult's index finger to the first crease in the finger. This amount should cover an area about the size of two adult palms. Using this as a guide, you can compare the area of the affected region and determine the amount of topical steroid recommended.

22.3 Prescription of Topical Steroids by Doctors in Japan

Doctors prescribing topical steroids in Japan do not necessarily have dermatological training. While doctors must examine patients before issuing a prescription, there is no legal obligation to provide an explanation about the medication's use or discuss its potential side effects. Some doctors may give patients detailed information, whereas others will provide virtually zero patient education. Some doctors may prescribe topical steroids where there is limited clinical indication for this treatment.

22.4 National Health Insurance System and Drug Price Margins Influence on Topical Steroid Prescriptions in Japan

In 1961 a National Health Insurance (NHI) system was introduced in Japan. Employees are covered by corporate insurance. Retirees and people who are self-employed are covered by citizen's health insurance which is provided by the local government. Cover is extended to families also. Insurers pay for 70–90% of the cost of medical consultations, investigations or medications. In 2013, the mean annual insurance premium paid by NHI patients was 70,000 Yen, while the medical benefits per patient averaged 300,000 Yen. Thus, the patient premium only partially offsets the cost of the programme which is largely paid for by the Japanese taxpayer.

Overservicing is rife in Japanese hospitals and private consulting rooms. There is a tendency to readily prescribe topical steroids even for minor skin conditions such as insect bites or benign self-limiting rashes.

The "drug price margin" is a unique issue in Japan. At present, medical practices are run separately from pharmacies. However, up till 1990, pharmacies were usually located within medical practices and run by the same company. This, in addition to the fact that patients experienced little out of pocket costs, meant overprescribing was rampant due to a push to increase company profits.

The drug price margin refers to the difference between the wholesale cost of the drug and the retail price for the patient. In the NHI system, the retail price of drugs is controlled at a national level at the time of the drug's approval. However, the wholesale price can be negotiated by the drug manufacturers and the pharmacy. Greater sales of drugs resulted in larger hospital profits, and thus in the 1970s and 1980s, overprescribing became a problem in Japan. This problem is becoming less of an issue now that pharmacies and medical practices are separate from one another.

Japan's total expenditure on topical steroids from 1992–1996 (source IMS Japan)

1992	39,256
1993	37,274
1994	35,257
1995	34,366
1996	33,252

Unit: 1,000,000 Yen

The table above clearly shows spending on topical steroids decreased steadily once the link between medical practices and pharmacies was removed.

22.5 The Media and Topical Steroid Use in Japan

Due to the issues with the NHI system and the previous drug price margin, overprescribing of medications was a hot topic in the Japanese media in the 1980s and 1990s. In 1992, the "News Station", a popular show in Japan, discussed the issue of overprescribing topical steroids. Dr. Takehara criticised the show repeatedly for their negative attitude towards the use of topical steroids. His views were widely published in newspaper articles, magazines, books and journals. He was particularly scathing towards the broadcaster of this programme for closing the programme with the line: "We know that, in the end, these topical steroids are drugs that will be used to the bitter end". However, the comment had actually been made by a pharmacology professor. Dr. Takehara later coauthored the Japanese Dermatological Association's atopic dermatitis guidelines.

22.6 Medical Malpractice Claims Regarding Topical Steroid Prescribing

Patients in Japan have sued over the management of their dermatological condition. The Kawasaki Steroid lawsuit [1] became famous. In this case, the patient experienced rosacea-like dermatitis to her face secondary to topical steroid use. Topical steroids had been prescribed over several years by multiple doctors in different medical facilities. The patient ultimately lost the case. Here is an extract of the expert opinion provided by Dr. Kawashima from Tokyo Women's Medical University:

It is easy for dermatologists to diagnosis atopic dermatitis if they focus on the itching, the characteristic skin eruption and the chronic clinical course. We believe misdiagnosis of this condition by a dermatologist with sufficient training is very unlikely. However, from the latter half of 1975, an increase in the number of patients with conspicuous facial erythema was observed and a diagnosis of atopic dermatitis was possible by considering skin eruptions at other sites. There is no consensus in determining whether facial lesions are (a) side effects of topical steroids, (b) the concomitant presence of atopic dermatitis and side effects or (c) symptoms of atopic dermatitis. We need to make clinical decisions based on the patient's history—including drug use history, current symptoms and examination findings. At that time, this facial erythema was suspected to be rosacea-like dermatitis, which was commonly seen in patients who had used topical steroids like make-up to healthy skin, but the facial skin eruptions in this condition and those in rosacea-like dermatitis are different. The former are eczematous lesions, while the latter are a mixture of acne and pustules and characterised by a burning sensation rather than itching. Most of the facial symptoms seen in this patient were of atopic dermatitis and we believe they should be considered to represent a case of atopic dermatitis.

Dr. Kawashima determined that "as there were no acne like pustules, we cannot diagnose this case as rosacea-like dermatitis and it should not be considered to be the result of an adverse effect of topical steroids". Currently, rosacea is commonly believed to present in two variants, one that is mainly erythema and the other that is erythema mixed with pustules [2]. Although there were some doubts with the expert testimony from Dr. Kawashima, it highlighted the difficulty of differentiating between the side effects of topical steroids and the primary condition (i.e. atopic dermatitis). Due to this fact, the ruling went in favour of the doctors.

22.7 Advocacy for Topical Steroid Withdrawal by Both Doctors and Alternative Health Practitioners

Under these conditions, Japanese doctors such as Dr. Tamaki [3], Dr. Sato [4] and Dr. Fujisawa began educating the public about the problems caused by overuse of topical steroids. Dr. Enomoto also reported several cases of patients with a history of long-term topical steroid use where they had ceased topical steroids and went on to experience marked systemic symptoms despite normal adrenocortical function [5]. This was the first report of systemic symptoms caused by the withdrawal of topical steroids. Dr. Hara and others published books aimed at the general public educating about the dangers of topical steroids overuse.

Meanwhile many "traditional" or alternative practitioners are treating "steroid withdrawal" in Japan. Topical steroid withdrawal does not generally require medical intervention unless complicated by infection. This is because the biggest factor in resolution of symptoms is time. As a result these traditional practitioners are able to generate a client load and income by "treating" these patients. Traditional practitioner manage-

ment has at times been counterproductive and deceitful. Some topical medications contained steroids despite being promoted to patients as a traditional (and steroid free) Chinese medication.

Thus management of steroid withdrawal in Japan has been a mixed bag since the 1990s.

22.8 The Development of the Japanese Dermatological Association Guidelines for Atopic Dermatitis

As a result of the above issues, guidelines for atopic dermatitis management in Japan were required for dermatologists, paediatricians and allergy medicine doctors. The Ministry of Health, Labour and Welfare (MHLF), in the interest of controlling health expenditure, has promoted the use of clinical guidelines.

However, as these guidelines were developed by doctors such as Dr. Kawashima and Dr. Takehara who have a history of taking a "pro topical steroid" stance, the guidelines contain little information about adverse effects of topical steroids and do not suggest precautions to avoid these. Instead, the guidelines serve to emphasise the safety of topical steroid treatment and promote strategies to counter so-called patient steroid phobia. Dr. Furue, who was chair of the committee who wrote the guidelines, went on to use a grant from MHLW to create a website campaigning introducing the phrase "standard treatment" and recommended all Japanese doctors strictly adhere to the guidelines. In Japan, most doctors feel compelled to follow this "standard treatment" and, reassured by these guidelines, do not consider potential side effects of topical steroids or the risks of topical steroid overuse.

22.9 Lessons from the Japanese Situation

Steps to reduce topical steroid overuse in Japan include the improvement of package inserts with OTC topical steroids and restriction of sales without a prescription. Neighbouring countries, especially in Southeast Asia, could potentially benefit from implementing similar measures. However, even with these strategies, the problem of topical steroid overuse remains in Japan. It is also difficult to differentiate atopic dermatitis from the adverse effects of topical steroid overuse. It does not help that terms such as red skin syndrome and topical steroid rebound are rejected by the Japanese Dermatological Association and are even considered taboo. There are concerns that if this condition was more widely recognised, there would be difficulties with prescribing topical steroids, which is currently a very common treatment. Calling patients steroid phobic is easier than dealing with the possibility that topical steroid overuse may have resulted in a problem for the patient.

However, now that Internet use has become widespread, it is evident that there are many patients around the world with symptoms fitting with red skin syndrome that state stopping topical steroids ultimately resulted in clinical improvement. Some of these patients may have had an exacerbation of a primary disease and healed with time, while others may genuinely have had severe side effects of topical steroid use similar to those cases reported by Enomoto. We cannot continue to ignore this problem.

In the future, there will be new drugs available for the treatment of atopic dermatitis. It may be beneficial for the drug companies promoting them to highlight the potential adverse effects of topical steroids so as to gain a market advantage. However, dermatologists must never forget first principles, namely, the treatment for contact dermatitis is the avoidance of irritants and allergens and the fact that atopic dermatitis can clear spontaneously and does not always require medical management. Treatment has financial implications for large drug companies and governments, but the doctor must always act in the best interests of their patient.

References

1. Case of Claiming Damages, Case Number (Wa) 448, Yokohama District Court Kawasaki Branch Civil Division, 1992.
2. Del Rosso JQ. Advances in understanding and managing rosacea: part 1: connecting the dots between pathophysiological mechanisms and common clinical features of rosacea with emphasis on vascular changes and facial erythema. J Clin Aesthet Dermatol. 2012;5(3):16–25.
3. Tamaki A, Ohashi T, Ishida T, Nakamura M. Treatment without steroid ointment for adult type atopic dermatitis. Jpn J Dermatol (Jpn). 1993;1:230–4.
4. Minami H, Sato K, Inui S, Maeda T. Withdrawal of topical steroids for the treatment of severe "adulttype" atopic dermatitis. Skin Research (JPMD). 1996;38:440–7.
5. Enomoto T, Arase S, Shigemi F, Takeda K. Steroid withdrawal syndrome by topical corticosteroid. J Jpn Cosm Sci Soc. 1991;15(1):17–24.

Topical Corticosteroid Abuse: Africa Perspective

23

Nejib Doss

Abstract

Even if topical corticosteroids (TCS) have contributed to manage many skin diseases, their wide use without prescription from the dermatologist has led to a myriad of complications.

Their misuse relies on two facts: the limited knowledge of general practitioners about these drugs and their long use and the patients' ignorance about these drugs since they are provided in local markets without any limitation.

To fight these complications, a clear health policy is needed (ban of importation of lightening products, regulation of dispensing of TCS, awareness sessions via media).

Keywords

Topical corticosteroids • Adverse effects • Misuse

Learning Points

1. Contribute to the dissemination of best practices in the field of topical corticosteroids (TCS)
2. To be more familiar with adverse effects of TCS, especially among clinicians
3. To raise the attention of political authorities about this scourge which is misuse of TCS
4. TCS should be issued only against a physician's prescription

Topical corticosteroids (TCS) are the corner stone in the management of a significant number of skin diseases due to their anti-inflammatory and antiproliferative effects. To avoid adverse effects, they should be prescribed appropriately taking into consideration their level of potency, the quantity of medication to be used, as well as the extent and location of the area to be treated.

When properly prescribed, their therapeutic effect is readily noticeable. Unfortunately, misuse of topical corticosteroids is becoming a major health problem in many countries, where they can be purchased over the counter or where they are freely sold in different market places. In these situations their complications are seen early (Fig. 23.1).

N. Doss
Department of Dermatology, Military Hospital of Tunis - Université de Tunis El Manar, 1089 Tunis, Tunisia
e-mail: nejib.doss@gmail.com

© Springer Nature Singapore Pte Ltd. 2018
K. Lahiri (ed.), *A Treatise on Topical Corticosteroids in Dermatology*,
DOI 10.1007/978-981-10-4609-4_23

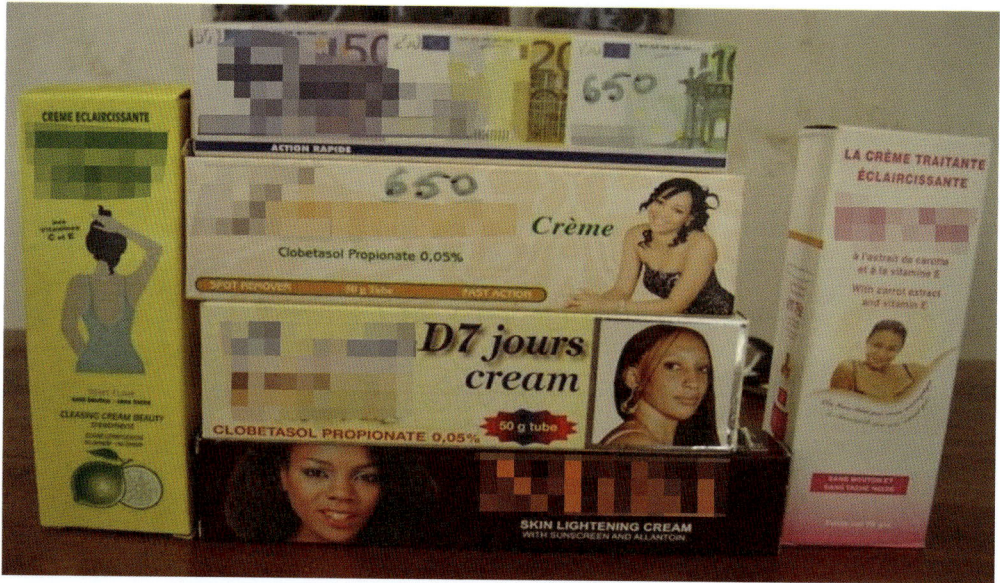

Fig. 23.1 Advertising for bleaching creams (Courtesy of Pr. M. Diallo (Senegal))

The complications vary according with the degree of potency of the topical corticosteroids, the location of their application, and the duration and the frequency of applications.

Adverse effects are classified into local and systemic effects.

23.1 Local Adverse Effects

A. Skin infections:
  1. Mycoses:
     • Especially tinea faciei which is an uncommon dermatophytosis affecting the glabrous skin of the face that is frequently misdiagnosed, especially the forms whose appearance has been modified by inappropriate treatment usually by a topical steroid leading to the so-called tinea incognita where the diagnosis is often difficult (Fig. 23.2). One specific form known as tinea pseudoimbricata starts with central erythematous, scaly, pruritic plaques from which one to three centrifugally spreading, concentric circles emerge (Fig. 23.3). The clinical manifestation is called tinea pseudoimbricata because of its resemblance to the infection typically

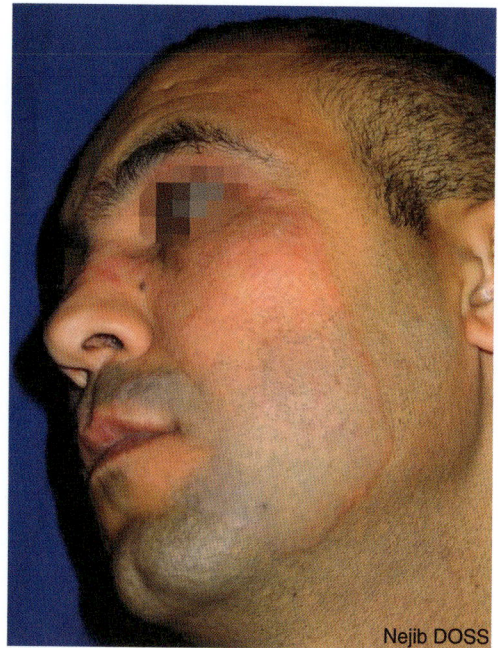

Fig. 23.2 Tinea incognita

caused by Trichophyton concentricum [1, 2].
     • Profuse or extensive dermatophytosis in any body location. Therefore, when examining patients with profuse mycosis (Figs. 23.4 and 23.5), one should

always inquire about the topical treatments used by the patient.

2. Parasites:
   - Crusted scabies: the unrestricted and inappropriate use of topical corticosteroids in some cases of undiagnosed scabies, especially in infants, may lead to the severe form which is called crusted scabies (Fig. 23.6) [3].
3. Bacterial:
   - Acneiform eruptions are the most frequent complications of abuse of TCS. These include the following:
     - Perioral dermatitis which is an erythematous-papular and sometimes papular-pustular disease localized in the perioral region (Fig. 23.7). Regardless of the variation of the etiologic factors of this disease, it is thought that the long-term use of TCS is considered a major factor in the pathogenesis of the disease or at least a trigger factor.
   - Rosacea is a disease of the face that manifests with erythema, papulopustules and telangiectasias. Among the different factors cited in the pathogenesis of rosacea, a prolonged use of topical and even systemic corticosteroids is one of them (Fig. 23.8).
   - Acne is one of the most frequent skin conditions especially in young persons.

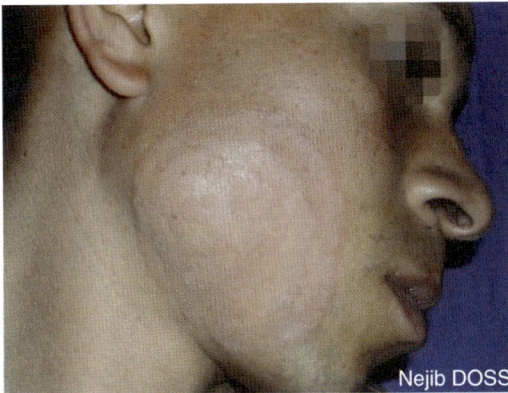

Fig. 23.3 Tinea pseudoimbricata

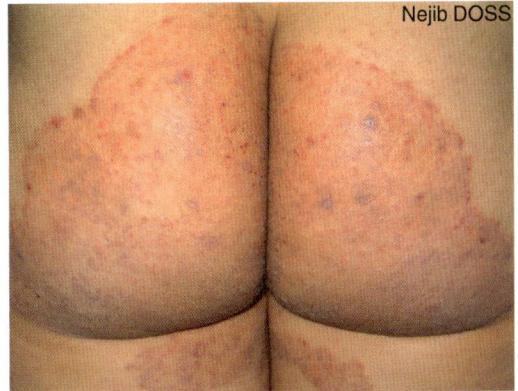

Fig. 23.5 Profuse tinea

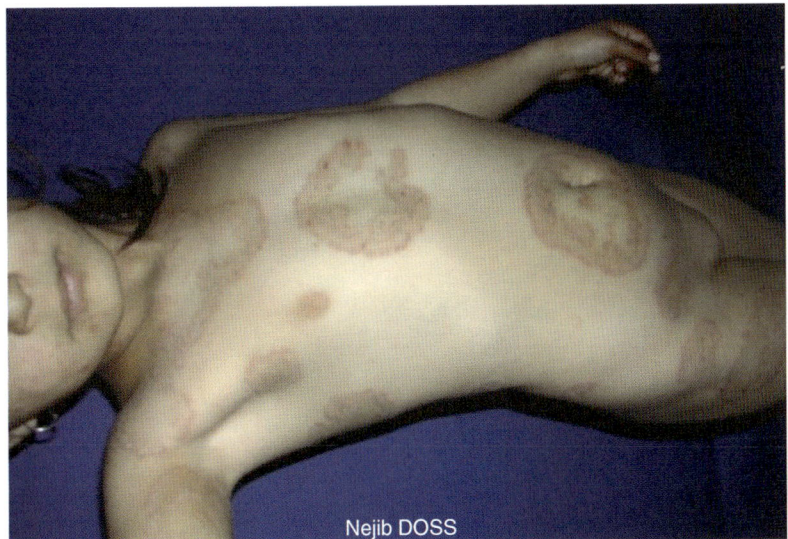

Fig. 23.4 Profuse tinea

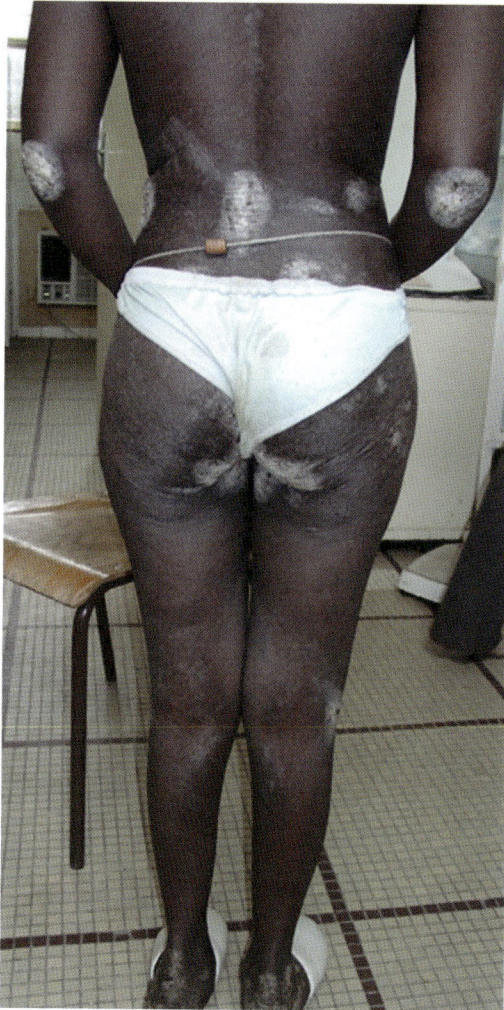

Fig. 23.6 Crusted scabies (Courtesy of Pr. M. Diallo-Senegal)

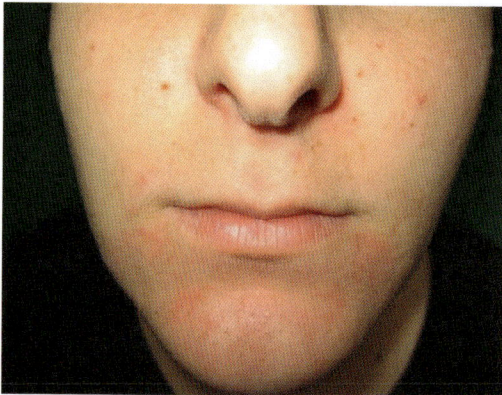

Fig. 23.7 Perioral dermatitis (Courtesy of Pr. A. Prohic - Bosnia)

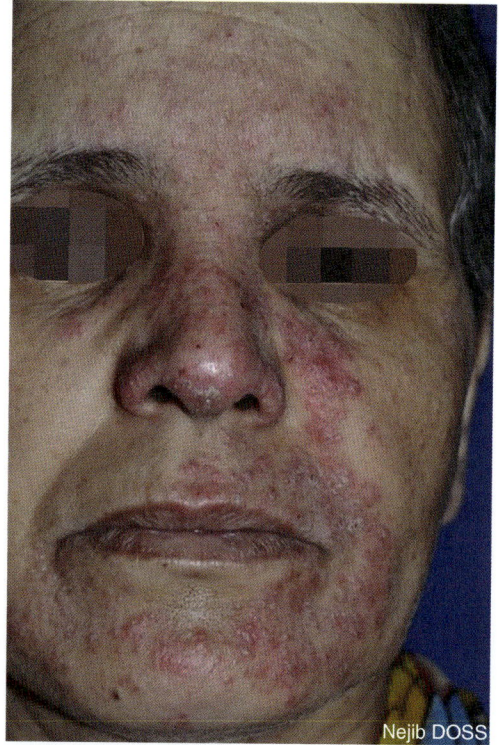

Fig. 23.8 Rosacea

Clinically it is characterized by a polymorphic pattern: open and closed comedones, papules, pustules, and even nodules. When the clinical picture turns to a monomorphous one (papules and pustules) especially when it is located on the back and chest, we should suspect a drug-induced acne and check for a misuse of topical corticosteroids (Fig. 23.9) [4, 5].

• Erysipelas: in Africa, TCS are used to bleach the skin, and many cases of erysipelas were reported after the use of topical corticosteroids. Corticosteroids potentiate the skin penetration of the bacterial pathogen causing erysipelas (Fig. 23.10) [6].

4. Viral: spreading and/or worsening of viral infections especially with herpes zoster virus and mollusca contagiosa.

B. Striae distensae is a well-known consequence of long use of topical and systemic corticosteroids. They are predominately

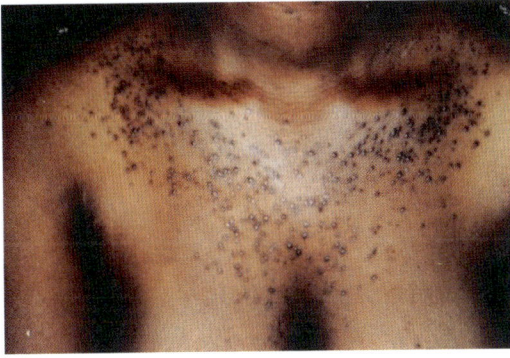

Fig. 23.9 Acne (courtesy of Pr. M. Diallo - Senegal)

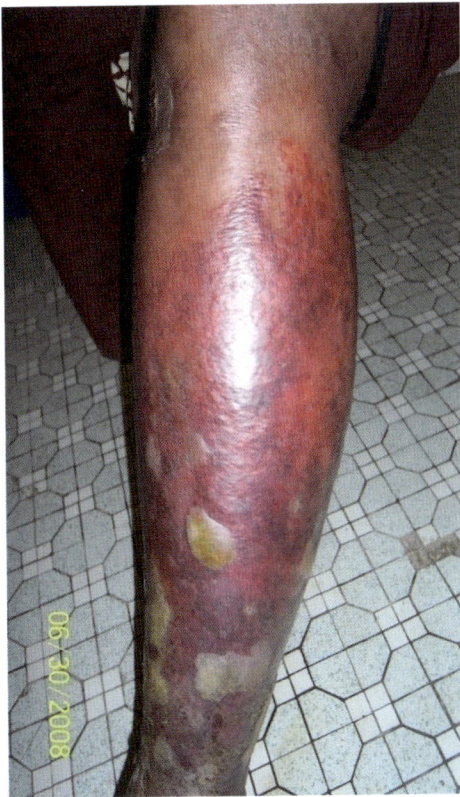

Fig. 23.10 Erysipelas (Courtesy of Pr. M. Diallo-Senegal)

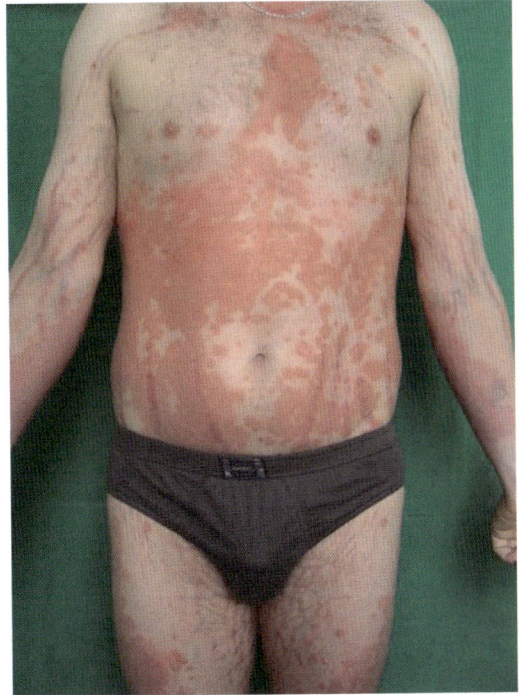

Fig. 23.11 Striae distensae (Courtesy of Pr. A. Prohic – Bosnia)

located on the trunk, arms, and legs. They are initially pink to purple in color and then become lighter or skin colored matching the color of the surrounding skin (Fig. 23.11) [7].

C. Skin atrophy is a major deleterious side effect of TCS, and it is thought that this atrophy is related to inappropriate occupancy of mineralocorticoid receptor in the epidermis by glucocorticoids. Skin atrophy could be seen also after use of intralesional injection of glucocorticoids. The skin is thin which easily bleeds and shows superficial erosions (Fig. 23.12). A delayed wound healing could be related to skin atrophy. Skin atrophy is usually reversible after stopping the treatment [8, 9].

D. Dyschromia:
  - Hypopigmentation: it is often reversible (Fig. 23.13) [10].
  - Hyperpigmentation: as seen in rare cases.

E. Allergic dermatitis: contact allergy to TCS is known to be gradually rising and represents a challenge for clinician to differentiate between the initial condition and the new one after the application of TCS. Hypersensitivity reactions can occur to the corticosteroid itself or to the additives and vehicles used in corticosteroid preparations. Patch testing can help to identify the causal agent (Fig. 23.14) [11].

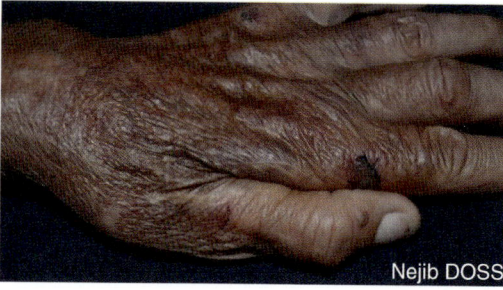

Fig. 23.12 Skin atrophy

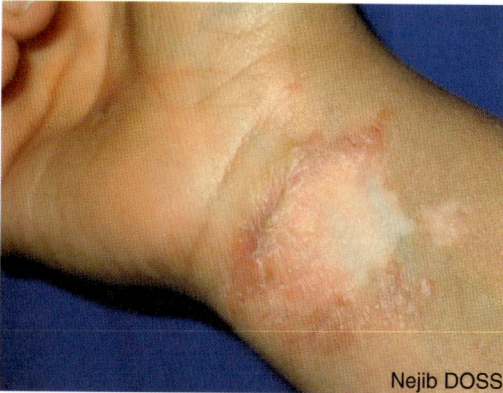

Fig. 23.13 Hypochromia

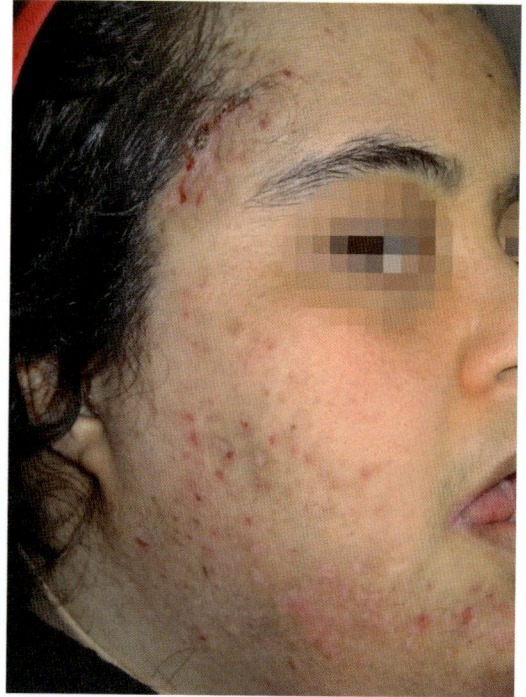

Fig. 23.15 Hypertrichosis and acne

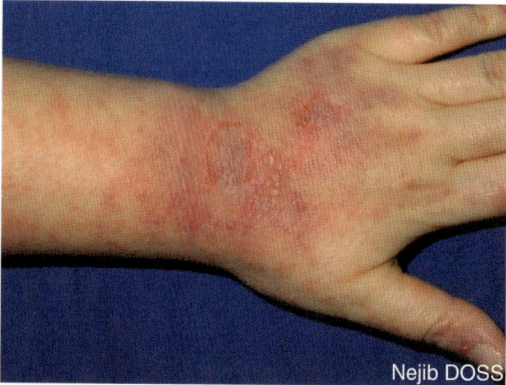

Fig. 23.14 Allergic dermatitis to TCS

F. Hypertrichosis has been reported as one of the TCS side effects, but it is mostly related to systemic corticosteroids (Fig. 23.15) [12].

G. Gluteal granuloma infantum is a benign granulomatous eruption, involving the gluteal region. Histopathologically, it shows a nonspecific dermal inflammatory infiltrate composed of neutrophils, lymphocytes, histiocytes, plasma cells, and eosinophils. It is important to recognize this condition, as it may clinically simulate a neoplastic process. It arises as a complication of primary irritant diaper dermatitis; however, it typically resolves without treatment [13, 14].

23.2 Systemic Adverse Effects

A. Cushing syndrome: an uncontrolled use of topical corticosteroids may cause immuno-suppression and iatrogenic's syndrome via hypothalamic-pituitary-adrenal axis. To avoid such complications, the patient's weight and serum cortisol should be checked regularly (Fig. 23.16).

B. Pustulosis psoriasis and the dermocorticoids: it is thought that corticosteroids (systemic or

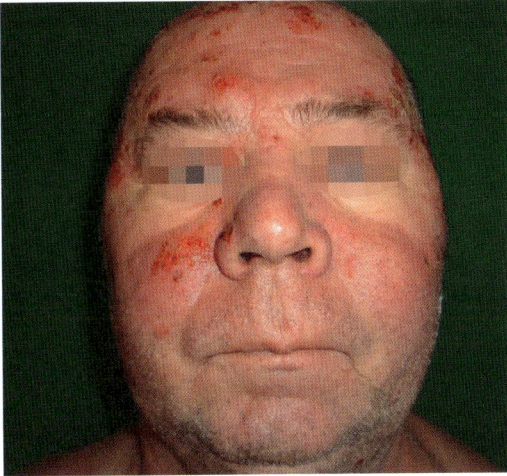

Fig. 23.16 Cushing syndrome (courtesy of Pr. A. Prohic from Bosnia)

topical) prescribed in psoriasis might be responsible for a pustulosis flare when they are stopped.

Conclusion

In African countries, corticosteroids are overused to treat inflammatory diseases and especially to bleach the skin.

They are used rather alone or in combination with other products such as hydroquinone and even mercurial products.

Most of these products are imported from Europe where they are banned!!!

A firm health policy is needed to ban these products or at least to limit their sell only in appropriate places.

All clinicians should have sufficient knowledge about TCS and their proper use.

Preventive measures and especially educational programs, should be settled, for patients receiving longterm glucocorticoids for chronic diseases.

Nanoencapsulation of topical glucocorticoids seems to bring a hope with minimization of their local and systemic adverse effects [15].

References

1. Verma S, Hay RJ. Topical steroid-induced tinea pseudoimbricata: a striking form of tinea incognito. Int J Dermatol. 2015;54:e192–3.
2. Quinones C, Hasbun P, Gubelin W. Tinea incognito due to *trichophyton mentagrophytes*: case report. Medwave. 2016;16(10):e6598.
3. Bilan P, Colin-Gorski AM, Chapelon E, Sigal ML, Mahé E. Crusted scabies induced by topical corticosteroids: a case report. Arch Pediatr. 2015;22(12):1292–4.
4. Gathse A, Ibara JR. Reasons for consulting related to skin-bleaching products used by 104 women in Brazzaville. Bull Soc Pathol Exot. 2005;98(5):387–9.
5. Dey VK. Misuse of topical corticosteroids: a clinical study of adverse effects. Indian Dermatol Online J. 2014;5:436–40.
6. Gathse A, Ntsiba H. Retrospective study of 53 erysipelas cases in Brazzaville University Hospital, Congo. Bull Soc Pathol Exot. 2006;99:3–4.
7. Ud-Din S, McGeorge D, Bayat A. Topical management of striae distensae (stretch marks): prevention and therapy of striae rubrae and albae. JEADV. 2016;30:211–22.
8. Maubec E. Topical mineralocorticoid receptor blockade limits glucocorticoid-induced epidermal atrophy in human skin. J Invest Dermatol. 2015;135:1781–9.
9. Barnes L, Kaya G, Rollason V. Topical corticosteroid-induced skin atrophy: a comprehensive review. Drug Saf. 2015;38(5):493–509.
10. Loopik MF, Winters M, Moen MH. Atrophy and depigmentation after pretibial corticosteroid injection for medial tibial stress syndrome: two case reports. J Sport Rehabil. 2016;25:380–1.
11. Guillot B. Glucocorticoid-induced cutaneous adverse events. Rev Med Interne. 2013;34:310–4.
12. Morand JJ, Ly F, Lightburn E, Mahe A. Complications of cosmetic skin bleaching in Africa. Med Trop. 2007;67:627–34.
13. Bluestein J, Fumer BB, Phillips D. Granuloma gluteale infantum: case report and review of the literature. Pediatr Dermatol. 1990;7:196–8.
14. Zeeuw D, Van Praag MC, Oranje AP. Granuloma gluteale infantum: a case report. Pediatr Dermatol. 2000;17:141–3.
15. Siddique MI, Katas H, Iqbal Mohd Amin MC, Ng SF, Zulfakar MH, Buang F, Jamil A. Minimization of local and systemic adverse effects of topical glucocorticoids by nanoencapsulation: in vivo safety of hydrocortisone-hydroxytyrosol loaded chitosan nanoparticles. J Pharm Sci. 2015;104(12):4276–86.

Topical Corticosteroid Use and Overuse: An Australian Perspective

24

Belinda Sheary

Abstract

Topical corticosteroids (TCS) are readily available and widely used in Australia. Low and moderate potency TCS may be purchased over the counter. Potent TCS are commonly prescribed in all age groups and have recently become easier to prescribe in large quantities. Australian TCS guidelines focus on TCS safety and under-treatment ('steroid phobia'). However, reported cases of 'steroid withdrawal syndrome' indicate TCS overuse exists in Australia too.

Keywords

Australia • Topical corticosteroids • Atopic dermatitis • Eczema • Over the counter

Learning Points
1. TCS are widely used in Australia.
2. Low and moderate potency TCS are available over the counter.
3. Potent TCS are commonly prescribed in all age groups and are now easier to prescribe in large amounts.
4. Australian TCS guidelines focus on TCS safety and underuse.
5. Evidence of TCS overuse is currently limited to reported cases of 'steroid withdrawal syndrome'.

24.1 Topical Corticosteroid Use in Australia

Topical corticosteroids (TCS) are readily available in Australia. Over the counter TCS are available in low and moderate potency forms: hydrocortisone 0.5% 30 g, hydrocortisone 1% 30 g and clobetasone butyrate 0.05% 30 g can be purchased without a script from Australian pharmacies.

TCS are frequently prescribed in Australia. In 2015–2016, 2.4% of general practitioner (GP) consults resulted in a prescription for TCS [1], and in a survey of 258 GPs, 66% reported prescribing TCS 1–5 times daily [2]. Most skin-related presentations are likely to be managed by GPs as while 17.4% of GP consults dealt with a skin complaint in 2015–2016, dermatological

B. Sheary
Royal Randwick Medical Centre,
70/73-115 Belmore Road, Randwick,
2031 NSW, Australia
e-mail: belinda.sheary@ipn.com.au

© Springer Nature Singapore Pte Ltd. 2018
K. Lahiri (ed.), *A Treatise on Topical Corticosteroids in Dermatology*,
DOI 10.1007/978-981-10-4609-4_24

referrals were provided in only 0.8 per 100 patient encounters [1].

Potent TCS are commonly prescribed in all age groups in Australia. In a 2014 survey of 198 Australian dermatologists, nearly all reported prescribing potent or superpotent TCS to treat paediatric eczema [3]. In an analysis of the 2008 Department of Veterans Affairs health claims, 73% of TCS scripts were for potent TCS [4].

24.2 Guidelines for Topical Corticosteroid Use in Australia

TCS prescribing recommendations vary slightly in Australia. An Australasian consensus statement on TCS in paediatric patients published in 2015 advised using TCS once or twice daily to all the inflamed skin until eczema is cleared [5]; and in a survey of GPs, 47% reported instructing patients to this effect [2]. In *Australian Prescriber,* the authors suggested the more specific recommendation of limiting TCS use to the face for 2 weeks and to the body for 3–4 weeks [6]. Similar explicit advice is provided by some GPs, with 41% reporting instructing patients to use TCS for a maximum of 2 weeks or less [2]. Australian Therapeutic Guidelines advise [7]: 'Do not give precise guidance about the number of days the topical corticosteroid can be used. Use the drug until the skin is completely clear (usually 7–14 days, but fewer in mild cases or more in severe cases or on thick skin)'. They also recommend: 'If the skin does not clear or the dermatitis continually recurs soon after clearance, refer for expert advice'.

Much of the discussion regarding TCS and eczema in Australia is focused on the safety of TCS [5] and TCS phobia [8], and so it is not surprising that Australian guidelines address under-treatment with TCS. No guidelines mention TCS overuse. The Australian Therapeutic Guidelines advise: 'Reassure patients and parents that the benefits of topical corticosteroids outweigh the harms and they should not be afraid to use them'. They also state: 'If topical corticosteroid therapy

fails, the most common reason is underuse due to misplaced fear about safety'. This emphasis on the problem of TCS under-treatment may be partially due to the death in Australia of a malnourished child from septicaemia secondary to infected atopic dermatitis, where the parents elected homoeopathic remedies over conventional medical management [9].

24.3 Research into Topical Corticosteroid Use in Australia

Research into TCS use in Australia is similarly focused on underuse and 'steroid phobia'—not TCS overuse. For example, Smith et al. researched pharmacists' knowledge about the use and safety of TCS in paediatric atopic dermatitis and concluded that '(pharmacists) advice to patients potentially contributes to poor treatment concordance' [10]. In another study looking at parent focus groups, the authors stated that 'corticosteroid phobia…is a fear generated by doctors (GPs), pharmacists, close acquaintances and information from the internet' [11].

24.4 Topical Corticosteroid Overuse in Australia

TCS overuse has not been studied in Australia, and evidence for this is limited. Factors which make overuse possible include the availability of over the counter TCS and more recently 'streamlined' authority scripts for increased amounts of potent TCS with multiple repeats.

Currently, the only indication that TCS overuse exists is the indirect evidence of case reports of TCS addiction and withdrawal, 'steroid withdrawal syndrome' and 'drug withdrawal syndrome' (as these conditions imply the patients had a history of TCS overuse). A single case report of an Australian child diagnosed with TCS addiction and withdrawal has been published [12], and 'steroid withdrawal syndrome' and 'drug withdrawal syndrome' cases have been reported to the Australian Therapeutic Goods Administration. Anyone in Australia can report a suspected adverse effect of a medication to the Therapeutic Goods Administration by completing the so-called 'blue card'. Over 16,500 such reports are received each year and entered into the Australian Adverse Drug Reactions System (ADRS) [13]. Three months later reports are entered into the ADRS database (which is publically accessible and searchable). A search for four commonly prescribed TCS, namely, hydrocortisone, betamethasone, methylprednisolone and mometasone furoate, for the period January 2014–November 2016, yields 16 case reports of either 'steroid withdrawal syndrome' or 'drug withdrawal syndrome'. Under-reporting is almost certain to occur due to the limited recognition [14] and acknowledgement [15, 16] of TCS addiction and withdrawal (or red skin syndrome) in Australia.

Only low and moderate potency TCS are over the counter in Australia so the risk of TCS overuse via this route has been mitigated; however, the incidence of TCS overuse could rise in Australia following recent changes which have made it quicker and easier for GPs to prescribe increased quantities of potent TCS with repeats. These 'streamlined' scripts may increase the risk of TCS overuse by normalising chronic regular (and possibly continuous) use of TCS and reducing medical supervision. Previously, doctors needed to call a government hotline to confirm the patient's medication usage requirements before being permitted to issue an 'authority' script for up to ten 15g tubes of potent TCS with five repeats. Since July 2016 this phone call has been replaced by the 'click of a button'. This plentiful supply, intended to last the patient 6 months, means patients can potentially use large amounts of potent TCS regularly (or continuously) long term without their condition or its management being reviewed by a doctor.

Thus, TCS overuse can easily occur in the Australian setting as patients have ready access to large amounts of TCS and—if the patient so chooses—only limited medical supervision.

24.5 Attitudes and Behaviour Regarding Topical Corticosteroid Use in Australia: A Personal Perspective

In the author's experience, potent TCS are now prescribed much more frequently and for younger patients than seen only 10 years ago. In 2006 it was surprising to learn a patient had been prescribed the moderately potent TCS triamcinolone acetonide 0.02% for their face. In the 1990s teaching had been that only mild TCS such as 1% hydrocortisone should ever be applied to the face. Fast forward to 2016 and it is not uncommon to see infants who have been prescribed the potent TCS methylprednisolone aceponate 0.1% for the face for up to 2 weeks and for older children to be prescribed potent TCS for the face twice a day with written advice to use 'as long as required' with no specific arrangements made for follow-up.

Many patients are blasé about TCS use on themselves and their children, and Australian patients regard TCS prescriptions as 'no big deal'. Requests for scripts to be left for the patient to collect from the reception desk are common, and the requirement that the patient come in for review is met with resistance as they do not consider this necessary. A lot of older patients ask for potent TCS scripts along with their other regular medications. On being questioned, they describe using it periodically for any itchy patch and have done so for many years. They like to keep a tube at home 'just in case'. Many patients see no issue in sharing their TCS with family members. Often on seeing a patient with a non-specific rash, they will report having already tried their partner's potent TCS, sometimes for a number of weeks, before presenting.

Some parents are comfortable using TCS on their young child without medical supervision or even a diagnosis. For example, in a case of an infant with a viral rash the mother had used 1% hydrocortisone the preceding 2 days. It hadn't helped. After discussing the (self-limiting) diagnosis, she asked whether she should continue to apply TCS. Infants are commonly treated for nappy rash with an over the counter cream containing both hydrocortisone 1% and an antifungal without being seen by a doctor.

Requests for oral steroids for eczema management were unheard of in my experience in 2006 but now occur on a semi-regular basis as patients report TCS no longer manage their symptoms. One woman in her 30s insisted that the eczema patch to her lateral ankle was persistent and she wanted it cleared in time for a holiday. One male in his 40s with a long history of eczema stated that he periodically took oral steroids to clear his eczema and volunteered: 'I don't care if oral steroids shorten my life span because eczema has literally ruined my life'. He declined a referral to a dermatologist as he believed a dermatologist would merely prescribe him more TCS (which he could obtain from a GP more readily and at a lower cost).

Conclusion

TCS are used a lot in Australia, and access to potent TCS has recently increased with the introduction of streamlined authority scripts. TCS underuse has received a lot of attention in Australia as evidenced by guidelines and published research. There is limited evidence of TCS overuse in Australia, but it is possible this is occurring to a greater extent than is currently recognised.

References

1. Britt H, Miler GC, Bayram C, Henderson J, et al. A decade of Australian general practice 2006–2007 to 2015–2016, General Practice Series Number 41. Sydney: Family Medicine Research Centre. The University of Sydney; 2016.
2. Smith SD, Lee A, Blaszczynski A, Fischer G. An assessment of Australian general practitioners' knowledge about use of topical corticosteroids in paediatric atopic dermatitis. Aust J Dermatol. 2016;57:17–8.
3. Smith S, Lee A, Blaszczynski A, Fisher G. Attitudes of Australian dermatologists to the use and safety of topical corticosteroids in paediatric atopic dermatitis. Aust J Dermatol. 2016;57:278–83. doi:10.1111/ajd.12402.
4. Topical issues—emollients and corticosteroids. Nov 2012. Australian Government Department of Veterans' Affairs www.veteransmates.net.au/topic-33-therapeutic-brief. Accessed 12 March 2017.
5. Mooney E, Rademaker M, Dailey R, Daniel BS, et al. Adverse effects of topical corticosteroids in paediatric eczema: Australian consensus statement. Aust J Dermatol. 2015;56(4):241–51.
6. Carlos G, Uribe P. Fernandez-Penas rational use of topical corticosteroids. Aust Prescr. 2013;36:5–6. doi:10.18773/austprescr.2013.063.
7. Dermatology Therapeutic Guidelines eTG. November 2016. Website: www.tg.org.au. Accessed 12 March 2017.
8. Smith SD, Dixit S, Fischer G. Childhood atopic dermatitis overcoming parental topical corticosteroid phobia. Med Today. 2013;14(6):47–52.
9. Smith SD, Stephens AM, Werren JC, Fischer GO. Treatment failure in atopic dermatitis as a result of parental health belief. MJA. 2013;199(7):467–9.
10. Smith SD, Lee A, Blaszczynski A, Fischer G. Pharmacists' knowledge about use of topical corticosteroids in atopic dermatitis: pre and post continuing professional development education. Aust J Dermatol. 2015;5:199–204. doi:10.1111/ajd.12339.
11. Smith SD, Hong E, Feams S, et al. Corticosteroid phobia and other cofounders in the treatment of childhood atopic dermatitis explored using parent focus groups. Aust J Dermatol. 2010;51(3):168–74.
12. Sheary B. Topical corticosteroid addiction and withdrawal in a 6 year old. J Prim Health Care. 2017; doi:10.1071/HC16049.
13. https://www.tga.gov.au/reporting-adverse-events. Accessed 12 March 2017.
14. Sheary B. Topical corticosteroid addiction and withdrawal—an overview for GPs. Aust Fam Physician. 2016;45(6):386–8.
15. Saxon S, Fischer G. Childhood atopic dermatitis: exploring the safety, efficacy and potential misinformation around topical corticosteroids. Australas J Pharm. 2016;97(1155):83–8.
16. Carter S. Topical steroids on old dry skin. Aust Pharm. 2016;35(8):20–1.

Systemic Side Effects of Topical Corticosteroids

25

Aparajita Ghosh and Arijit Coondoo

Abstract

Corticosteroids are the most commonly used topical anti-inflammatory and immunosuppressive drugs in dermatology. If used injudiciously, significant amounts of these drugs can be absorbed into the circulation. The systemic side effects that occur from such an exposure are similar to those seen with systemic administration of glucocorticoids, varying only in severity. Awareness regarding these adverse effects and knowledge regarding proper use of topical corticosteroids among both physicians and patients is of utmost importance to prevent these potentially serious side effects. Selective glucocorticoid receptor agonists (SEGRAs) are newer drugs which are being developed to overcome this problem.

Keywords

Topical corticosteroids • Adverse effects • Selective glucocorticoid receptor agonists

Learning Points

1. Topical corticosteroids can be absorbed into the circulation to produce systemic side effects.
2. These side effects are similar to those seen with systemic (oral or parenteral) administration of glucocorticoids but are often less severe.
3. Majority of these side effects can be prevented with judicious use of the drug.
4. These side effects are underreported and can range from mild and reversible HPA axis suppression to serious and life-threatening infections.
5. Systemic side effects are more common at the extremes of age (pediatric and the geriatric population).

A. Ghosh (✉) • A. Coondoo
Department of Dermatology, KPC Medical College and Hospital, Raja S.C. Mullick Road, Jadavpur, Kolkata 700032, West Bengal, India
e-mail: dr.aparajitaghosh@gmail.com

25.1 Introduction

Glucocorticoids are an important class of anti-inflammatory and immunosuppressive agents. However, their systemic use is often limited by their generalized adverse effects.

© Springer Nature Singapore Pte Ltd. 2018
K. Lahiri (ed.), *A Treatise on Topical Corticosteroids in Dermatology*,
DOI 10.1007/978-981-10-4609-4_25

The development of topically effective gluco-corticoid molecule in 1950 revolutionized the treatment of skin disorders, providing for the first time effective drugs which could be applied directly to the site of cutaneous lesion [1]. This in many cases obviated the need of systemic steroid therapy.

An ideal topical drug should be effective at the site of application without any local side effects. It should not be absorbed systemically or should become deactivated when absorbed into the circulation thus causing no systemic effects. However, the currently available topical corticosteroids (TCs) are far from ideal and have often been reported to cause adverse effects both systemic and local, on inappropriate use.

25.1.1 Mechanism of Percutaneous Drug Absorption

To cause systemic effects, a significant amount of the drug applied on the skin should first be absorbed into the circulation.

Percutaneous absorption of topically applied drug is a complex process, and various mathematical models have been proposed to predict the absorption of various molecules through human skin.

One of the most common to be used is the Fick's second law of diffusion which calculates the diffusion of a molecule along its concentration gradient across a semipermeable membrane [2].

$$[J = Kp \times \Delta Cs = (Dm \times Km) / L \times \Delta C$$

J, flux; *Kp, permeability constant*; *ΔCs, concentration gradient*; *Dm, diffusion constant*; *Km, partition coefficient*, and *L, length of the diffusion pathway or thickness of the membrane*.]

In spite of its simplicity, the usefulness of this law is limited by the human skin having multiple layers of varying composition and being structurally far more complex than a simple semipermeable membrane.

The application of a topical drug to the skin to its absorption into the system is a sum total of the following steps [3]:

- *Release* of the drug from its vehicle
- *Penetration* into the stratum corneum which acts as the first and the most important barrier
- *Permeation* of the drug through various layers of skin
- *Resorption or uptake* of the drug into the circulation by the capillary walls of the cutaneous blood vessels and lymphatic channels

Routes for cutaneous absorption may be "transcellular" involving passage of the drug through the layers of epidermis and "transfollicular or transappendageal" which involves penetration of the drug via openings of hair follicles or sweat glands [4, 5]. The transcellular route appears to be the most important. However, contrary to the earlier concept of the relative insignificance of the transappendageal route, it is now considered to contribute significantly to percutaneous drug absorption especially in areas of high follicular density [6].

25.1.2 Factors Affecting Systemic Adverse Effects

Systemic adverse effects due to topical corticosteroids are less common than local reactions but are far more serious. To give rise to these effects, the drug must be present in the systemic circulation in adequate amounts for a reasonably prolonged period of time. The various factors which determine the type and severity of the systemic effects caused by TC are summarized in Table 25.1:

Table 25.1 Factors affecting magnitude of systemic adverse effects caused by TC application

Factors affecting severity of systemic adverse effects			
Duration of systemic exposure to the drug: This is mostly determined by the duration of topical therapy [7]	*Nature of the drug*: More potent TC molecules are known to produce more severe systemic adverse effects compared to less potent ones, even with similar duration of therapy [8]. Clobetasol ointment in doses of 7.5 g/week can cause HPA axis suppression as compared to 49 g/week of betamethasone dipropionate [9, 10]	*Amount of drug absorbed into the system*: Multiple factors determine the quantity of drug that gets absorbed percutaneously into the systemic circulation • *Amount of drug applied*: Repeated or frequent applications or application of large quantities of drug locally increases the total quantity and contact time of the drug applied and hence absorbed into the system [11] • *Total surface area of drug application*: A large surface area of application increases the total amount of drug required and also the area available for drug absorption, thus increasing systemic drug levels. Compared to adults, children have larger body surface area-to-mass ratio and hence show increased chances of adverse effects [12]. Similarly, enhanced absorption is also seen in the geriatric age group with decreased skin thickness • *Site of application*: Stratum corneum is the predominant barrier to drug penetration; hence, variation in stratum corneum thickness causes wide variation in drug absorption form various sites. Drug absorption through scrotal skin and eyelids is the highest (almost 300 times) compared to skin of palms and soles [13] • *Condition of the skin*: Defective epidermal barrier increases drug absorption. Hence, diseases like atopic dermatitis, which damage the epidermal barrier, lead to greater absorption [14] • *Occlusion* increases hydration of the skin and consequent absorption [15]. It assumes significance in areas which are naturally occluded like the intertriginous areas or the diaper area in case of infants • *Chemical properties of TC molecule or its formulation*: 1. Higher concentration of steroid in the formulation increases flux for absorption 2. More lipophilic molecules likely show enhanced penetration [11] 3. Vehicle in which the drug is formulated affects absorption [16]. It is significantly more when the TC is formulated in an ointment base, possibly due to increased hydration of the skin and occlusive effect of the base [17] 4. Simultaneous use of keratolytic agents can damage the stratum corneum thus increasing penetration	*Clearance of drug from the body*: Most corticosteroid molecules are metabolized in the liver and finally excreted through the kidneys [18]. Hence, absorbed corticosteroids may accumulate to cause adverse effects in patients with deranged hepatic and renal function and in pediatric age group especially preterms and neonates with decreased ability for hepatic and renal clearance

Table 25.2 Systemic adverse effects due to TC absorption

Systemic adverse effects due to TC absorption	
Ocular	Glaucoma, ocular hypertension, posterior subcapsular cataract, blindness
Endocrine	HPA axis suppression, iatrogenic Cushing's syndrome, delayed puberty
Metabolic	Glucose intolerance, diabetes mellitus, electrolyte imbalance (sodium retention, hypokalemia, hypocalcemia), hypertension, edema and water retention, dyslipidemia, benign intracranial hypertension
Musculoskeletal	Osteoporosis, growth retardation, osteonecrosis (avascular necrosis of femur head), muscle atrophy
Immune function	Decreased immunity, recurrent pyogenic infections, disseminated systemic infections
Cutaneous	Atrophy of skin, striae, delayed wound healing
Neuropsychiatric	Worsening of previous psychiatric disorders, psychosis and mania, depression (may also occur on withdrawal), psychologic dependence on topical steroid

25.2 Systemic Adverse Effects Due to Topical Agents

There is paucity of data regarding the exact incidence of systemic side effects due to TC application, though it appears to be relatively uncommon. Reported adverse effects range from slight reversible suppression of hypothalamic-pituitary-adrenal (HPA) axis [19, 20] to fatal generalized cytomegalovirus infection in infant [21, 22]. These are similar to those seen with systemic administration of corticosteroids but are often less severe. Table 25.2 summarizes the systemic adverse effects due to TC absorption.

25.2.1 HPA Axis Suppression and Iatrogenic Cushing's Syndrome

These constitute the most commonly reported systemic adverse effects [23]. The HPA axis is a finely regulated, interlinked system of hormones with widespread effects on body metabolism including maintenance of blood glucose levels and response to stress. Almost all TC molecules have the ability to suppress the HPA axis; however, the menace is more with the class I molecules especially clobetasol (0.05% ointment) which can cause suppression at doses as less as 2 g/day within a few days of use. Continuous use leads to increase in bodyweight, development of moon face, buffalo hump, striae, delayed wound healing, and other features of Cushing's syndrome. Exogenous TC molecules suppress the release of CRH and ACTH leading to decreased stimulation of the adrenal glands and consequent low levels of endogenously produced cortisol. This results in a form of secondary adrenal insufficiency. Sudden stoppage of TC application in such patients may lead to Addisonian crisis. Recovery of the HPA axis occurs spontaneously once the TC application stops. The recovery period of HPA axis suppression was reported to be 3.49 ± 2.92 and 3.84 ± 2.51 months in children and adult, respectively [23]. Laboratory investigations recommended for assessment of HPA axis function are enlisted in Table 25.3.

25.2.2 Musculoskeletal System

Growth retardation and delayed puberty are seen in children especially those with atopic dermatitis who are exposed to long duration of TC therapy [7]. Delayed puberty and decreased bone age are often because of low growth hormone (GH) and thyroid hormone levels as a result of a generalized suppression of hypothalamic and pituitary function. However, premature closure of the epiphyses resulting in a small but significant diminution of final height has been reported in children exposed to systemic corticosteroid [7].

In adults, glucocorticoid-induced osteoporosis mostly affects the cancellous bones; hence, vertebral bodies and ribs are most commonly affected.

Table 25.3 Laboratory investigations for assessment of HPA axis function

Evaluation of HPA axis function [24–26]
• *Early morning cortisol test*:
– Measures the plasma levels of cortisol at 8 am. Values <110 mmols/L indicative of HPA axis suppression
– Simple but limited sensitivity must be followed by an assessment of serum ACTH levels and/or the ACTH stimulation test
• *ACTH stimulation test*:
– Measures the responsiveness of the adrenal glands to exogenous ACTH. 1 μg (low-dose test) or 250 μg (conventional-dose test) *synthetic ACTH* is injected. Plasma cortisol levels assessed at 0 (baseline), 30, and 60 min
– In healthy individuals, cortisol level should double from baseline (20–30 μg/dL) within 60 min
– In secondary adrenal insufficiency, ACTH may dramatically stimulate cortisol release from the adrenals by several folds from the low baseline
– Often inconclusive especially in case of partial adrenal failure due to long-standing HPA suppression
• *Insulin tolerance test (ITT)*:
– Gold standard for functional assessment of entire HPA axis including partial adrenal insufficiency or recent onset adrenal suppression
– Blood glucose and cortisol levels at baseline measured, followed by injection of 0.1–0.15 units of short-acting insulin. Blood glucose and cortisol levels are measured again at 30, 45, 60, 90, and 120 min after the insulin injection
– Adequate response—rise of cortisol >550 nmol/L on achieving adequate hypoglycemia (blood glucose <2.2 mmol/L)
– Cushing's syndrome—rise <170 nmol/L above the fluctuations of basal levels of cortisol
– Limitation—potential for serious hypoglycemia
• *Metyrapone test*:
– Safer than the ITT
– Reversible inhibitor of steroid 11β-hydroxylase and blocks cortisol synthesis. Stimulates ACTH secretion, in turn increasing plasma 11-deoxycortisol levels
– Metyrapone administered orally at midnight. The plasma cortisol and 11-deoxycortisol are measured next morning at 8:00 am
– Secondary adrenal insufficiency—plasma cortisol <220 nmol/L indicates adequate inhibition of 11β-hydroxylase. 11-deoxycortisol <7 μg/dL (202 nmol/L) suggestive of impaired HPA axis at the level of pituitary or hypothalamus
• *Serum ACTH*—alone this test is of limited diagnostic value. May be used in conjunction with other stimulation tests
• *Dexamethasone suppression test*
• *Urinary cortisol test*
• *Midnight salivary cortisol*

Vertebral fractures and hip fracture may occur after several years of therapy with large amounts of potent TC [27, 28]. Females especially postmenopausal, geriatric patients and those with concurrent disease like COPD are at higher risk of developing such complications [7]. The mechanism of corticosteroid-induced bone loss is complex and is schematically depicted in Fig. 25.1.

High level of systemic glucocorticoids is one of the most important causes of avascular bone necrosis (AVN) or osteonecrosis [29]. It involves bones with a single terminal blood supply and leads to progressive destruction of the bone as a result of compromise of bone vasculature, the femoral head being the most commonly affected. The mechanism of glucocorticoid-induced AVN is not fully understood till date. Several hypotheses exist which include fat cell hypertrophy, fat embolization, intravascular coagulation, and osteocyte apoptosis, all resulting in compromise of bone vasculature and marrow, leading to ischemic necrosis of the femoral head and subsequent collapse of the bone [29].

Glucocorticoid causes muscle atrophy due to overall catabolic effect on muscles [30]. It inhibits glucose uptake and utilization by the skeletal muscles and also increases the breakdown of muscle proteins and decreases protein synthesis. The effect is more pronounced in the proximal muscle groups with the muscles around the hip joint and quadriceps being more severely involved [31].

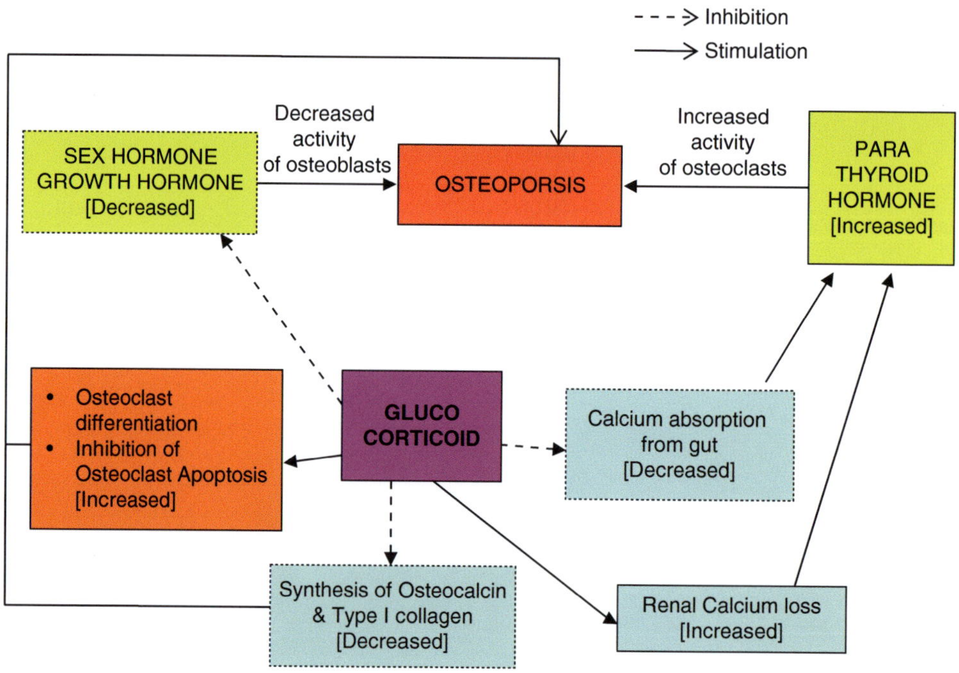

Fig. 25.1 Schematic depiction of mechanism of corticosteroid-induced bone loss

25.2.3 Hyperglycemia and Metabolic Disorders

Glucocorticoids can induce diabetes in previously nondiabetic patients or may worsen the glycemic control in persons with preexisting diabetes [7]. It works synergistically with glucagon pathway, inhibits insulin release from the beta cells of pancreas, and promotes insulin resistance resulting in decreased glucose uptake and utilization in target organs (muscles and fatty tissue) [32].

It increases gluconeogenesis (synthesis of glucose from amino acids) by increasing the activity of cytoplasmic aspartate aminotransferase enzyme in liver cells. Glucose 6-phosphatase is another enzyme which is similarly affected, thus increasing glucose synthesis. The raised amount of glucose leads to increased synthesis of glycogen and its deposition in the liver [32].

Hypertension and hyperlipidemia can also occur as part of Cushing's syndrome [33]. The cause of hypertension is complex and is not only because of the sodium retaining mineralocorticoid effect of the corticosteroid molecule. Most of the TC molecules except hydrocortisone have no significant mineralocorticoid effect [18].

25.2.4 Ocular Adverse Effects

Percutaneous absorption of TC through eyelids and facial skin is high. Application of TC for long duration on these areas has been reported to increase intraocular tension in some cases leading to glaucoma and blindness [22, 34]. This effect is possibly due to glucocorticoid-induced morphological and functional changes in the trabecular meshwork as a result of accumulation of polymers of glycosaminoglycans and alterations in composition of extra cellular matrix [35].

Cataract especially the posterior subcapsular type can occur associated with Cushing's syndrome and hyperglycemia induced by corticosteroid [36].

25.2.5 Cutaneous Adverse Reactions

Skin atrophy, striae, and delayed wound healing are known to occur not only at and around the site of TC application but also in a more generalized pattern as part of systemic hypercortisolism. Steroid-induced atrophy of the skin affects all the layers of the skin [37]. There is a reduction in proliferation of keratinocytes and dermal fibroblasts. Decrease in synthesis of collagen I and III, elastin, hyaluronic acid, and sulfated glycosaminoglycans has been described [38, 39].

Corticosteroid-induced downregulation of proinflammatory cytokines, proteases, and growth factors and decreased chemotaxis of inflammatory cells result in inhibition of the early phase of inflammation which appears to be important for wound healing [7, 40]. Decrease in collagen synthesis especially collagen VII which is the major component of anchoring fibrils has also been reported further hampering the healing process [41].

25.3 Special Concerns Regarding TC Use in Pediatric and Geriatric Population

Patients at the two extremes of age are more prone to develop TC-induced systemic side effects.

Children have a much larger surface area compared to their body mass. This results in higher systemic concentration of corticosteroid as compared to adults for the same amount of TC absorbed through the skin. Also the percutaneous absorption of the drug is greater as infant skin has thinner epidermis and stratum corneum, and corneocytes are smaller. The water-handling properties are not fully developed till the second year of life [42]. The renal and hepatic functions in them are also not adequately mature to handle the systemic corticosteroid resulting in higher incidence of systemic adverse effects. The use of diapers in infants and toddlers not only predisposes to intertrigo and diaper dermatitis which is often treated with TC but also results in occlusion and higher absorption of TC from this area.

In the geriatric population because of age-related atrophy, the skin is thinner leading to greater percutaneous absorption [43]. Also underlying renal and hepatic compromise may coexist predisposing them to greater systemic side effects.

Precautions for TC application:

- Use of TC of appropriate potency according to area of application.
- Use of appropriate potency of TC required for disease control, with subsequent change to less potent drug or once the disease is under control.
- Application of TC in an intermittent fashion (e.g., alternate day application or twice in a week application) instead of daily application is preferable as it has been shown to be associated with less chances of HPA axis suppression [44, 45].
- Use of less potent TCs under occlusion may produce an effect equivalent to potent steroid without occlusion and has the advantage of much less systemic effects even on absorption [46, 47].
- When potent steroid is used, the use should be restricted to less than 50 g/week [22].
- Educating the patient regarding FTU (fingertip unit) and the amount of drug to be applied to various body sites can prevent both excess and inadequate application of the drug.

Conclusion

There is an increasing concern regarding the systemic adverse effects of TCs. However, a large number of these effects are preventable. The solution lies in judicious use of TC by both the physician and the patient. The adverse effect profile of this very useful class of drugs has fueled the search for molecules with a similar but more selective mechanism of action. The development of molecules called selective glucocorticoid receptor agonists (SEGRAs) is a step in that direction. Unlike the traditional corticosteroid molecules which act by transactivation and transrepression, the SEGRAs act majorly via transrepression and are reported to possess a better safety profile [47]. The current molecules like GSK866, mapracorat, and

PF-04171327 belong to this category and are still at various phases of clinical trials [48]. Efforts are on to develop topically effective SEGRA which will be useful in dermatologic therapy [49].

References

1. Sulzberger MB, Witten VH. The effect of topically applied compound F in selected dermatoses. J Invest Dermatol. 1952;19:101–2.
2. Kubota K, Dey F, Matar SA, Twizell EH. A repeated-dose model of percutaneous drug absorption. Appl Math Model. 2002;26(4):529–44.
3. Göpferich A, Lee G. An improved diffusion/compartmental model for transdermal drug delivery from a matrix-type device. Int J Pharm. 1991;71(3):237–43.
4. Lauer AC, Lieb LM, Ramachandran C, Flynn GL, Weiner ND. Transfollicular drug delivery. Pharm Res. 1995;12(2):179–86.
5. Meidan VM, Bonner MC, Michniak BB. Transfollicular drug delivery—is it a reality? Int J Pharm. 2005;306(1–4):1.
6. Ogiso T, Shiraki T, Okajima K, Tanino T, Iwaki M, Wada T. Transfollicular drug delivery: penetration of drugs through human scalp skin and comparison of penetration between scalp and abdominal skins in vitro. J Drug Target. 2002;10(5):369–78.
7. Schäcke H, Döcke WD, Asadullah K. Mechanisms involved in the side effects of glucocorticoids. Pharmacol Ther. 2002;96(1):23–43.
8. Scott M, Malmsten LA, Thelin I. Effect on plasma cortisol level and urinary cortisol excretion, in healthy volunteers, after application of three different topical steroid ointments under occlusion. Acta Derm Venereol. 1980;61(6):543–6.
9. Ohman EM, Rogers S, Meenan FO, McKenna TJ. Adrenal suppression following low-dose topical clobetasol propionate. J R Soc Med. 1987;80(7):422–4.
10. Weston WL, Fennessey PV, Morelli J, Schwab H, Mooney J, Samson C, Huff L, Harrison LM, Gotlin R. Comparison of hypothalamus-pituitary-adrenal axis suppression from superpotent topical steroids by standard endocrine function testing and gas chromatographic mass spectrometry. J Invest Dermatol. 1988;90(4):532–5.
11. Dhar S, Seth J, Parikh D. Systemic side-effects of topical corticosteroids. Indian J Dermatol. 2014;59(5):460.
12. Coondoo A, Phiske M, Verma S, Lahiri K. Side-effects of topical steroids: a long overdue revisit. Indian Dermatol Online J. 2014;5(4):416.
13. Feldmann RJ, Maibach HI. Regional variation in percutaneous penetration 14C cortisol in man. J Invest Dermatol. 1967;48:181–3.
14. Turpeinen M, Lehtokoski-Lehtiniemi E, Leisti S, Salo OP. Percutaneous absorption of hydrocortisone during

15. Zhai H, Maibach HI. Effects of skin occlusion on percutaneous absorption: an overview. Skin Pharmacol Physiol. 2001;14(1):1–0.
16. Wiedersberg S, Leopold CS, Guy RH. Bioavailability and bioequivalence of topical glucocorticoids. Eur J Pharm Biopharm. 2008;68(3):453–66.
17. Ayres PJ, Hooper G. Assessment of the skin penetration properties of different carrier vehicles for topically applied cortisol. Br J Dermatol. 1978;99(3):307–17.
18. Czock D, Keller F, Rasche FM, Häussler U. Pharmacokinetics and pharmacodynamics of systemically administered glucocorticoids. Clin Pharmacokinet. 2005;44(1):61–98.
19. Gilbertson EO, Spellman MC, Piacquadio DJ, Mulford MI. Super potent topical corticosteroid use associated with adrenal suppression: clinical considerations. J Am Acad Dermatol. 1998;38(2):318–21.
20. Walsh P, Aeling JL, Huff L, Weston WL. Hypothalamus-pituitary-adrenal axis suppression by superpotent topical steroids. J Am Acad Dermatol. 1993;29(3):501–3.
21. Güven A, Karadeniz S, Aydin O, Akbalik M, Aydin M. Fatal disseminated cytomegalovirus infection in an infant with Cushing's syndrome caused by topical steroid. Horm Res Paediatr. 2005;64(1):35–8.
22. Hengge UR, Ruzicka T, Schwartz RA, Cork MJ. Adverse effects of topical glucocorticosteroids. J Am Acad Dermatol. 2006;54:1–15.
23. Tempark T, Phatarakijnirund V, Chatproedprai S, Watcharasindhu S, Supornsilchai V, Wananukul S. Exogenous Cushing's syndrome due to topical corticosteroid application: case report and review literature. Endocrine. 2010;38(3):328–34.
24. Chrousos GP, Kino T, Charmandari E. Evaluation of the hypothalamic-pituitary-adrenal axis function in childhood and adolescence. Neuroimmunomodulation. 2009;16(5):272–83.
25. Schmidt IL, Lahner H, Mann K, Petersenn S. Diagnosis of adrenal insufficiency: evaluation of the corticotropin-releasing hormone test and basal serum cortisol in comparison to the insulin tolerance test in patients with hypothalamic-pituitary-adrenal disease. J Clin Endocrinol Metab. 2003;88(9):4193–8.
26. Ospina NS, Al Nofal A, Bancos I, Javed A, Benkhadra K, Kapoor E, Lteif AN, Natt N, Murad MHACTH. Stimulation tests for the diagnosis of adrenal insufficiency: systematic review and meta-analysis. J Clin Endocrinol Metab. 2015;101(2):427–34.
27. Manelli F, Giustina A. Glucocorticoid-induced osteoporosis. Trends Endocrinol Metab. 2000;11(3):79–85.
28. Van Staa TP, Leufkens HG, Cooper C. The epidemiology of corticosteroid-induced osteoporosis: a meta-analysis. Osteoporos Int. 2002;13(10):777–87.
29. Chan KL, Mok CC. Glucocorticoid-induced avascular bone necrosis: diagnosis and management. Open Orthop J. 2012;6(1):449–57.
30. Decramer M, De Bock V, Dom R. Functional and histologic picture of steroid-induced myopathy in

chronic obstructive pulmonary disease. Am J Respir Crit Care Med. 1996;153(6):1958–64.

31. Pereira RM, De Carvalho JF. Glucocorticoid-induced myopathy. Joint Bone Spine. 2011;78(1):41–4.

32. Hwang JL, Weiss RE. Steroid-induced diabetes: a clinical and molecular approach to understanding and treatment. Diabetes Metab Res Rev. 2014;30(2):96–102.

33. Wang M. The role of glucocorticoid action in the pathophysiology of the metabolic syndrome. Nutr Metab. 2005;2(1):3.

34. Kersey JP, Broadway DC. Corticosteroid-induced glaucoma: a review of the literature. Eye. 2006;20(4):407–16.

35. Tripathi RC, Parapuram SK, Tripathi BJ, Zhong Y, Chalam KV. Corticosteroids and glaucoma risk. Drugs Aging. 1999;15(6):439–50.

36. James ER. The etiology of steroid cataract. J Ocul Pharmacol Ther. 2007;23(5):403–20.

37. Pérez P, Page A, Bravo A, del Río M, Giménez-Conti I, Budunova I, Slaga TJ, Jorcano JL. Altered skin development and impaired proliferative and inflammatory responses in transgenic mice overexpressing the glucocorticoid receptor. FASEB J. 2001;15(11):2030–2.

38. Oikarinen A, Haapasaari KM, Sutinen M, Tasanen K. The molecular basis of glucocorticoid-induced skin atrophy: topical glucocorticoid apparently decreases both collagen synthesis and the corresponding collagen mRNA level in human skin in vivo. Br J Dermatol. 1998;139:1106–10.

39. Schoepe S, Schäcke H, May E, Asadullah K. Glucocorticoid therapy-induced skin atrophy. Exp Dermatol. 2006;15(6):406–20.

40. Wicke C, Halliday B, Allen D, Roche NS, Scheuenstuhl H, Spencer MM, Roberts AB, Hunt TK. Effects of steroids and retinoids on wound healing. Arch Surg. 2000;135(11):1265–70.

41. Gras MP, Verrecchia F, Uitto J, Mauviel A. Downregulation of human type VII collagen (COL7A1) promoter activity by dexamethasone. Exp Dermatol. 2001;10(1):28–34.

42. Stamatas GN, Nikolovski J, Mack MC, Kollias N. Infant skin physiology and development during the first years of life: a review of recent findings based on in vivo studies. Int J Cosmet Sci. 2011;33(1):17–24.

43. Couturaud V, Coutable J, Khaiat A. Skin biomechanical properties: in vivo evaluation of influence of age and body site by a non-invasive method. Skin Res Technol. 1995;1(2):68–73.

44. Hanifin J, Gupta AK, Rajagopalan R. Intermittent dosing of fluticasone propionate cream for reducing the risk of relapse in atopic dermatitis patients. Br J Dermatol. 2002;147(3):528–37.

45. Thomas KS, Armstrong S, Avery A, Po AL, O'Neill C, Young S, Williams HC. Randomised controlled trial of short bursts of a potent topical corticosteroid versus prolonged use of a mild preparation for children with mild or moderate atopic eczema. BMJ. 2002;324(7340):768.

46. Bewley A. Expert consensus: time for a change in the way we advise our patients to use topical corticosteroids. Br J Dermatol. 2008;158(5):917–20.

47. Stahn C, Löwenberg M, Hommes DW, Buttgereit F. Molecular mechanisms of glucocorticoid action and selective glucocorticoid receptor agonists. Mol Cell Endocrinol. 2007;275(1):71–8.

48. Lesovaya E, Yemelyanov A, Swart AC, Swart P, Haegeman G, Budunova I. Discovery of compound A: a selective activator of the glucocorticoid receptor with anti-inflammatory and anti-cancer activity. Oncotarget. 2015;6(31):30730–44.

49. Ryabtsova O, Joossens J, Van Der Veken P, Berghe WV, Augustyns K, De Winter H. Novel selective glucocorticoid receptor agonists (SEGRAs) with a covalent warhead for long-lasting inhibition. Bioorg Med Chem Lett. 2016;26(20):5032–8.

Topical Side Effects of Topical Corticosteroids

Rashmi Sarkar and Nisha V. Parmar

Abstract

Topical corticosteroids (TCS) are the most commonly used drugs by dermatologists around the globe. Their use is many times abused by patients resulting in unwanted and sometimes irreversible side effects. Majority of these adverse events go unreported in the dermatology literature leading to paucity of data regarding this subject. This chapter discusses the cutaneous side effects of TCS.

Keywords

Topical steroids • Cutaneous side effects • Topical side effects • Cutaneous atrophy • Easy bruisability • Steroidinduced rosacea • Acneiform eruption • Rebound phenomenon • Red scrotum syndrome

Learning Points

1. Topical corticosteroids are the most frequently prescribed medications by dermatologists. In spite of this, a database of their adverse cutaneous reactions is virtually non-existent.
2. Factors promoting the cutaneous side effects of topical corticosteroids are potency, site of application, duration of their application and application under occlusion.
3. The topical side effects of topical corticosteroids are broadly clubbed into the following categories: atrophy and related changes, pigmentary changes, follicular changes, vascular changes, infections and miscellaneous side effects.
4. Few of the uncommon side effects such as red scrotum syndrome and Majocchi's granuloma need a high index of suspicion for their diagnosis and hence dermatologists need to be aware of their presentation.
5. Steroid abuse is an active and massive societal problem in the world today with significant psychosocial impact on the patients affected.

R. Sarkar (✉)
Department of Dermatology, Maulana Azad Medical College and Lok Nayak Hospital, New Delhi, India
e-mail: rashmisarkar@gmail.com

N.V. Parmar
Aster Medical Centre, Dubai, United Arab Emirates

© Springer Nature Singapore Pte Ltd. 2018
K. Lahiri (ed.), *A Treatise on Topical Corticosteroids in Dermatology*,
DOI 10.1007/978-981-10-4609-4_26

26.1 Introduction

Topical corticosteroids (TCS) are the dermatologist's first-line armamentarium in the treatment of various skin disorders. A variety of compounds were isolated by Mason, Meyers and Kendall in 1935 from bovine adrenal glands and named compounds A–F [1]. Kendall's compound E (cortisone) and compound F (hydrocortisone) were found to be active in human subjects. Compound F was first used by Sulzberger and Witten in 1952 for the treatment of dermatological conditions [2]. Since then, a wide range of topical corticosteroids have been formulated by fluorination and halogenation at various carbon positions. As the number of compounds increases, the ease of their prescription by dermatologists also increases, and so does the frequency of their side effects. This chapter focuses on the side effects of TCS pertaining to the skin itself.

26.2 Topical Side Effects

The first report of a side effect surfaced in 1955 when Fitzpatrick et al. reported the occurrence of oedema and sodium retention secondary to topically applied fludrocortisone acetate [3]. Although this was a systemic side effect, it highlighted the protean effects that could result secondary to a topically applied substance.

Factors predicting the occurrence of cutaneous side effects of TCS include site of application, duration of application, potency of the steroid used and the presence of occlusion.

The site influences the thickness of the epidermis and hence the percutaneous penetration of the TCS. An inverse relationship exists between the epidermal thickness and the percutaneous penetration of the topical corticosteroid. The eyelid and scrotal skin is the thinnest; hence, they are sites of maximum percutaneous penetration and in turn potential side effects, whereas the palmoplantar skin is the thickest and hence allows minimal penetration (Fig. 26.1) [4]. The facial skin has

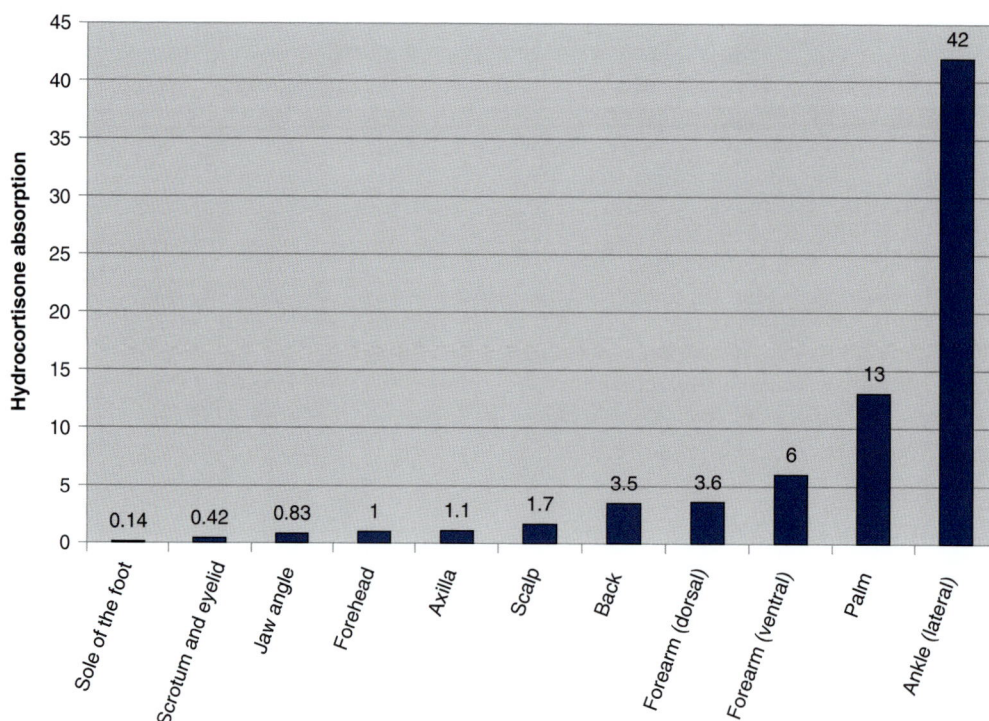

Fig. 26.1 Regional variation in the percutaneous penetration of hydrocortisone in men. Adapted from Feldman and Maibach

a thinner stratum corneum, and numerous sebaceous glands hence account for the maximum percutaneous penetration. It has been shown that only 1% of a topically applied corticosteroid has essentially therapeutic activity, whereas the rest 99% is usually subjected to rubbing, being washed off or exfoliated with the stratum corneum [5]. Under occlusion, the therapeutic activity of TCS increases to 10% due to enhanced percutaneous penetration.

The duration of application of the TCS also contributes significantly to the occurrence of side effects. The frequency of side effects is minimized when the duration of treatment is limited to a few days to a few weeks or via the use of intermittent therapy rather than continuous therapy when prolonged treatment is indicated.

The most important factor that is linked directly to the occurrence of cutaneous side effects however is the potency of the TCS, which is derived at after subjecting it to the vasoconstrictor assay, designed by McKenzie and Stoughton [6]. Most of the classifications of TCS, including the American classification into seven classes, and the British National Formulary classification are based on the assessment of the compound using the vasoconstrictor assay. In this assay, the TCS is applied to the skin of normal human volunteers. It then penetrates the stratum corneum and causes pallor of the skin as a result of its capacity to constrict the dermal blood vessels. The degree of vasoconstriction is then evaluated instrumentally as well as objectively using a visual grading scale and the compound classified. Characteristically, pallor secondary to the TCS reaches a maximal intensity around 9–12 h after application and fades initially rapidly over the next 10 h and slowly thereafter [7].

Cutaneous side effects of TCS are commoner than systemic side effects of TCS [5]. They can be classified into atrophy and related changes, pigmentary changes, follicular changes, vascular changes, infections and miscellaneous (Table 26.1). The side effects listed are usually confined to the sites of application of the TCS.

Table 26.1 Topical side effects of topical corticosteroids

Cutaneous adverse effects of topical corticosteroids
Atrophy and related changes
• Steroid atrophy
• Striae
• Easy bruising
• Ulceration
• Telangiectasia
• Purpura
• Stellate pseudoscars
Pigmentary changes
• Hypopigmentation
• Hyperpigmentation
Follicular changes
• Hypertrichosis
• Acneiform eruption
Vascular effects
• Rosacea
• Rebound phenomenon
• Facial erythema
• Red scrotum syndrome
Infections and Infestations
• Bacterial infections: folliculitis, furuncles
• Viral infections: herpes
• Fungal infections:
– Tinea incognito
– Majocchi granuloma
– Candidiasis
– Granuloma gluteale infantum
• Infestations: scabies incognito
Miscellaneous
• Perioral dermatitis
• Contact sensitization
• Delayed wound healing

26.3 Atrophy and Related Changes

Steroid atrophy is the most common cutaneous side effect of TCS [5]. Atrophy is also an irreversible side effect particularly when the TCS has been applied for a prolonged period. Steroid atrophy is most likely to occur at sites where the skin is inherently thinner such as the face especially the eyelids and flexures. Both fluorinated and non-fluorinated TCS can cause cutaneous atrophy. All atrophic changes secondary to application of TCS are reminiscent of actinically damaged skin and the ageing skin. Cutaneous atrophy secondary to TCS is classified into epidermal atrophy and dermal atrophy. Subcutaneous atrophy can rarely occur.

26.3.1 Epidermal Atrophy

In the first few days after commencing therapy with TCS, the metabolic activity of the keratinocyte is reduced [8]. Following protracted or rigorous exposure to the compound, the overall thickness of the epidermis decreases, as evidenced by thinning of the stratum corneum and almost complete loss of the underlying stratum granulosum. Ultrastructurally these changes occur as a result of decreased synthesis of keratohyalin granules, stratum corneum lipids and corneodesmosomes that are vital for the integrity of the stratum corneum [9].

Epidermal atrophy is clinically evident as fine 'cigarette paper' wrinkling of the skin at the site of application of the TCS.

26.3.2 Dermal Atrophy

This occurs as a result of diminution in the synthesis of dermal collagen via inhibition of the enzyme hyaluronan synthase 2 in the dermis [10]. In addition, the size of dermal fibroblasts as well as the number of mast cells is also significantly reduced [11, 12]. Research using capillaroscopic studies has demonstrated prolonged ischemia as another factor leading to dermal atrophy [13, 14]. These effects are heightened when the TCS is applied under occlusion. Collagen synthesis was found to be decreased as early as the third day of application of a potent TCS like betamethasone valerate and persisted for more than 2 weeks after discontinuation of the compound [12].

26.3.3 Striae

Striae are visible linear scars which form in areas of dermal damage. Striae occurring due to TCS application occur as a result of cutaneous atrophy and are observed at the site of prolonged TCS application. Histologically they are characterized by thinning of the epidermis and arrangement of the dermal collagen in fine thin lines parallel to the surface of the skin. Striae initially have an inflammatory phase in which they may be elevated and tender. Subsequently they flatten and become violaceous and smooth [15].

26.3.4 Purpura and Easy Bruisability

Secondary to TCS-induced loss of glycosaminoglycans in the dermis, the dermal blood vessels lose their supportive framework and hence rupture when subjected to even trivial trauma, leading to easy bruisability and subsequent purpura formation [16]. Frank cutaneous ulceration has also been rarely documented [17].

26.3.5 Telangiectasia

Telangiectasia refers to chronically dilated capillaries or venules. The word is derived from Latin, *tel* = end; Greek, *angos* = vessel; and Greek, *ectasis* = expansion. Due to loss of surrounding dermal substance and overall cutaneous atrophy, the blood vessels become more prominent and are visible to the naked eye [16]. Endothelial cell proliferation by TCS is also another mechanism which leads to formation of telangiectasia [18].

26.3.6 Stellate Pseudoscars

These are another consequence of TCS-induced cutaneous atrophy. They appear as hypopigmented star-shaped or linear scars with irregular margins [19]. They mostly occur on the skin of the extremities, sometimes at the sites of resolved purpura.

26.4 Pigmentary Changes

TCS inhibit melanin synthesis by hindering normal function of melanocytes [20]. This is pronounced when the TCS is applied under occlusion and results in hypopigmentation. This effect is reversible and normal pigmentation is restored within a few weeks after discontinuation of the TCS application [21].

26.5 Follicular Changes

26.5.1 Hypertrichosis

Hypertrichosis is defined as increase in the growth of hair which is thicker, denser and longer for the age, sex and race of the individual at a particular site. It has to be differentiated from hirsutism in which there is increase in terminal hair in the androgen-dependant areas of the body in women. TCS are iatrogenic causes of localized hypertrichosis; they stimulate growth of the vellus hair after prolonged application [22]. The hair persists as long as the TCS is continued. Upon stopping, the hair will be shed only after the anagen stage is over, an average of 2–3 years [5].

26.5.2 Acneiform Eruption

Acneiform eruption is an inflammatory follicular reaction characterized by erythematous monomorphic papules and pustules. Unlike acne vulgaris, the lesions here are monomorphic and lack comedones and cysts. The commonest cause is steroids, both systemic and topical, although various other drugs can also cause it [23]. The most common sites affected include the face, chest and upper back. Histopathologically a steroid-induced acneiform eruption demonstrates focal necrosis in the follicular infundibulum with extrusion of the follicular contents into the surrounding dermis and neutrophilic infiltrate in the perifollicular and intrafollicular arcas [24]. A drug-induced acneiform eruption should be suspected when there is a sudden occurrence of the lesions in a patient who has never had acne before, abrupt flare of acne in a patient with pre-existing acne, or late-onset of acne [25]. The treatment of acneiform eruption is similar to acne vulgaris.

26.6 Vascular Side Effects

They include steroid-induced rosacea, perioral dermatitis, red scrotum syndrome and rebound phenomenon. They occur more commonly with the use of fluorinated TCS [26].

26.6.1 Rosacea and Perioral Dermatitis

These side effects were first observed in 1957 after topical steroids were in use for 7 years. The terminology steroid rosacea has undergone numerous revisions; it was initially termed 'light sensitive seborrheid' by Frumess and Lewis as it resembled seborrhoeic dermatitis [27]. It was later named 'perioral dermatitis' by Mihan and Ayres [28]. Following this in 1969, Sneddon labelled it 'rosacea-like dermatitis' [29], and in 1974, the term 'steroid rosacea' was introduced by Leydon et al. [30]. Both the later terminologies are used in the current dermatology literature.

The time of onset of these varies greatly and can range between 2 months and 7 years but usually lies within 2–6 months [31]. TCS are used with or without prescription for a wide range of facial dermatoses. Following initial use, the patient notes dramatic improvement in the concerned dermatosis and continues using the TCS without consultation. After temporary discontinuation, flaring of the dermatosis results, and the TCS restarted by the patient. Hence, the vicious cycle continues before a patient lands at a dermatology OPD with full-blown steroid rosacea.

The symptoms include burning, stinging, facial flushing, skin dryness, persistent redness, photosensitivity and sometimes immense pruritus, similar to the symptoms of classical rosacea. On examination, telangiectasia, papules and pustules are seen on a background of erythema. Increased dermal populations of the commensal mite *Demodex folliculorum* are particularly noted in steroid rosacea and are postulated to cause blockage of the hair follicle leading to an inflammatory response [32].

The clinical picture is classified into three morphological types: perioral, centrofacial and diffuse [30].

The perioral form, also referred to as perioral dermatitis, is characterized by erythematous papulopustules in the perioral area with a rim of sparing immediately adjacent to the vermilion border of the lips. The centrofacial type affects the convexities of the face including the cheeks, chin and forehead with sparing of the perioral area. The diffuse type affects the entire face and is the severe form. Untreated, steroid rosacea can progress to fibrotic changes in the dermis and irreversible lymphedema secondary to prolonged inflammation.

The first step in the management of steroid rosacea is discontinuation of the offending agent, the TCS. In a patient who has been using a potent TCS for more than 2 months, tapering of the potency for the first few weeks followed by slow tapering of the low-potency steroid is initiated. In one who has been using a low-potency steroid for a prolonged duration, using it initially on alternate days, followed by twice weekly, once weekly and finally discontinuation, is advised. Tapering the TCS in the above manner is done to avoid the rebound phenomenon. In addition to this, low-dosed doxycycline at a dose of 40–100 mg daily for 3–4 months is prescribed. This is done to act against the increased populations of *Propionibacterium acnes* that are observed in a chronic steroid-exposed face [33]. The treatment regimen is changed after 3–4 months if adequate response is not achieved; low-dose isotretinoin at a dose of 5–20 mg is then introduced and continued for 3–4 months [31].

26.6.2 Red Scrotum Syndrome

This syndrome is analogous to rosacea and occurs due to repeated application of TCS on the scrotum [33]. It is characterized by chronic bright red erythema, itching, hyperalgesia and a burning sensation. A neuropsychiatric aetiology compounded by repeated application of TCS is implicated in the pathogenesis [34, 35]. Withdrawal of the TCS and response to tetracyclines favour the latter, whereas a response to gabapentin in a few patients favours the neuropsychiatric theory.

26.6.3 Rebound Phenomenon

This is characterized by the worsening of the dermatosis when the TCS is withdrawn. It is commoner in chronic dermatoses such as psoriasis and rosacea. On withdrawal of the TCS application on psoriatic plaques, pustulation can be precipitated, localized usually, but rarely generalized [36]. This phenomenon occurs with the use of potent TCS, application under occlusion, use of large quantities and sudden withdrawal. Mommers et al. demonstrated that an almost complete block of proliferation of basal cells occurs after use of clobetasol-17-propionate ointment, a superpotent TCS, under occlusion in psoriatic patients, and a rebound increased proliferation resulted after withdrawal [37].

26.7 Infections and Infestations

TCS decrease the overall immunity of the skin, both cell-mediated and humoral. Hence, bacterial, viral, fungal infections as well infestations can resurface or be aggravated.

26.7.1 Bacterial Infections

Colonization of *Staphylococcus aureus* on atopic skin due to diminished levels of surface antimicrobial peptides is a well-known fact; hence, these subjects are more prone to impetigo, folliculitis and furuncles. However, evidence suggests that treatment of atopic dermatitis with TCS of higher potencies significantly decreases the density of *Staphylococcus aureus* [38].

26.7.2 Viral Infections

The use of TCS is contraindicated in areas of the skin where there is an active viral infection such as herpes simplex, molluscum contagiosum or viral warts for fear of exacerbation of the infection [39].

26.7.3 Fungal Infections

Fungal infections are masked by the use of TCS. There is typically initial improvement with clearance of the infection followed by sudden flare on discontinuation. A classical example of this is tinea incognito (unrecognized tinea) in which repeated application of TCS to a dermatophyte infection leads to marked flare and spread of infection upon discontinuation of the TCS [40].

The other dermatophyte infection perpetuated by the use of TCS is Majocchi granuloma, a deep form of dermatophytosis in which the fungus is introduced to the dermis via minor breeches in the epidermis. The follicular form of Majocchi granuloma affects women who shave their legs and individuals who have used TCS for prolonged periods [41]. It presents as follicular nodules and pustules that do not respond to oral antibiotics. A high index of suspicion is required for its diagnosis.

Nodular granulomatous candidiasis or infantile gluteal granuloma represents a granulomatous cutaneous response to *Candida albicans* in the diaper area of infants in whom TCS are applied for conditions such as diaper dermatitis, atopic dermatitis or intertrigo [42]. The diaper area is more prone to the side effects of TCS due to the naturally occlusive effect of the folds, as well as diapers in addition to the inherently thinner infantile skin. It presents as bluish brown nodules occasionally up to 2 cm in size on the buttocks, upper thighs, mons pubis and groin folds. They occur due to a suppressed inflammatory immune response to *Candida species* by the TCS [43]. They are not a common occurrence nowadays.

26.7.4 Infestations

Ordinary scabies can be converted to crusted scabies by the use of potent TCS [44]. Its clinical picture can also be modified when it is referred to as scabies incognito [45]. The itching and skin lesions temporarily wither, while the mites multiply and infestation persists.

26.8 Contact Sensitization

It is quite ironical that a compound as beneficial in the treatment of allergic dermatitis as a TCS can itself produce an allergic dermatitis secondary to sensitization. This represents a delayed hypersensitivity reaction and occurs on prolonged use of the TCS. Coopman and colleagues classified TCS into four classes based on the groups of sensitization; cross-reactivity is most likely to occur among compounds within a single group (Table 26.2) [46]. Tixocortol pivalate and budesonide are the compounds of choice for screening of allergic contact dermatitis to TCS.

Allergic contact dermatitis to TCS is commoner with the use of fluorinated compounds such as hydrocortisone, budesonide and hydrocortisone-17-butyrate, than with the use of

Table 26.2 Classification of topical corticosteroids by cross-reactivity (Coopman et al. [46])

Group A
Hydrocortisone, hydrocortisone acetate, cortisone acetate, tixocortol pivalate, prednisolone, methylprednisolone, prednisone
Group B
Triamcinolone acetonide, triamcinolone alcohol, amcinonide, budesonide, desonide, fluocinonide, fluocinolone acetonide, halcinonide
Group C
Betamethasone, betamethasone sodium phosphate, desoximetasone, dexamethasone, dexamethasone sodium phosphate, fluocortolone
Group D
Hydrocortisone-17-butyrate, hydrocortisone-17-valerate, alclometasone dipropionate, betamethasone valerate, betamethasone dipropionate, prednicarbate, clobetasol-17-butyrate, clobetasol-17-propionate, fluocortolone caproate, fluocortolone pivalate, fluprednidene acetate

non-fluorinated TCS [47]. A requirement for the occurrence of the allergic contact dermatitis to TCS is the binding to the amino acid arginine to the human skin proteins [48].

Allergic contact dermatitis to TCS is often missed and requires a high index of suspicion for the diagnosis. Initially thought to be rare, it is now known to have a prevalence of 0.2–6% by various contact dermatitis groups [49, 50]. A suspicion of allergic contact dermatitis should occur in a patient who with known dermatitis but who is not responding to the TCS or when there is initial response followed by no decline in response. Patch testing with the TCS series is warranted in this group of patients [5].

26.9 Miscellaneous

26.9.1 Delayed Wound Healing

Delayed wound healing due to corticosteroids is multifactorial. Cutaneous atrophy, delay in formation of granulation tissue and vasoconstriction secondary to TCS application are some of the factors that contribute to delayed wound healing [51].

26.10 How to Prevent the Cutaneous Adverse Effects of Topical Steroids: Tips for Dermatologists

The following points should be kept in mind when prescribing a TCS.

1. Prolonged application of TCS should be discouraged in steroid-responsive dermatoses. Once the dermatosis shows signs of response, intermittent therapy, weekend therapy and slow taper of the potency of the TCS should be undertaken. Duration of application on the face should be limited to 10–14 days and rest 3–4 weeks for the rest of the body.
2. Occlusion should be limited to the palms and soles and dermatoses with thicker lesions. It should never be used on the face and flexures due to their naturally occlusive effect.
3. Caution should be taken in certain age groups. In the paediatric age group, the surface area to volume ratio is high; hence, more absorption of the TCS occurs with higher chances of HPA axis suppression. The skin is relatively thinner in infants and children; hence, the likelihood of developing the cutaneous side effects is higher. Similarly, in the geriatric age group, the skin is generally fragile and thinner and they are hence more vulnerable to the side effects of TCS.
4. When the TCS has to be applied to larger areas, duration should be limited and potency should be lower.
5. Finally it is our duty as dermatologists to report any side effect or adverse events secondary to TCS as trivial as it may be.

In conclusion, it is pertinent to be aware of the cutaneous side effects of TCS including age-related effects as few of them may be masked by the TCS itself. Conditions such as steroid rosacea and Majocchi granuloma need a high index of suspicion for their diagnosis.

References

1. Mason HL, Meyers CS, Kendall HC. The chemistry of crystalline substances isolated from the suprarenal gland. J Biol Chem. 1936;114:613–31.
2. Sulzberger MB, Witten VH. The effect of topically applied compound F in selected dermatoses. J Invest Dermatol. 1952;19(2):101.
3. Fitzpatrick TB, Griswold HC, Hicks JH. Sodium retention and edema from percutaneous absorption of fludrocortisone acetate. J Am Med Assoc. 1955;158:1149–52.
4. Feldman RJ, Maibach SR. Regional variation in percutaneous penetration of 14C cortisol in man. J Invest Dermatol. 1967;48:181–3.
5. Robertson DB, Maibach HI. Topical corticosteroids. Int J Dermatol. 1982;21:59–67.
6. McKenzie AW, Stoughton RB. Method for comparing percutaneous absorption of steroids. Arch Dermatol. 1962;86:608–10.
7. Barry BW, Woodford R. Comparative bio-availability and activity of proprietary topical corticosteroid preparations: vasoconstrictor assays on thirty one ointments. Br J Dermatol. 1975;93:563–71.

8. Delforno C, Holt PJ, Marks R. Corticosteroid effect on epidermal cell size. Br J Dermatol. 1978;98:619–23.

9. Lehmann P, Zheng P, Lavker RM, Kligman AM. Corticosteroid atrophy in human skin. A study by light, scanning and transmission electron microscopy. J Invest Dermatol. 1983;81:69–76.

10. Averbeck M, Gebhardt C, Anderegg U, Simon JC. Suppression of hyaluronan synthase 2 expression reflects the atrophogenic potential of glucocorticoids. Exp Dermatol. 2010;19:757–9.

11. Oikarinen A, Haapasaari KM, Sutinen M, Tasanen K. The molecular basis of glucocorticoid-induced skin atrophy: topical glucocorticoid apparently decreases both collagen synthesis and the corresponding collagen mRNA level in human skin in vivo. Br J Dermatol. 1998;139:1106–10.

12. Haapasaari KM, Risteli J, Karvonen J, Oikarinen A. Effect of hydrocortisone, methylprednisolone aceponate and mometasonefuruoate on collagen synthesis in human skin in vivo. Skin Pharmacol. 1997;10:261–4.

13. Hoffman K, Auer T, Stucker M, Hoffmann A, Altmeyer P. Comparison of skin atrophy and vasoconstriction due to mometasonefuroate, methylprednisolone and hydrocortisone. J Eur Acad Dermtol Venereol. 1998;10(2):137–42.

14. Barnes L, Kaya G, Rollason V. Topical corticosteroid-induced skin atrophy: a comprehensive review. Drug Saf. 2015;38(5):493–509.

15. Ammar NM, Rao B, Schwartz RA, Janniger CK. Cutaneous striae. Cutis. 2000;65:69–70.

16. Stevanovic DV. Corticosteroid-induced atrophy of the skin with telangiectasia. A clinical and experimental study. Br J Dermatol. 1972;87:548–56.

17. Kligman AM. Letter: topical steroid addicts. JAMA. 1976;235(15):1550.

18. Hettmannsperger U, Tenorio S, Orfanos CE, Detmar S. Corticosteroids induce proliferation but do not influence TNF or IL-1 beta-induced ICAM expression of human dermal microvasculature endothelial cells in vitro. Arch Dermatol Res. 1993;285:347–51.

19. Colomb D. Stellate spontaneous pseudoscars. Senile and presenile forms: especially those forms caused by prolonged corticoid therapy. Arch Dermatol. 1972;105(4):551.

20. Arnold J, Anthonioz P, Marchand JP. Depigmenting action of corticosteroids. Dermatologica. 1975;151:274–80.

21. Hengge UR, Ruzicka T, Schwartz RA, Cork MJ. Adverse effects of topical glucocorticoids. J Am Acad Dermatol. 2006;54:1–15.

22. Takeda K, Arase S, Takahasi S. Side effects of TCS and their prevention. Drugs. 1988;5:15–23.

23. Du-Thanh A, Kluger N, Bensalleh H, Guillot B. Drug-induced acneiform eruption. Am J Clin Dermatol. 2011;12:233–45.

24. Kiadbey KH, Kligman AM. The pathogenesis of topical steroid acne. J Invest Dermatol. 1974;62:31–4.

25. Plewig G, Kligman AM. Induction of acne by topical steroids. Arch Dermatol Forsch. 1973;247:29–52.

26. Sneddon I. Adverse effect of topical fluorinated corticosteroids in rosacea. Br Med J. 1969;1:671–3.

27. Frumess GM, Lewis HM. Light-sensitive seborrheid. Arch Dermatol. 1957;75:245–8.

28. Mihan R, Ayres S Jr. Perioral dermatitis. Arch Dermatol. 1964;89:803–5.

29. Sneddon I. Iatrogenic dermatitis. Br Med J. 1969;4:49.

30. Leyden SJ, Thew M, Kligman AM. Steroid rosacea. Arch Dermatol. 1974;110:619–22.

31. Ljubojević S, Basta-Juzbasić A, Lipozeneić J. Steroid dermatitis resembling rosacea. J Eur Acad Dermatol Venereol. 2002;16:121–6.

32. Basta-Juzbasić A, Subić JS, Ljubojević S. Demodex folliculorum in development of dermatitis rosaceiformissteroidica and rosacea-related diseases. Clin Dermatol. 2002;20:135–40.

33. Shibata M, Katsuyama M, Onodera T, Ehama R, Hosoi J, Tagami H. Glucocorticoids enhance toll-like receptor 2 expression in human keratinocytes stimulated with propionobacterium acnes or proinflammatory cytokines. J Invest Dermatol. 2009;129(2):375–82.

34. Narang T, Kumaran MS, Dogra S, Saikia UN, Kumar B. Red scrotum syndrome: idiopathic neurovascular phenomenon or steroid addiction? Sex Health. 2013;10(5):452–5.

35. Wollina U. Red scrotum syndrome. J Dermatol Case Rep. 2011;5(3):38–41.

36. Baker H. Corticosteroids and pustular psoriasis. Br J Dermatol. 1976;94(Suppl 12):83–8.

37. Mommers JM, van Erp PE, van De Kerkhof PC. Clobetasol under hydrocolloid occlusion in psoriasis results in a complete block of proliferation and in a rebound of lesions following discontinuation. Dermatology. 1999;199(4):323–7.

38. Nilsson EJ, Henning CG, Magnusson J. Topical corticosteroids and Staphylococcus aureus in atopic dermatitis. J Am Acad Dermatol. 1992;27:29–34.

39. Hellier FF. Profuse molluscacontagiosa of face induced by corticosteroids. Br J Dermatol. 1971;85:398.

40. Arenas R, Moreno-Coutino G, Vera L, Welsh O. Tinea incognito. Clin Dermatol. 2010;28(2):137–9.

41. Molina-Leyva A, Perez-Parra S, Garcia-Garcia F. Case for diagnosis. Majocchi granuloma. An Bras Dermatol. 2014;89(5):839–40.

42. Bluestein J, Furner BB, Phillips D. Granuloma glutealeinfantum: case report and review of the literature. Pediatr Dermatol. 1990;7(3):196–8.

43. Bonifazi E, Garofalo L, Lospalluti M. Granuloma glutealeinfantum with atrophic scars: clinical and histological observations in eleven cases. Clin Exp Dermatol. 1981;6:23–9.

44. Wishart J. Norwegian scabies, a Christ Church epidemic. Aust J Dermatol. 1972;13:127.

45. Marliere V, Raul S, Labreze C, Taieb A. Crusted (Norwegian) scabies induced by use of TCS and treated successfully with ivermectin. J Pediatr. 1999;135:122–4.

46. Coopman S, Degreff H, Dooms-Goossens A. Identification of cross-reaction patterns in allergic contact dermatitis from topical steroids. Br J Dermatol. 1989;121:27–34.

47. Thomson KF, Wilkinson SM, Powell S, Beck MH. The prevalence of corticosteroid allergy in two U.K. centres: prescribing implications. Br J Dermatol. 1999;141:863–6.

48. SM JMF. Corticosteroid usage and binding to arginine: determinants of corticosteroid hypersensitivity. Br J Dermatol. 1996;135:225–30.

49. Lutz ME, el-Azhary RA. Allergic contact dermatitis due to topical application of corticosteroids: review and clinical implications. Mayo Clin Proc. 1997;72:1141–4.

50. Isaksson M, Andersen KE, Brandao FM, Bruynzeel DP, Bruze M, Camarasa JG, et al. Patch testing with corticosteroid mixes in Europe. A multicentre study of the EECDRG. Contact Dermatitis. 2000;42:27–35.

51. Marks JG Jr, Cano C, Leitzel K, Lipton A. Inhibition of wound healing by topical steroids. J Dermatol Surg Oncol. 1983;9:819–21.

Topical Corticosteroid Addiction

Arijit Coondoo, Koushik Lahiri,
and Aparajita Ghosh

Abstract

Topical corticosteroids have been rampantly used, misused and abused down the years in various ways. Topical steroid abuse may lead to a couple of psychosomatic problems particularly topical corticosteroid addiction. Topical steroid addiction was recognised about a decade after the introduction of the molecule. It is manifested as psychological distress due to continuous and unsupervised use and misuse of the drug as well as a rebound phenomenon occurring when the drug is stopped. The ill effects of topical corticosteroid addiction and rebound occur both as cutaneous and systemic manifestations and may in some cases be irreversible particularly in the face and genitalia. "Topical corticosteroid addiction/dependence" implies the cutaneous and psychological dependence of the patient on the drug (topical corticosteroid), which results in rebound phenomenon and psychological distress on stoppage of its application. It is this psychological aspect which differentiates this condition from the other topical corticosteroid-induced skin reactions.

Keywords

Topical corticosteroid • Addiction • Dependence

A. Coondoo (✉) • A. Ghosh
Department of Dermatology, K.P.C. Medical College and Hospital, Raja S.C. Mullick Road, Jadavpur, Kolkata 700032, West Bengal, India
e-mail: acoondoo@gmail.com;
dr.aparajitaghosh@gmail.com

K. Lahiri
Department of Dermatology, Apollo Gleneagles Hospitals and WIZDERM, Kolkata, India
e-mail: doctorlahiri@gmail.com

Learning Points
1. Topical corticosteroids were introduced in 1952 and since then have been used extensively in various inflammatory disorders.
2. Physical side effects and addiction to topical corticosteroids may occur due to overuse and misuse of the drug.

3. The phenomenon of "TSDF" which is an acronym for "topical steroid damaged/dependent face" has been recently described.
4. TSDF is a disease entity which encompasses a plethora of physical signs and symptoms as well as steroid addiction due to unsupervised overuse and misuse of the drug for an unspecified period of time.
5. Topical steroid is easily available in India over the counter and is often applied on the advice of people who are unaware of the ill effects of such misuse.
6. Withdrawal of the drug causes physical and psychological symptoms.

27.1 Introduction

The introduction of topical corticosteroids (TCs) in the form of hydrocortisone in 1952 completely revolutionised dermatologic therapy [1]. Later from the same decade onwards, more potent TCs were introduced making the treatment of dermatological disorders easier and simpler. However, more than 10 years after the introduction of TC, the first reports of cutaneous adverse effects of TC misuse started appearing in the literature [2]. Moreover, the addictive potential of TC came to light when Burry reported cases of addiction to TC in 1973 [3]. The term "steroid addiction" was coined by Kligman and Frosch in 1979 when they first described in detail the parameters of the condition [4]. TC addiction has also been later reported under various names such as light-sensitive seborrheic dermatitis [5], red skin syndrome [6], steroid-induced rosacea-like dermatitis [7] and topical corticosteroid damaged face [8], each of which describes a particular manifestation of TC addiction. "Topical corticosteroid addiction/dependence" implies the cutaneous and psychological dependence of the patient on the drug (TC), which results in rebound phenomenon and psychological distress

on stoppage of its application. The psychological aspect differentiates this condition from the other TC-induced adverse effects.

27.2 Addiction

The term addiction implies an excessive liking or fondness for any substance. Addiction, therefore, leads to repeated use of the substance resulting in overuse, misuse and finally a dependence on that item. Dependence on a psychoactive substance is characterised by certain distinctive features. Once the person starts using the substance, e.g. a drug, he might lose control of amount and duration of intake. This further leads to an intense craving for the drug. Withdrawal of the drug leads to a set of withdrawal symptoms. The patient may experience a tolerance to the substance—progressive increase in the amount of the substance may be required to produce the desired physiological and psychological effect. Dependence is also characterised by a continuous use of a substance in spite of being aware of its harmful physical, social or legal consequences. A person is officially diagnosed with dependence on a substance if three or more of these features are present together at a particular period of time [9]. Dependence, addiction, abuse or harmful use all imply that the person is harmfully and helplessly attached to the substance for a substantial period and hence are essentially synonymous [10].

27.3 Topical Corticosteroid Addiction (TCA)

TCA is a condition which results from chronic misuse of TC causing intense psychological and physical (cutaneous) dependence on the drug. Stoppage of the TC results in a rebound or flare in the symptoms which causes physical and psychological distress to the patient and a craving for the culprit TC. The quality of life of the patient is affected in such a manner that the individual starts using the TC again to maintain normal or near-normal social functioning. Further attempts to withdraw it are resisted by the patient. Most of the studies on TC misuse are hospital based and have assessed the incidence of side effects and the magnitude of TC misuse among dermatology OPD patients. However, no population-based study to assess the prevalence of TC misuse in the society at large is as yet available. Hence, it is difficult to assess the number of patients of chronic TC misuse who develop the rebound phenomenon [9]. The largest multicentric study on TC misuse on the face conducted in India found that 15% of such patients were addicted to it [8]. A hospital-based study in Iraq found 94% of patients with steroid-induced rosacea to experience a rebound [11]. The face is the commonest site of TCA [12]. TC addiction is also manifested at other sites of the body such as the flexures, perianal area and genital area in both males and females [6]. However, irrespective of the site, the basic clinical features of TCA remain the same, though the clinical features may vary depending on the site.

27.4 TCA of Face

TC misuse on the face has often been reported in cases of chronic atopic dermatitis or seborrheic dermatitis [6, 13, 14]. The patient starts applying the TC, which may be of the wrong potency for the treatment of a disease which may or may not be steroid responsive. As the disease becomes increasingly resistant to the drug, the treating physician or the patient himself may step up the potency of the TC or increase the frequency of application. This results in a vicious cycle as the patient becomes increasingly addicted to the TC [9]. TCs are also commonly misused as fairness creams or for self-treatment of acne by the lay public [8]. As the misuse continues, various side effects of TC such as pustules, acneiform lesions and erythematous papules start appearing on the face. These lesions tend to flare up on stopping the TC. Clinically the patient presents with diffuse facial erythema (which is the hallmark of TC misuse) along with papules, pustules, dryness and telangiectasia [8]. Additionally many patients may exhibit photosensitivity [15]. Sometimes the

rebound phenomenon may involve an area larger than the area of TC misuse. Distant sites may also be affected [16]. In many cases there may be symptoms resembling status cosmeticus or repeated flares of photosensitivity with erythema resembling chronic actinic dermatitis [6].

27.5 TCA of Genitalia and Perianal Area

TCA of the male genitalia and perineal area has been reported by various authors [4, 6]. The patient experiences a burning erythema of the entire region along with scrotal pain followed by atrophy of the glans in some cases. TC abuse may also result in the condition known as red scrotum syndrome [6]. As in the case of TCA of the face, the erythema and pain flare up on stopping the TC and may be so intense that the patient starts reapplying the drug. TCA of the genitalia causes intense psychological distress, depression and anxiety which may be so intense that it may even lead to impotence. Misuse of TC on the female genitalia for control of nonspecific discomfort or pruritus may also cause TCA. Persistent pruritus vulvae and vulvodynia may occur and may worsen on withdrawal. The labia and vestibule usually appear erythematous and glazed, and the normal daily functioning of the patient may be affected [6]. On the perianal area, TCA presents as persistent perianal burning, erythema and perianal atrophoderma on long-term use [6].

27.6 Pathogenesis

TCs of higher potencies have a greater potential for causing TCA. However, long-term use of TCs of lower potencies may also be risky. The time period needed to produce symptoms of TCA depends on the potency of the TC, to a large extent. More potent TCs produce side effects after a relatively shorter period of use as compared to TCs of lower potencies. Similarly the management of cases of TCA caused by more potent molecules is more difficult and more time-consuming [9]. Some workers have reported that a period from 2 to 4 months of TC abuse is required to produce symptoms of TCA [7, 15]. Withdrawal of the TC results in stoppage of the vasoconstrictive effect of TC. This causes the fixed erythema which is the hallmark of the rebound phenomenon. This process is probably mediated by nitric oxide (NO) [6]. Repeated application of TC causes inhibition of action of NO resulting in chronic vasoconstriction. On withdrawal of TC, the endothelial NO is released resulting in hyperdilatation of the blood vessel. This is further worsened by the TC-induced dermal atrophy and lack of support to the cutaneous vasculature [15]. An alternative hypothesis regarding the pathogenesis of the rebound phenomenon is that the chronic immunosuppression caused by the TC results in overgrowth of microorganisms which may act as superantigens. TC withdrawal also results in withdrawal of the TC-induced immunosuppression causing in an antigen-mediated inflammatory reaction of the skin. This inflammatory reaction is manifested as inflammatory papules and pustules which occur as a part of the rebound phenomenon [17]. Atopic individuals are more prone to developing TCA because of inherent vasomotor instability. In a study involving more than 800 patients of TC of the face, 90% of the patients were atopic [6].

27.7 Management

The aim of treatment is complete withdrawal of the TC, alleviation of the symptoms caused by the withdrawal and reversal of the skin damage due to TC misuse. Counselling of patients regarding the symptoms and distress which accompany rebound on withdrawal is of primary importance. The patients need a good amount of psychological support at this stage. There is a disagreement among workers regarding the mode of withdrawal of TC. While some advocate a sudden and total cessation of TC along with supportive measures [6], the other school advocates slower withdrawal by tapering the potency of TC, to prevent the extremely distressing rebound [7, 17]. Some workers have found topical calcineurin inhibitors to be quite useful as therapy for the TC-induced rosacea

and erythema [18, 19]. However, others found them to be ineffective as well as to cause further increase of the burning sensation [6]. Some drugs which have been suggested to be helpful are doxycycline, minocycline and metronidazole [20]. Supportive measures such as repeated ice compress, Burrow's compress for wet weepy lesions and use of bland emollients to alleviate dryness may be helpful [6]. Oral antihistamines may be required to control the associated pruritus [15]. Sulfonated shale oil cream 4% which has both anti-inflammatory and antibacterial properties has been used as a safe alternative to TC in cases of atopic eczema affecting the face [21, 22]. Some patients may also need anxiolytics [6].

References

1. Sulzberger MB, Witten VH. Effect of topically applied compound F in selected dermatoses. J Invest Dermatol. 1952;19:101–2.
2. Epstein NM, Epstein WL, Epstein H. Atrophic striae in patients with inguinal intertrigo. Arch Dermatol. 1963;87:450.
3. Burry N. Topical drug addiction. Adverse effects of fluorinated corticosteroid creams and ointments. Med J Aust. 1973;1:393–6.
4. Kligman AM, Frosch PJ. Steroid addiction. Int J Dermatol. 1979;18:23–31.
5. Frumess GM, Lewis HM. Light sensitive seborrheid. Arch Dermatol. 1957;75:245–8.
6. Rapaport MJ, Rapaport V. The red skin syndromes: corticosteroid addiction and withdrawal. Expert Rev Dermatol. 2006;1:547–61.
7. Rathi SK, Kumrah L. Topical corticosteroid-induced rosacea-like dermatitis: a clinical study of 110 cases. Indian J Dermatol Venereol Leprol. 2011;77:42–6.
8. Saraswat A, Lahiri K, Chatterjee M, Barua S, Coondoo A, Mittal A, et al. Topical corticosteroid abuse on the face: a prospective, multicenter study of dermatology outpatients. Indian J Dermatol Venereol Leprol. 2011;77:160–6.
9. Ghosh A, Sengupta S, Coondoo A, Jana AK. Topical corticosteroid addiction and phobia. Indian J Dermatol. 2014;59:465–8.
10. American Psychiatric Association. Diagnostic and statistical manual of mental disorders. 5th ed. Arlington, VA: American Psychiatric Association; 2013.
11. Hameed AF. Steroid dermatitis resembling rosacea: a clinical evaluation of 75 patients. ISRN Dermatol. 2013;2013:491376.
12. Lahiri K, Coondoo A. Topical steroid damaged/dependent face (TSDF): An entity of cutaneous pharmacodependence. Indian J Dermatol. 2016;61:265–72.

13. Hajar T, Leshem YA, Hanifin JM, Nedorost ST, Lio PA, Paller AS, et al. A systematic review of topical corticosteroid withdrawal ("steroid addiction") in patients with atopic dermatitis and other dermatoses. J Am Acad Dermatol. 2015;72(3):541–9.

14. Fukaya M, Sato K, Sato M, Kimata H, Fujisawa S, Dozono H, et al. Topical steroid addiction in atopic dermatitis. Drug Health Patient Saf. 2014;6:131–8.

15. Fisher M. Steroid-induced rosacealike dermatitis: case report and review of the literature. Cutis. 2009;83:198–204.

16. Xiao X, Xie H, Jian D, Deng Y, Chen X, Li J. Rebounding triad (severe itching, dryness and burning) after facial corticosteroid discontinuation defines a specific class of corticosteroid-dependent dermatitis. J Dermatol. 2015;42(7):697–702.

17. Ljubojeviae S, Basta-Juzba Siae A, Lipozeneiae J. Steroid dermatitis resembling rosacea: aetiopathogenesis and treatment. J Eur Acad Dermatol Venereol. 2002;16: 121–6.

18. Goldman D. Tacrolimus ointment for the treatment of steroid-induced rosacea: a preliminary report. J Am Acad Dermatol. 2001;44:995–8.

19. Chu CY. An open-label pilot study to evaluate the safety and the efficacy of topically applied pimecrolimus cream for the treatment of steroid-induced rosacea-like eruption. J Eur Aca Dermatol Venereol. 2007;21:484–9.

20. Narang T, Kumaran MS, Dogra S, Saikia UN, Kumar B. Red scrotum syndrome: idiopathic neurovascular phenomenon or steroid addiction? Sex Health. 2013;10(5):452–5.

21. Warnecke J, Wendt A. Anti-inflammatory action of pale sulfonated shale oil (ICHTHYOL pale) in UVB erythema test. Inflamm Res. 1998;47(2):75–8.

22. Korting HC, Schöllmann C, Cholcha W, Wolff L, The Collaborative Study Group. Efficacy and tolerability of pale sulfonated shale oil cream 4% in the treatment of mild to moderate atopic eczema in children: a multicentre, randomized vehicle-controlled trial. J Eur Acad Dermatol Venereol. 2010;24:1176–82.

Topical Corticosteroid Phobia

28

Arijit Coondoo, Koushik Lahiri,
and Sujata Sengupta

Abstract

Since their discovery in 1952, topical corticosteroids have been one of the most frequently used drugs in dermatology. Due to their overtly beneficial effects and over-the-counter availability, these drugs have been rampantly misused leading to an epidemic of ill effects. This has recently given rise to a surge of pharmacophobia particularly in parents and caregivers of atopic children as well as patients who genuinely need the application of topical corticosteroids for their steroid-responsive diseases. Topical corticosteroid phobia is defined as an extreme fear of side effects of topical corticosteroids and reluctance to use the drug even when prescribed by the treating physician.

Keywords

Topical corticosteroid • Phobia • Corticophobia • Atopic dermatitis

Learning Points
1. Topical corticosteroid phobia is defined as a fear regarding application of the TC.
2. This phobia occurs due to rampant, widespread and sometimes irrational TC use.
3. Topical corticosteroid phobia occurs particularly among parents of atopic children.
4. Recently, a questionnaire-based scale called **TOPICOP** has been developed to measure TC phobia among parents of atopic children.
5. Psychological counselling of patients and their parents and caregivers is the mainstay of management of TCP.
6. Educating non-dermatologists and pharmacists and counteracting negative information in the electronic, print and social media are necessary to halt the growing menace of TC phobia.

A. Coondoo (✉) • S. Sengupta
Department of Dermatology, K.P.C. Medical College and Hospital, Raja S.C. Mullick Road, Jadavpur, Kolkata 700032, West Bengal, India
e-mail: acoondoo@gmail.com

K. Lahiri
Department of Dermatology, Apollo Gleneagles Hospitals and WIZDERM, Kolkata, India
e-mail: doctorlahiri@gmail.com

© Springer Nature Singapore Pte Ltd. 2018
K. Lahiri (ed.), *A Treatise on Topical Corticosteroids in Dermatology*,
DOI 10.1007/978-981-10-4609-4_28

28.1 Introduction

Corticosteroids form the backbone of topical therapy in many dermatological diseases. Many of these drugs are easily available as over-the-counter medications in India and are widely used by dermatologists, general physicians, physicians of other specialities especially paediatricians, doctors practising alternative medicine as well as quacks. This rampant use has led to the phenomenon of misuse or abuse of these drugs resulting in addiction and the various side effects which are sometimes irreversible. However, this rampant misuse and the resultant side effects have resulted in a flood of misgivings regarding TC in the minds of a large number of people causing a phenomenon known as topical corticosteroid phobia (TCP). TCP lies at the opposite end of the pole of addiction and is gradually growing into a menace of epidemic proportions.

28.2 Aetiology

The word phobia is defined as an extreme irrational fear, leading to aversion and deliberate avoidance. The person concerned often agrees that the fear is irrational but still cannot help avoiding it [1]. TCP is defined as a fear regarding application of the TC, rational or not [2]. Most researchers agree that TCP is a result of rampant, widespread and sometimes irrational TC use. The common side effects of these compounds such as acne, striae, atrophy and hypopigmentation often initiate this phobia. Abuse of the drug by dermatologists, non-dermatologists and laymen plays a significant role in the development of these side effects to a large extent. Physicians and patients often shun the drug due to the problems that arise from its indiscriminate use. The press, the electronic media and the pharmaceutical industry further confuse the ill-informed patient. Hearsay among laymen, package inserts of medicines, the Internet, media publicity and sometimes the overcautious non-dermatologist physician may add to this fear. These physicians are often unaware of the intricate nuances of TC use including the indications, potency, duration and amount of application of TCs [3]. Ironically the phobia occurs mostly in cases where TC use is actually beneficial, for example, in inflammatory diseases like atopic dermatitis. TC phobia, among patients and doctors, was first reported from Germany in 1992 [3]. Later, Charman et al. published the first study of TCP in patients of atopic dermatitis [4]. The study was based on a questionnaire for 200 patients of atopic dermatitis or their caregivers. 72% of them worried about using the steroid because of possible side effects, and 24% were already non-compliant. Steroid phobia was more commonly found in the female sex, in cases of paternal history of atopic dermatitis and a history of frequent change of clinics [5]. A reluctance to use steroids was seen in 38% of these subjects. Hon et al., in a study of childhood eczema, found that 50% parents requested non-steroidal prescriptions due to concerns about skin atrophy and growth retardation [6]. To measure such TC phobia among parents of children with atopic dermatitis, a questionnaire-based scale called TOPICOP has been developed recently [7].

28.3 Consequences of TCP

The consequences of TCP can be harmful in steroid-responsive dermatoses because it may lead to inadequate use of the medication in both amount and frequency of application. Sometimes the phobia may result in complete abstinence as well. The resulting therapeutic failure lures the patient towards alternative and indigenous medications [8]. In the latter forms, steroids are often used indiscriminately without the patient's knowledge. In one such form of alternative therapy, Chinese medications and herbs were used. Paradoxically, some of these medications themselves were found to contain TCs [6].

28.4 Management

Management of TCP involves various steps that need to be taken simultaneously to counteract the ignorance, misinformation and improper advice that leads to it. TCP leads to refusal to apply, irregular application (haphazardly as and when the patient feels) or less than useful application (e.g. only one application per day when the patient is asked to apply the drug twice) [9].

Hence, the patients and their parents/caregivers need to be counselled properly regarding the use of TC. That the TC basket includes several drugs which differ in their potency is a fact little known to most patients, their caregivers and even some physicians necessitating counselling regarding proper use of TC. The potency determines the efficacy and the safety of the medication. A more potent one requires a shorter duration of application and vice versa. Systemic steroids are much more likely to produce side effects than their topical counterparts. It has been proposed that the labels on the packets and tubes of topical corticosteroids should clearly identify the potency and side effects of the various classes of the drug. This labelling shall raise awareness and remove irrational fears about the side effects of the medication and reinforce the counselling by doctors [10].

Pharmacists contribute significantly towards TCP by passing on wrong information to patients. Hence, counselling of pharmacists by dermatologists may help by removing misconceptions and prevent passing of misinformation by the pharmacists [11].

Similarly there is a negative awareness about the benefits and side effects of corticosteroids among many non-dermatologist doctors including general practitioners [12]. General practitioners and paediatricians frequently treat AD patients, many of whom trust them solely for health-related advice. Hence, better education and counselling of general practitioners regarding the safety of topical corticosteroids are necessary to dispel wrong notions about the drug [8].

To ensure TC therapy compliance, the dermatologist should establish a strong relationship with the patient to remove all doubts and anxiety in the minds of the patients and their caregivers. The nature of the disease and the reason for the necessity of TC therapy should be impressed upon them. The potencies of different steroids with their benefits and side effects can be explained. Oral and written advice regarding the method of application (fingertip unit), frequency and duration should be very clear. It should be emphasized that side effects are unlikely if the given instructions are followed strictly. A regular follow-up to ensure the patient's wellbeing is very important in removing any apprehension that may occur during the course of therapy. All this would go a long way in improving the compliance and lowering the morbidity and mortality due to TCP [12].

References

1. American Psychiatric Association. Diagnostic and statistical manual of mental disorders. 5th ed. Arlington, VA: American Psychiatric Association; 2013.
2. Aubert H, Barbarot S. Non adherence and topical steroids. Ann Dermatol Venereol. 2012;139(Suppl 1): S7–12.
3. Drosner M. Paths to a rational cortisone therapy via urea supplements-countering cortisone phobia. Hautarzt. 1992;43(Suppl 11):23–9.
4. Charman CR, Morris AD, Williams HC. Topical corticosteroid phobia in patients with atopic eczema. Br J Dermatol. 2000;142:931–6.
5. Kojima R, Fujiwara T, Matsuda A, Narita M, Matsubara O, Nonoyama S, et al. Factors associated with steroid phobia in caregivers of children with atopic dermatitis. Pediatr Dermatol. 2013;30:29–35.
6. Hon KL, Kam WY, Leung TF, Lam MC, Wong KY, Lee KC, et al. Steroid fears in children with eczema. Acta Paediatr. 2006;95:1451–5.
7. Moret L, Anthoine E, Aubert-Wastiaux H, Le Rhun A, et al. TOPICOP©: a new scale evaluating topical corticosteroid phobia among atopic dermatitis outpatients and their parents. PLoS One. 2013;8:e76493.
8. Coondoo A, Sengupta S. Topical corticophobia among parents and caregivers of atopic children. Indian J Paediatr Dermatol. 2016;17:255–7.
9. Ghosh A, Sengupta S, Coondoo A, Jana AK. Topical corticosteroid addiction and phobia. Indian J Dermatol. 2014;59:465–8.
10. Bewley A, Dermatology Working Group. Expert consensus: time for a change in the way we advise our patients to use topical corticosteroids. Br J Dermatol. 2008;158:917–20.
11. Raffin D, Giraudeau B, Samimi M, Machet L, Pourrat X, Maruani A. Corticosteroid phobia among pharmacists regarding atopic derma-titis in children: a national french survey. Acta Derm Venereol. 2016;96: 177–80.
12. Ponnambath M, Pynn E. How to reassure patients with topical steroid phobia. Prescriber. 2014;25(5):21–3.
13. Aubert-Wastiaux H, Moret L, Le Rhun A, Fontenoy AM, Nguyen JM. Topical corticosteroid phobia in atopic dermatitis: a study of its nature, origins and frequency. Br J Dermatol. 2011;165:808–14.

Treatment of Topical Corticosteroid-Damaged Skin

29

Omid Zargari

Abstract

Topical corticosteroids (TCSs) are the mainstay of anti-inflammatory treatments and are used in a variety of skin conditions. TCS abuse is particularly common in countries where these products are easily available as over-thecounter drugs. The most frequent adverse effects of TCS abuse are skin atrophy, striae, rosacea, perioral dermatitis and pigmentary changes. Dermatologists should be aware of early diagnosis and proper management of these adverse effects.

Keywords

Steroid-induced rosacea • Lipoatrophy • Striae distance • Treatment • Saline injection

Learning Points
1. After reading this chapter, participants should be able to recognize and treat the cutaneous complications of topical corticosteroid abuse.

29.1 General

With introduction of compound F (hydrocortisone) in 1952, a modern era began in dermatologic therapies [1]. Once the molecular secret was revealed, stronger versions of steroids have been made, as Albert Kligman once said: "larger benefits obtained at the cost of greater hazard" [2].

Nowadays, topical corticosteroids (TCSs) are the mainstay of anti-inflammatory treatments and are used in a variety of skin conditions including different kinds of dermatitis, psoriasis, lichen planus and many other steroid-responsive dermatoses. On the other hand, TCSs are one of the most commonly abused drugs. They are misused for different conditions such as acne, melasma

O. Zargari
Consultant Dermatologist, Rasht, Iran
e-mail: ozargari@gmail.com

© Springer Nature Singapore Pte Ltd. 2018
K. Lahiri (ed.), *A Treatise on Topical Corticosteroids in Dermatology*,
DOI 10.1007/978-981-10-4609-4_29

and fungal infections and sometimes merely as a cosmetic product.

The two most important factors in determining the rate of these adverse effects are the potency of the applied TCS and the location of application.

Application of high-potency TCS is restricted in areas such as the thin-skinned eyelids, periocular area, face, neck, axillae and genitals due to an increased risk of adverse events. The structure of the skin in these areas, characterised by a thin epidermis, extensive vascularisation or many epidermal appendages and nerve endings, causes it to be more absorbent. In fact, scrotum and eyelids have the highest percutaneous penetration for steroids [3, 4].

It should be kept in mind that in some dermatologic conditions, the penetration of steroids is even higher. Particularly, in atopic dermatitis—where the epidermal barrier is impaired—the penetration of TCS is 2–10 times greater than that through healthy skin [5].

Also, children are more prone to develop systemic reactions to topically applied medication because of their higher ratio of total body surface area to body weight [6].

In general, local adverse events of corticosteroid use are far more prevalent than systemic reactions [7]. TCS can produce a myriad of adverse effects including skin atrophy, striae, telangiectasia, purpura, stellate pseudoscars, folliculitis, acne and rosacea-like eruptions, focal hypertrichosis, hypo- and hyperpigmentation, allergic contact dermatitis, infections, glaucoma and papilloedema [2, 6].

TCS abuse is particularly a common practice in countries where these products are easily available as over-the-counter drugs. Dermatologists, especially in these countries, should be aware of early diagnosis and proper management of TCS-induced damaged skin.

excessive topical steroid application to facial areas [8]. Application of topical corticosteroids causes immediate vasoconstriction and reduces the symptoms of many skin conditions such as different kinds of dermatitis, rosacea and even acne. For this reason, patients frequently abuse these products for a variety of facial skin conditions. However, when patients discontinue usage of the topical corticosteroid, symptoms immediately reappear even worse than the original condition, and this forces them to restart using them which finally leads to steroid addiction.

SIR is usually characterised by pruritic papules and pustules on an erythematous background. It primarily affects young to middle-age women, although it has been reported both in men and in children. It can be classified to three different types depending on the location of the eruption: perioral, centrofacial and diffuse.

The exact pathogenesis of SIR remains unclear. Rebound vasodilatation and pro-inflammatory cytokine release by chronic steroid exposure are among the responsible mechanisms. Also, the immunosuppressive effect of corticosteroids may facilitate the overgrowth of various bacteria, yeast or other organisms including *Demodex*. It remains controversial whether these organisms are triggers of rosacea and SIR or act merely as a secondary phenomenon [9].

As in other forms of steroid-induced damaged skin, discontinuation of steroid is the first step in treatment of SIR. However, this usually leads to severe rebound reaction. Therefore, a temporary decrease to a lower-potency steroid prior to discontinuation remains an option in such situation.

Medical treatment of SIR is not very different from classic rosacea. In milder forms, topical calcineurin inhibitors are usually effective and well tolerated [10–12]. In more severe cases, the best choice is oral tetracycline in a subantimicrobial dose until complete remission is achieved [13].

29.2 Steroid-Induced Rosacea

Steroid-induced rosacea (SIR) or rosacea-like dermatitis, which was first described in 1969 by Sneddon, is a relatively common side effect of

29.3 Steroid-Induced Atrophy

Skin atrophy is the most common adverse effect of topical steroids [14]. It can occur with all steroids and is particularly common in intertriginous areas of the body. Skin atrophy manifests as increased transparency and shininess of the skin.

Combining vitamin D analogues probably reduce the rate of steroid-induced atrophy. These analogues act by restoring epidermal barrier function, which is impaired with corticosteroid use, and counteract steroid-induced skin atrophy [15].

Also, topical tretinoin can be combined to TCSs to prevent skin atrophy induced by long-term use of topical corticosteroids, without diminishing their anti-inflammatory effects [16, 17].

Another option would be thyroid hormone analogues. A study has shown that topical triiodothyroacetic acid may have a therapeutic effect on steroid-induced dermal atrophy in mouse skin and a direct stimulatory effect on dermal proliferation [17].

29.4 Steroid-Induced Striae

Striae distensae (SD), or stretch marks, are linear atrophic dermal scars covered with flat atrophic epidermis. SD commonly occurs during growth spurts in adolescence and in pregnancy. It can happen in certain endocrine disorders such as Cushing's syndrome. Also, SD is a known side effect of both systemic and topical steroids. In fact, SD can be considered as the advance stage of steroid-induced skin atrophy.

There are two forms of SD: striae rubrae and striae albae. The acute stage (striae rubrae) is characterised by the initial erythematous, red and stretched lesions which are aligned perpendicular to the direction of skin tension, whilst the chronic stage (striae albae) is classified when SD has faded and appears atrophic, wrinkled and hypopigmented [18].

There are various treatment modalities for SD; however, no method of prevention or treatment has shown satisfactory results. In general, striae rubra are more responsive to treatment; therefore, it is important to recognise the situation as early as possible, and if it is caused by steroid misuse, the first step should be stopping it.

Among the topical agents, tretinoin is perhaps the most effective treatment for SD [19].

In the last two decades, various types of light and laser systems have been studied for the treatment of striae rubra and striae alba, or both, with different results. Practically, in striae rubra, the targets are blood vessels, and in striae alba, the aim is induction of collagen and elastin.

Intense pulsed light (IPL), pulsed dye laser (PDL), neodymium-doped yttrium aluminium garnet (Nd:YAG) laser, fractional CO_2 laser and many other systems have shown partial response in SD [20–22].

In a study done by El-Taieb on 40 patients with SD, both IPL and fractional CO_2 laser were effective in treating SD, but the latter was more effective than IPL in the same duration of treatment and with lesser treatment sessions [20].

Overall, fractional lasers seem to be the most promising choice [22].

29.5 Steroid-Induced Lipoatrophy

Steroid-induced lipoatrophy (SIL), commonly associated with hypopigmentation, usually occurs after intralesional injection of non-diluted corticosteroids.

A variety of techniques have been reported to be effective in treating SIL. Both autologous fat injection and intralesional poly-L-lactic acid have been used in treating SIL [23, 24]. However, in my experience on over 30 cases of SIL, intralesional injection of normal saline or distilled water is a practical and convenient way in dealing with SIL, and there is usually no need for above-mentioned expensive treatments (Fig. 29.1). The mechanism of SIL is probably the continuous acting of remnants of steroid crystals at the site of injection. It is hypothesised that injecting saline would put these crystals back into suspension, where they could then be recognised as foreign bodies and naturally removed from the body [25].

Serial saline injections on weekly or bimonthly basis effectively resolve SIL within 4–8 weeks of the initial saline injection [26].

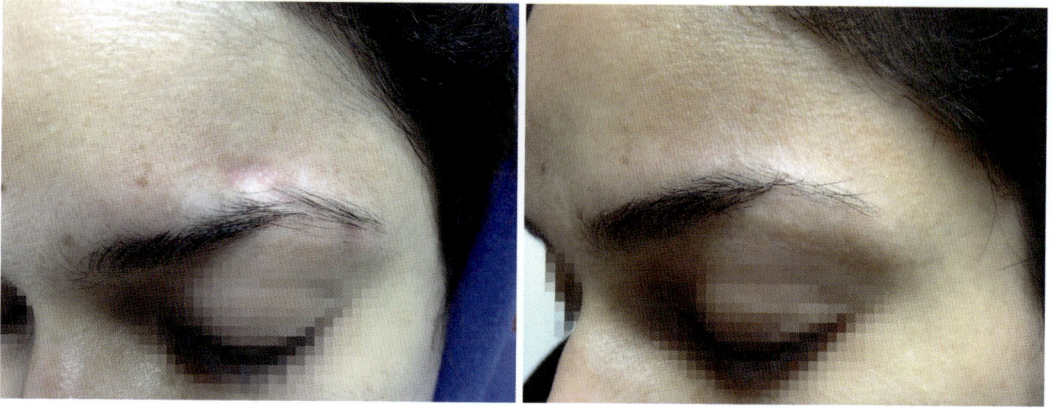

Fig. 29.1 Complete recovery of steroid-induced lipoatrophy after three times saline injections, two weeks apart

References

1. Sulzberger MB, Witten VH. Effect of topically applied compound F in selected dermatoses. J Invest Dermatol. 1952;19:101–2.
2. Kligman AM, Frosch PJ. Steroid addiction. Int J Dermatol. 1979;18(1):23–31.
3. Feldmann RJ, Maibach HI. Regional variation in percutaneous penetration of 14C cortisol in man. J Invest Dermatol. 1967;48:181–3.
4. Wester RC, Maibach HI. Dermatopharmacokinetics in clinical dermatology. Semin Dermatol. 1983;2: 81–4.
5. Turpeinen M, Lehtokoski-Lehtiniemi E, Leisti S, Salo OP. Percutaneous absorption of hydrocortisone during and after the acute phase of dermatitis in children. Pediatr Dermatol. 1988;5:276–9.
6. Hengge UR, Ruzicka T, Schwartz RA, Cork MJ. Adverse effects of topical corticosteroids. J Am Acad Dermatol. 2006;54(1):1–15.
7. Lagos BR, Maibach HI. Frequency of application of topical corticosteroids: an overview. Br J Dermatol. 1998;139:763–6.
8. Sneddon I. Adverse effect of topical fluorinated corticosteroids in rosacea. Br Med J. 1969;1:671–3.
9. Two AM, Wu W, Gallo RL, Hata TR. Rosacea: part I. Introduction, categorization, histology, pathogenesis, and risk factors. J Am Acad Dermatol. 2015;72(5): 749–58. quiz 759–60
10. Goldman D. Tacrolimus ointment for the treatment of steroid-induced rosacea: a preliminary report. J Am Acad Dermatol. 2001;44(6):995–8.
11. Bhat YJ, Manzoor S, Qayoom S. Steroid-induced rosacea: a clinical study of 200 patients. Indian J Dermatol. 2011;56(1):30–2.
12. Lee DH, Li K, Suh DH. Pimecrolimus 1% cream for the treatment of steroid-induced rosacea: an 8-week split-face clinical trial. Br J Dermatol. 2008;158(5): 1069–76.
13. Mokos ZB, Kummer A, Mosler EL, Čeović R, Basta-Juzbašić A. Perioral dermatitis: still a therapeutic challenge. Acta Clin Croat. 2015;54(2):179–85.
14. Ponec M, De Haas C, Bachra BN, Polano MK. Effects of glucocorticosteroids on cultured human skin fibroblasts. III. Transient inhibition of cell proliferation in the early growth stages and reduced susceptibility in later growth stages. Arch Dermatol Res. 1979;265: 219–27.
15. Segaert S, Ropke M. The biological rationale for use of vitamin d analogs in combination with corticosteroids for the topical treatment of plaque psoriasis. J Drugs Dermatol. 2013;12(8):e129–37.
16. Kwon HB, Choi Y, Kim HJ, Lee AY. The therapeutic effects of a topical tretinoin and corticosteroid combination for vitiligo: a placebo-controlled, paired-comparison, left-right study. J Drugs Dermatol. 2013; 12(4):e63–7.
17. Yazdanparast P, Carlsson B, Sun XY, Zhao XH, Hedner T, Faergemann J. Action of topical thyroid hormone analogues on glucocorticoid-induced skin atrophy in mice. Thyroid. 2006;16(3):273–80.
18. Elson ML. Treatment of striae distensae with topical tretinoin. J Dermatol Surg Oncol. 1990;16(3): 267–70.
19. Ud-Din S, McGeorge D, Bayat A. Topical management of striae distensae (stretch marks): prevention and therapy of striae rubrae and albae. J Eur Acad Dermatol Venereol. 2016;30(2):211–22.
20. El Taieb MA, Ibrahim AK. Fractional CO2 laser versus intense pulsed light in treating striae distensae. Indian J Dermatol. 2016;61(2):174–80.

21. Goldman A, Rossato F, Prati C. Stretch marks: treatment using the 1064-nm Nd:YAG laser. Dermatol Surg. 2008;34(5):686–91.
22. Aldahan AS, Shah VV, Mlacker S, et al. Laser and light treatments for striae distensae: a comprehensive review of the literature. Am J Clin Dermatol. 2016; 17(3):239–56.
23. Imagawa KA. Case of fat injection for treating subcutaneous atrophy caused by local administration of corticosteroid. Tokai J Exp Clin Med. 2010;35(2):66.
24. Brodell DW, Marchese Johnson S. Use of intralesional poly-L-lactic acid in the treatment of corticosteroid-induced lipoatrophy. Dermatol Surg. 2014;40(5):597–9.
25. Shiffman MA. Letter: treatment of local, persistent cutaneous atrophy after corticosteroid injection with normal saline infiltration. Dermatol Surg. 2010; 36(3):436.
26. Shumaker PR, Rao J, Goldman MP. Treatment of local, persistent cutaneous atrophy following corticosteroid injection with normal saline infiltration. Dermatol Surg. 2005;31(10):1340–3.

Procedural Techniques in Management of Topical Corticosteroid Abuse

30

Niti Khunger

Abstract

Topical steroids are one of the most abused creams among dermatological products because of their strong anti-inflammatory action being misused for acne and fungal infections and hypomelanotic activity where they are misused as "fairness creams." This leads to adverse effects such as skin atrophy, striae, acneiform eruptions, telangiectasia, hypertrichosis, and masking of skin infections. Management of these adverse effects is a long-drawn process due to steroid dependence and difficulty in reversing the cutaneous side effects. Most of these are managed with medical treatment, but occasionally procedural treatments are required to expedite therapy. Chemical peels for the treatment of acne, lasers, and light systems for the treatment of telangiectasia, striae, and hypertrichosis are the common procedures that can be of benefit, if chosen wisely and according to patient's skin type. The need of the hour is appropriate patient and society education regarding the potential adverse effects of topical corticosteroids following inappropriate use to stem the epidemic of steroid misuse.

Keywords

Topical steroid • Adverse effects • Chemical peels • Lasers • Acne • Striae • Telangiectasia • Hypertrichosis

Learning Points

1. Comedone extraction and chemical peels are useful for recalcitrant steroid aggravated acne.

2. Intense pulsed light (IPL) systems with a cutoff filter between 525–595 nm, pulsed dye lasers (PDL 585 nm), and 1064 nm long-pulsed Nd:YAG lasers are useful for steroid-induced rosacea and telangiectasia.

3. Diode laser (850 nm), Nd:YAG laser (1064 nm), and the IPL systems can be used for hypertrichosis and hirsutism.

N. Khunger
Department of Dermatology and STD, Vardhman Mahavir Medical College, Safdarjang Hospital, New Delhi, India
e-mail: drkhungerniti@gmail.com

© Springer Nature Singapore Pte Ltd. 2018
K. Lahiri (ed.), *A Treatise on Topical Corticosteroids in Dermatology*,
DOI 10.1007/978-981-10-4609-4_30

4. Stria can be minimized by pulsed dye laser in the initial erythematous phase, chemical peels in the pigmented phase and fractional CO_2 laser, and fractional nonablative erbium glass laser in the late atrophic stage.

30.1 Introduction

Topical corticosteroids are one of the most widely used products, and their sale accounts for almost 82% of total dermatological product sale in India [1]. The use of topical steroids has become a double-edged sword due to constantly rising instances of abuse and misuse leading to serious local, systemic, and psychological side effects [2, 3]. Topical corticosteroids are commonly misused because they give dramatic results due to their strong anti-inflammatory and hypomelanotic activity. They are commonly misused by patients as "fairness creams," contrarily for reducing acne and to alleviate itch and redness in topical fungal, bacterial infections, and undiagnosed skin rashes. These prescriptions are mostly by non-physicians on the advice of friends, chemists, and non-registered or unqualified practitioners. Management of topical steroid abuse consists of withdrawal of the steroid accompanied with constant counseling of the patient during the rebound phase, treatment of the underlying condition, and obvious adverse effects arising due to prolonged topical steroid therapy. Most of these can be controlled by medical treatment and are discussed elsewhere. This chapter focuses on the procedural treatment of adverse effects of topical steroids.

30.2 Common Manifestations of Steroid Abuse

The common manifestations of topical corticosteroid abuse and their management are given in Table 30.1. The details of the adverse effects are described elsewhere in the book.

30.2.1 Procedural Techniques for Steroid Abuse

30.2.1.1 Acne and Acneiform Eruptions

Topical steroid abuse in patients with preexisting acne is common as it leads to a quick reduction in erythema and edema giving an

Table 30.1 Common side effects of topical corticosteroids and their management

Side effect	Medical treatment	Procedural treatment
Acne/acneiform eruptions	Topical anti-acne treatment as per severity of acne—benzoyl peroxide, adapalene	Comedone extraction Chemical peels Intense pulsed light
Telangiectasia and rosacea	Topical brimonidine Systemic doxycycline	Intense pulsed light Pulsed dye laser KTP laser Nd:YAG laser
Hypertrichosis/hirsutism	Eflornithine	Long-pulsed Nd:YAG laser Diode laser Intense pulsed light
Atrophy/striae	Tretinoin, glycolic acid	Chemical peels, pulsed dye laser, fractional CO_2 laser, intense pulsed light, excimer lamp/laser
Subcutaneous atrophy	Topical retinoid. Self-resolving in the early stages may become irreversible in later stages	Hyaluronic acid fillers or autologous fat transfer in irreversible cases at cosmetically important sites
Hypopigmentation	Topical tacrolimus	Excimer lamp/laser

appearance of instant improvement. With prolonged use, patients present with monomorphic erythematous papular and pustular lesions. However the presence of numerous, multiple open and closed comedones, giant comedones, and cysts is not uncommon (Fig. 30.1a, b). In such patients comedone extraction with a comedone extractor leads to faster improvement. In the case of multiple closed comedones, light electrodessication or piercing with a sterile disposable no. 26 G needle, under topical anesthesia, followed by comedone extraction leads to gratifying improvement over a short period. Multiple sessions may be required for complete clearance. Topical and systemic anti-acne medication as appropriate for the severity of acne should be continued. Topical retinoids should be used judiciously as they can cause further irritation to an inflamed erythematous face, due to the steroid withdrawal.

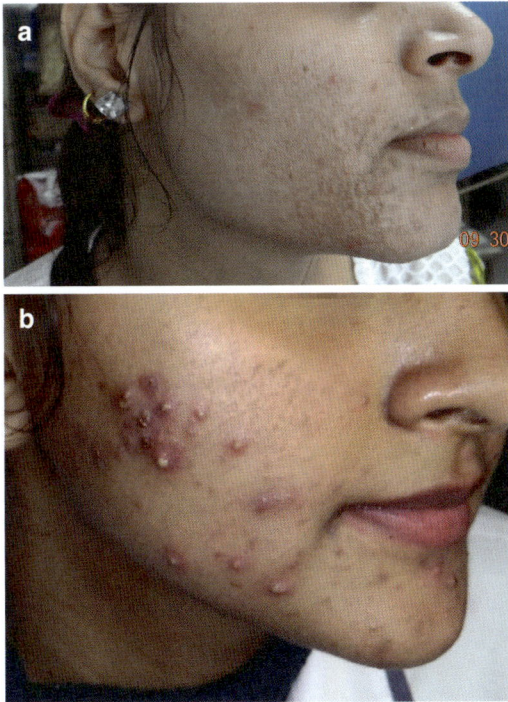

Chemical peel with a salicylic-mandelic acid combination in a gel base is another useful procedure in resistant cases. The advantage is that salicylic acid leads to reduction in erythema due to its anti-inflammatory effect, and mandelic acid has an antibacterial and skin-lightening effect (Fig. 30.2a, b). The patient should be primed well with a sunscreen before performing peels as photosensitivity is common in patients with steroid abuse. Gel base peels are better tolerated as compared to alcoholic solutions in sensitive skins. Interval between peeling

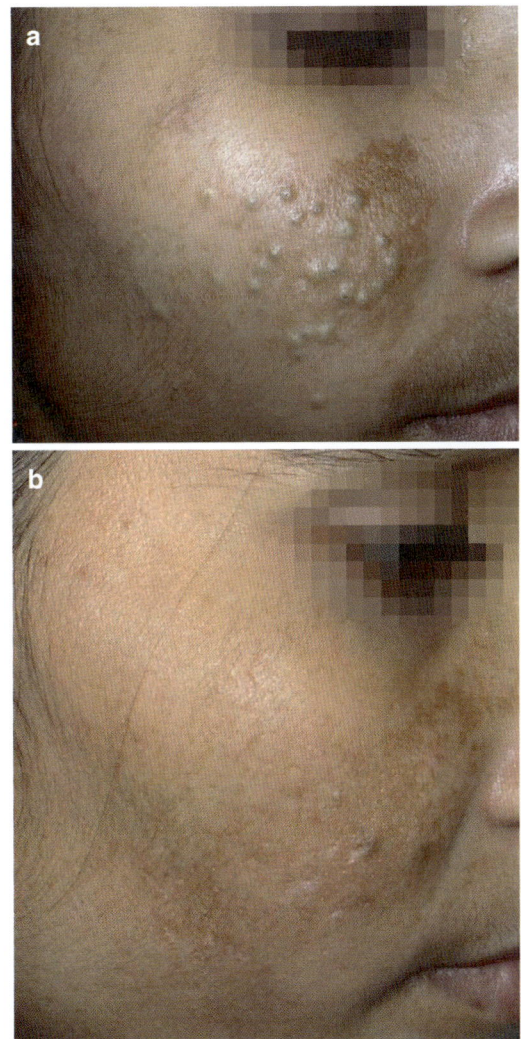

Fig. 30.1 Topical steroid induced acne. (a) Multiple closely packed visible and submarine comedones. (b) erythematous papules and pustules

Fig. 30.2 Improvement of acne with comedone extraction followed by combination salicylic -mandelic acid peels

sessions should be longer at 3–4-week intervals to allow for complete healing of the skin between the sessions.

30.2.1.2 Telangiectasia and Steroid-Induced Rosacea

Steroid-induced telangiectasia is a common manifestation of steroid abuse and can be picked up very early with dermoscopy (Fig. 30.3a, b). It is caused by stimulation of release of nitric oxide by the steroid from the endothelial cells of the dermal vessels, leading to abnormal dilatation of capillaries [4]. It can present as redness and close examination on stretching the skin will reveal the dilated capillaries. Treatment is difficult and depends on the size of the vessel. The older procedures used were cauterization of individual vessels with electrosurgery. This was tedious and painful and sometimes led to scarring. The advent of next-generation intense pulsed light (IPL)

systems and pulsed dye lasers (PDL) has given rise to better treatment options [5]. Though these lasers do not penetrate deeply, they are effective since most of the vessels are superficial and small (0.5–1 mm) in diameter. Wavelengths used are between 525 and 595 nm. Purpura can occur due to rupture of small vessels during treatment. This can be a problem but usually clears in 1–2 weeks. Using large spot sizes and effective cooling can make side effects less frequent. A typical treatment would include the use of an 8–10 mm spot size, fluence of 6.5–8.5 J/cm^2, and 6 ms pulse width. The number of treatments required can vary from one to four done at 4–6-week intervals. Prominent and slightly larger vessels can be treated individually with a 1 mm spot size and short pulses, moving slowly along the vessel. The diffuse redness of rosacea is better treated with the 595 nm pulsed dye laser. Though brimonidine tartrate gel helps in reducing redness, the effect is temporary and only lasts for 12 hours. The other lasers that can be used are the 532 nm KTP and 1064 nm long-pulsed Nd:YAG lasers.

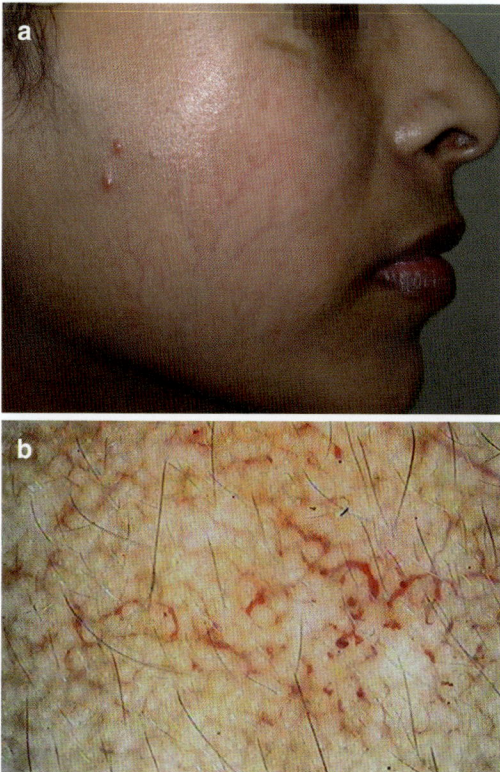

30.3 Hypertrichosis and Hirsutism

Prolonged application of topical steroids, particularly on the face, causes hypertrichosis. This is most evident on the cheeks and forehead but can also develop on the upper lip (Fig. 30.4). The hair are typically fine, long vellus hair in nonandrogen-dependent areas as opposed to hirsutism where they are thick, dark, terminal hair in androgen-dependent areas such as the chin, sideburns, and lower face. In most patients it reverses after the application of steroids is stopped. However cosmetic procedures such as bleaching or waxing will help to reduce the anxiety associated with the appearance. In patients with persistent and marked hypertrichosis, laser hair removal is an option. However it may not be very efficacious for the fine vellus hair that is seen with topical steroids. Various lasers have been used such as the diode laser (850 nm), the Nd:YAG laser (1064 nm), and the IPL. In darker pigmented skins, the Nd:YAG laser is safer [6]. A recent report of using black eyelash mascara as an

Fig. 30.3 Steroid induced telangiectasia: (**a**) Clinical image (**b**) Dermoscopic image showing dilated vessels and hypertrichosis

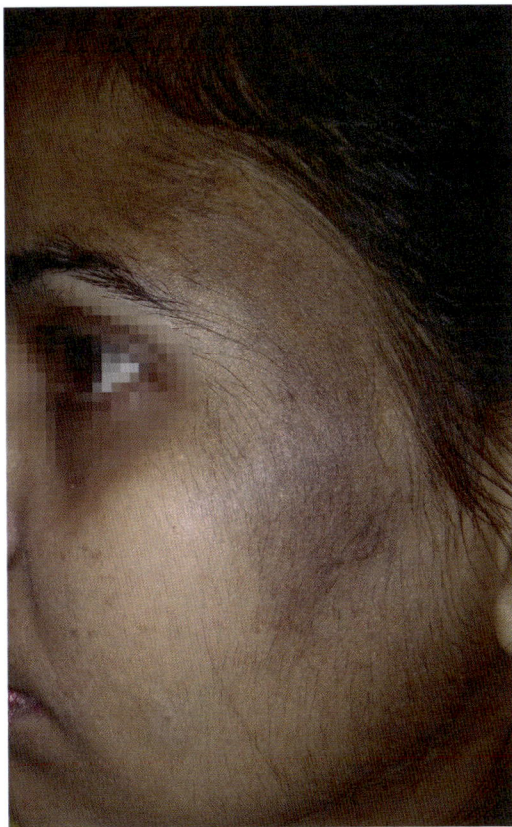

Fig. 30.4 Hypertrichosis on the cheek and mandibular area following application of triple combination cream containing mometasone furoate 0.1%, hydroquinone 2% and tretinoin 0.025% for 3 months

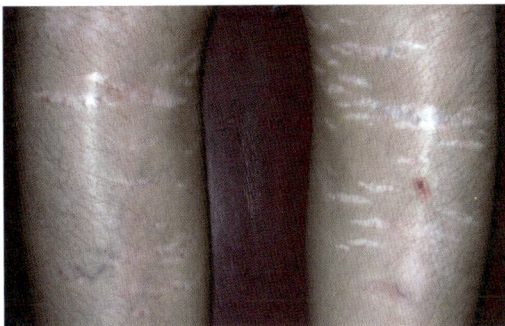

Fig. 30.5 Striae on the legs following application of high potent clobetasol proprionate for vitiligo

adjunct to alexandrite laser (755 nm) and Nd: YAG laser applications for removing thin and white-colored facial and axillary *hair reported good results on the painted* sites [7].

30.4 Striae

Striae are linear atrophic scars that occur with topical and systemic steroid use. They are common in the flexural areas like the axillae, groin, popliteal fossa, lower abdomen, and lower back (Fig. 30.5). They occur due to dermal atrophy due to reduction in the extracellular matrix as well as reduction in collagen and elastin induced by topical steroids. Initially they appear as reddish or purplish streaks and later turn white with thin papery skin. Treatment is difficult and it is not possible to recover normal skin. However they can be made less prominent. In the initial phases, topical retinoids such as tretinoin 0.1% have been used [8]. In the later white atrophic stage, procedural treatment may help partially. Chemical peels have also reported to be beneficial. A study compared topical 20% glycolic acid and 0.05% tretinoin versus 20% glycolic acid and 10% L-ascorbic acid for the treatment of striae albicans [9]. It was reported that both regimens improved the appearance of striae alba.

Laser therapy has also been reported to be of benefit [10]. Various lasers have been used, depending on the appearance and stage of the striae. The 585 nm pulsed dye laser is moderately effective in the treatment of early striaerubra [11]. The 308 nm excimer laser has been used for treating striae alba [12]. Intense pulsed light and fractional CO_2 laser are also moderately efficacious with minimal side effects [13]. Multiple treatments at 4–6-week intervals are required.

Conclusion

Adverse effects of prolonged or inappropriate corticosteroid use are myriad as steroids have an extensive effect on all the layers of the skin. Acne and acneiform eruptions, telangiectasia and rosacea, hypopigmentation, hypertrichosis, and striae are the most common, besides topical fungal, viral, and bacterial infections. These effects may not always be reversible on stopping the steroid such as telangiectasia and striae. Procedural techniques, chiefly the use of lasers and light sources, are of benefit, if chosen wisely and according to patients' skin type. The need of the hour is appropriate patient and society education regarding the potential adverse effects of topical corticosteroids following inappropriate use to stem the epidemic of steroid misuse.

References

1. Verma SB. Sales, status, prescriptions and regulatory problems with topical steroids in India. Indian J Dermatol Venereol Leprol. 2014;80:201–3.
2. Coondoo A, Phiske M, Verma S, Lahiri K. Side-effects of topical steroids: a long overdue revisit. Indian Dermatol Online J. 2014;5:416–25.
3. Saraswat A, Lahiri K, Chatterjee M, Barua S, Coondoo A, Mittal A, et al. Topical corticosteroid abuse on the face: a prospective, multicenter study of dermatology outpatients. Indian J Dermatol Venereol Leprol. 2011;77:160–6.
4. Hengge UR, Ruzicka T, Schwartz RA, Cork MJ. Adverse effects of topical glucocorticosteroids. J Am Acad Dermatol. 2006;54:1–18.
5. Hare McCoppin HH, Goldberg DJ. Laser treatment of facial telangiectases: an update. Dermatol Surg. 2010;36(8):1221–30.
6. Gan SD, Graber EM. Laser hair removal: a review. Dermatol Surg. 2013;39(6):823–38.
7. Üstüner P, Balevi A, Özdemir M. Efficacy and safety of mascara dyeing as an adjunct to alexandrite and Nd: YAG laser applications for removing thin and white-colored facial and axillary hair. J Cosmet Laser Ther. 2016;18(8):459–66.
8. Kang S, Kim KJ, Griffiths CE, et al. Topical tretinoin (retinoic acid) improves early stretch marks. Arch Dermatol. 1996;132:519–26.
9. Ash K, Lord J, Zukowski M, McDaniel DH. Comparison of topical therapy for striae alba (20% glycolic acid/0.05% tretinoin versus 20% glycolic acid/10% L-ascorbic acid). Dermatol Surg. 1998;24:849–56.
10. McDaniel DH. Laser therapy of stretch marks. Dermatol Clin. 2002;20:67–76.
11. Jimeenez GP, Flores F, Berman B, Gunja-Smith Z. Treatment of striaerubra and striae alba with the 585 nm pulsed dye laser. Dermatol Surg. 2003;29:362–5.
12. Alexiades-Armenakas MR, Bernstein LJ, Friedman PM, Geronemus RG. The safety and efficacy of the 308 nm excimer laser in pigment correction of hypopigmented scars and striae alba. Arch Dermatol. 2004;140:955–60.
13. Hernandez-Perez E, Colombo-Charrier E, Valencia-Ibiett E. Intense pulsed light in the treatment of striaedistensae. Dermatol Surg. 2002;28:1124–30.

Topical Corticosteroids: Regulatory Aspects

31

Rajetha Damisetty and Shyamanta Barua

Abstract

Topical steroids are the keystones of dermatologic therapy. When used rationally, for the right indications, they are extremely effective and cause minimal effects. Sadly, their (mis)use is often fraught with adverse effects. Their potential for causing addiction has led to enormous psycho-socio-economic burden, in addition to long term and, at times, permanent disfiguring physical sequelae. Rampant abuse of irrational combinations of topical steroid-antifungal, with or without antibiotics, has led to the epidemic of recalcitrant steroid modified dermatophytosis in India. Regulatory aspects related to permissions to sell irrational steroid containing topical fixed drug combinations, drug dispensing without valid prescriptions, lack of control over who can prescribe steroid preparations and advertisements to lay public promoting steroid-hydroquinone-tretinoin creams as fairness creams have led to the menace of topical steroid abuse. If these flaws in the system are not corrected on a war-footing, the nightmare would worsen rapidly.

Keywords

Topical steroids • Rational usage • "Prescription drugs" • Fixed drug combinations • Drug control authorities

Learning Points

1. Topical steroids are safe when used rationally, by physicians who possess understanding of skin, steroid potency, and patients' psyche.
2. They are frequently used without appropriate prescriptions, as fairness or acne creams or relief of itching secondary to varied etiologies; they cause numerous short- and long-term adverse events and, at times, addiction.

R. Damisetty (✉)
Consultant Dermatologist and Additional Medical Director, Oliva Chain of Skin and Hair Clinics, Hyderabad, India
e-mail: drrajethadamisetty@gmail.com

S. Barua
Assistant Professor, Department of Dermatology, Assam Medical College and Hospital, Dibrugarh, Assam, India
e-mail: drshyamanta@gmail.com

© Springer Nature Singapore Pte Ltd. 2018
K. Lahiri (ed.), *A Treatise on Topical Corticosteroids in Dermatology*,
DOI 10.1007/978-981-10-4609-4_31

3. Easy availability of irrational topical steroid containing FDCs has led to their rampant abuse in dermatophytosis in India.
4. Control of new drug licenses, ban of irrational topical steroid containing FDCs and strict implementation of drug dispensing rules ensuring that dispensing against valid prescriptions are the need of the day.

31.1 The Dark Side of Topical Steroids

Sulzberger and Witten in 1952 introduced compound F (hydrocortisone), the first topical steroid to the world of dermatology [1]. Hydrocortisone and later, its most more potent analogues seemed like the holy grail of dermatology, a means to quell inflammation of the integument [2]. A decade passed before the adverse events first report of adverse events surfaced [3]. Another decade passed before addiction to topical steroids was reported in 1973 [4]. Kligman and Frosch [5] coined the term "steroid addiction" and gave a poignant description of the physical, psychological and social trauma that patients "hooked" to topical steroids go through.

A spate of articles on misuse and addiction continued to pour in over the next four decades [6–16]. The unabated accumulation of literature on the subject is merely a sign of the growing menace of topical steroid abuse.

31.2 Regulatory Aspects Related to Topical Steroid Abuse

Drug control authorities of a country are responsible for issuing drug licenses for manufacture and sale and approving indications and that can be treated with the drug. They may also decide to cap the price of certain drugs. Laws of the land decide which drugs can be sold over-the-counter, without prescriptions. They also decide which drugs may be advertised to lay people, if at all. The law machinery needs to implement the laws and check how stringently rules are being honored.

In the context of topical steroids, the controversy lies around issuing licenses to irrational fixed drug combinations that contain antibiotics and antifungals, in addition to steroid molecules. Use of mid-potent steroids like mometasone in modified Kligman's formula is also a case in point.

31.3 Focus on India, the Hotbed of Topical Steroid Abuse

Failure of regulatory authorities in India has no small role to play in the topical steroid menace that the nation is fighting. The major chinks in the armor of relevant law are:

1. Exclusion of all topical steroids from schedule H of drugs and cosmetics act.
2. Approval of numerous irrational topical steroid containing FDCs
3. Price control on betamethasone
4. Lack of will and means to implement laws to regulate sales.

Indian Association of Dermatologists, Venereologists and Leprologists (IADVL) has constituted a task force, the IADVL Taskforce Against Topical Steroid Abuse (ITATSA) to fight the growing menace of topical steroid abuse.

31.3.1 The Indian Drug Regulation Scene

An article in Lancet [17] said "To say that India's drug regulatory authority, the Central Drugs Standard Control Organization (CDSCO)— whose remit includes new drug approval, licensing of manufacturing facilities, and regulation of drug trials—is not fit for the purpose seems a gross understatement. A damning 118-page report from the Indian Parliamentary Standing Committee on Health and Family Welfare documents its successive failings. It describes a vast, geographically disseminated organization that is dangerously understaffed: "nine officers at headquarters deal with 20,000 applications, more than 200 meetings, 700 parliamentary questions, and 150 court cases per year. There is also a dearth of medically qualified staff, poor support infrastructure, a seeming lack of coordination between departments, and a scarcity of decent computer systems." Medication misuse in India has been termed a public health problem [18].

31.3.2 The Schedule H Tragedy and Legislation to Regulate Marketing and Sales of Topical Steroids

Schedule H is an appendix to the Drugs and Cosmetics Rules, India 1945 [19]. It includes a class of drugs, which cannot be purchased over the counter without the prescription of a qualified doctor. The manufacture and sale of all drugs are covered under the Drugs and Cosmetics Act and Rules. Four steroid molecules have been listed in this schedule, viz. clobetasol propionate, clobetasone 17-butyrate, fluticasone propionate, and mometasone furoate. The former two are available only for topical use on skin while the latter two are available for intranasal use too.

A footnote in the schedule H of the D&C Act stated that "The salts, esters, derivatives and preparations containing the above substances excluding those intended for topical or external use (except ophthalmic and ear/nose preparations containing antibiotics and/or steroids) are also covered by this Schedule" [19]. After incessant lobbying by ITATSA, this is slated to be modified.

Thus, topical steroids were not in the purview of schedule H. This is the root of topical steroid abuse in India. In most countries, no topical steroid may be purchased without a valid prescription. In a few countries, mildest of steroids, 1% hydrocortisone is available over the counter.

After extensive lobbying by IADVL, the drug technical advisory board decided to amend the footnote to include topical steroids on May 13th 2016 [20]. A notification of the same was published in the gazette of government of India on 12th Aug, 2016 [21]. No objections to this amendment were received within the stipulated six weeks apparently. Yet, till May 2017, the final

notification regarding implementation is still to be issued.

Even if the amendment is carried out (without further modification), potent steroid molecules like halobetasol and betamethasone dipropionate remain outside the schedule. The Drug Controller General of India took cognizance of this fact and called for reassessment of list of drugs in schedule H; he acknowledged the role of IADVL in initiating this change of attitude [22].

If the government of India intends to safeguard the skin health of its citizens, amendment of schedule H to include all steroid molecules and implementation of this change in letter and spirit has to be initiated. Till then, the strongest of steroid creams can be legally sold to the Indian consumer without prescriptions. Advertisements promoting these potentially dangerous products will continue to lure hapless people into the steroid addiction trap.

31.4 Plethora of Irrational Steroid Containing FDCs in India

Topical steroid-antifungal ± antibacterial combinations account for 43% of all topical steroid preparations sold, contributing to a staggering Rs. 753 crore, out of the total Rs. 1.716 billion of all topical steroid sales [23]. Most of these preparations are irrational and unscientific. Widespread use of topical steroids in conjunction with antifungals has led to the emergence of recalcitrant and atypical fungal infections [24]. The use of these FDCs has become so commonplace that most of the dermatophytosis seen by dermatologists is now steroid modified. As patients feel relief within just a few days of usage of these creams, they stop the topical preparation. Local immune suppression caused by the steroid component of the cream allows spread of the infection. Intermittent exposure to antifungals makes the organism resistant to its action. The medication is restarted when the itching and redness return, usually with a vengeance. Steroid part of the cream provides some symptom relief but the antifungal fails to do any good, resulting in the infection spreading rapidly. This vicious cycle has made treating steroid modified tinea a frustrating and expensive exercise. As it is contagious, family members frequently acquire recalcitrant tinea and end up spending money they can ill-afford to.

Unless urgent action is initiated, irrational topical steroid containing FDCs are all banned and strong legislation implemented to stop the unsupervised sale of steroid creams, this nightmare will turn more sinister. It might be years before the sensitivity of dermatophytes returns to normal even if effective steps are taken.

31.4.1 The COOT Cocktail

The largest contribution to this market is by a combination of clobetasol-ofloxacin-ornidazole and terbinafine (the COOT cocktail) which accounted for Rs. 262 crores. Panderm + cream, the top selling brand in this category alone accounted for Rs. 172 crore in the year 2015 [25].

Not a single study exists to support its usage in any indication. There isn't a single skin disease that requires this combination. Though it is considered "new drug," like all combinations are, it was given a license without the DCGI's approval. The safety and efficacy data that are required do not exist. No other country in the world has this combination. Yet, India has numerous such brands that accounted for revenue of Rs. 2.72 billion.

The Govt. of India appointed Kokate committee recognized the irrationality of this combination and recommended its ban, along with a ban of almost 350 other irrational fixed dose combinations (FDCs) including 27 topical steroid containing ones [26]. The ban had been overthrown by the Delhi High Court and is currently being examined by the supreme court of India.

31.4.2 Other Steroid Cocktails

These may be described as yet another Indian innovation; very few countries in the world have more than a handful of steroid-anti-microbial combinations. Almost none have antibiotics and/or antifungals in combination with potent steroids. Over-the-counter sales of all but the most

banal of antibiotic creams is prohibited not just in the developed world but in cash strapped countries like Bangladesh and Nepal too.

The availability of steroid-antifungal-antibiotic combinations makes people of various walks of life brave enough to attempt to treat undiagnosed skin ailments with shotgun therapy. They presume that one of the components in the cocktail would take care of the problem, be it a bacterial or fungal infection or an inflammatory condition like psoriasis or eczema; they imagine, erroneously, that the other components of the cream are harmless. Sadly, every component acts on skin and the mixture has disastrous consequences that none of the components could produce by themselves.

Indian Association of Dermatologists, Venereologists, and Leprologists prepared a consensus statement on topical steroid containing FDCs and shared it with the drug controller general of India on 12th August, 2016 (Personal Communication: Dr. Shyamanta Barua, Dept. of Dermatology, Assam Medical College, Dibrugarh, Assam, India). They recommended that all combinations other than the followed be banned at the earliest.

1. Any steroid with salicylic acid/urea/lactic acid and similar penetration enhancers and keratolytics/humectants.
2. Antibiotic-steroid combinations Mupirocin with hydrocortisone butyrate/acetate or fluticasone propionate. Fusidic acid with betamethasone valerate/0.1%/0.12%/hydrocortisone. 1% Dexamethasone with framycetin
3. Modified Kligman's formula containing Fluocinolone acetonide 0.01%, Hydrocortisone 1%/hydrocortisone acetate 1%.

31.4.3 The Imitators

While the ban recommended by Kokate committee on 27 irrational topical steroid containing combinations was being contested in court, many pharmaceutical companies came up with alternative formulations with similar sounding names so that brand value of the contentious best sellers was not lost. A case in point is Panderm NM+, with "NM" written in a miniscule font, which contains clobetasol-neomycin-miconazole combination. Panderm super, containing clobetasol, clotrimazole, and fusidic acid was approved by the DCGI himself in 2015.

31.4.4 Need for a Blanket Ban of Combinations of Classes of Drugs

Unless a blanket ban is imposed naming classes of drugs that should not be combined (e.g., Class A should never be combined with class B or C), rather than specific combinations (drug A + B + C), success in stemming this menace of topical steroid abuse will not be achieved. Indian pharmaceutical industry, renowned world over for their innovations, will come up with new permutations that defeat the purpose and spirit of the ban.

31.4.5 The Price Control Angle

In 2012, betamethasone was included under the list of drugs subject to price control by the national pharmaceutical pricing authority [27]. That is when the avalanche of steroid abuse started, with more potent clobetasol propionate replacing betamethasone in almost all preparations. Pharmaceutical industry was not keen on selling these products at Rs. 30 (0.4 USD) or less and quickly reformulated their wares with a minimal or no change in the name of the products. Indian dermatologists believe that this was the game changer that initiated the epidemic of recalcitrant tinea that fails to respond to prolonged therapy even with double doses of oral antifungals.

A 10 g tube of clobetasol-gentamicin cream can be bought for Rs. 5.60 (<0.1 USD) as gentamicin was brought under price control.

31.4.6 Misuse of Steroid Creams for Fairness

Misuse of topical steroids as "fairness" creams is rampant in India; the use of the COOT cocktail at the behest of the "pharmacist," Betnovate C's role in daily skincare [10], extensive use of mometasone-hydroquinone-tretinoin combinations such as "Skinlite," "Skinbrite," and "Noscar" to the veiled use of steroids in supposedly herbal creams like Pearl cream and Meglow fairness cream for women have ensured that the average Indian's fairness quest is paved with steroid creams. Lightening of skin color was the main reason for using topical corticosteroids in 50.39% patients in the absence of any primary skin condition in a study in central India.

Blanket ban of dangerous steroid containing lightening creams, along with abolition of advertisements in the media and strict control of sale of steroid preparations would be required to stop innumerable Indian fairness seekers from becoming a statistic in the epidemic of "topical steroid damaged face" [12].

Blatant advertising of fluocinolone and mometasone containing formulae "UBfair" and "Noscar" in newspapers led Maharastra branch of IADVL to complain to the state federal drug authorities who seized stocks of the drug. Torque pharma, the manufacturers of UB fair and Noscar filed a case against the Maharastra FDA. IADVL Maharastra had joined as an intervenor in the case. Indian laws prohibit direct-to-consumer advertisements of drugs. Fairness of skin is listed at number 18 in Schedule J of the Drugs and Cosmetics Rules, 1945 of India. Schedule J contains a list of diseases and ailments which a drug may not claim to prevent or cure. Under Rule 106 of the Drugs and Cosmetics Act, 1940, a drug cannot make claims to treat or prevent any of the diseases or reform the conditions listed.

Yet Indian pharma industry continues to sell its fairness inducing wares with little regard for the law of the land.

31.4.7 A Glimpse of the Point of Sale in India

A person manning the pharmacy counter, usually with minimal formal education of any sort, not to mention lack of understanding of drug science, is the one who dispenses medical advice to a vast majority of the Indian populace. Even educated people are not averse to taking this advice.

31.5 The African Scene: Jungle of the Law

In Africa, a fascination for lighter skin has led to rampant abuse of steroid-hydroquinone-mercurials mix. More than half the adult women attending dermatology out-patient department were found to be using "skin bleaching creams" in Dakar, Senegal [28]. Their skin diseases "appeared to be induced, aggravated or modified by this practice." Super-potent topical glucocorticoids seemed to be the culprits in most cases. The victims were mostly black women who were unaware of the risk factors and were advised to use topical steroid containing creams by their friends [29].

In addition to the adverse events caused by topical steroids in these spurious preparations, the renal and neuro-pyschiatric risks posed by mercury have to be considered. A study conducted on imported products in Cape town [30] revealed that 79.5% of the 29 products tested in this study contained banned or illegal substances including betamethasone, clobetasol, mercury, and hydroquinone in strengths higher than 2%. At least four of the products, manufactured in Democratic Republic of Congo (DRC), France, India and Italy contained both clobetasol and betamethasone. One each, manufactured in India and DRC, had all four of the ingredients tested. Another study found banned or illegal substances in 90% of the 10 top-selling skin-lightening creams in Durban, South Africa [31]. Law enforcement officials in SA had seized massive quantities of skin-lightening products containing hydroquinone and its monobenzyl, monoethyl, and monomethyl ethers, illegally imported from India, DRC, Cote d'Ivoire, the UK, and the EU [32].

It is ironic that European Union, in spite of its strict regulations, continues to manufacture and export harmful products to less developed countries. Their unrestricted availability in South Africa reveals the non-existent control on imports of "cosmetics" and underlines the need for law enforcement, random testing of skin lightening products, and appropriate penal action.

31.6 The First World Scenario

European Union legislation [33] has prohibited the usage of glucocorticoids in cosmetic products. In most developed countries, all steroid preparations except 1% hydrocortisone are dispensed only against valid prescriptions. Few combinations of topical steroids with antibiotics, antifungals, or rarely both exist but do not contain potent or super-potent steroid molecules. Illegal production of "cosmetics" containing topical steroids is known but these are mostly exported to underdeveloped countries.

31.7 The Way Forward

The actions needed to stop the menace of topical steroid abuse [34] are

1. A comprehensive and meaningful legislation to control production, import, and sale of topical steroid containing preparations.
2. Effective implementation of the modified rules, with sale against valid prescriptions.
3. A blanket ban on all existing irrational topical steroid containing FDCs
4. Regulation of permissions to new combinations
5. Clear labeling of all topical steroid preparations so that consumers may be wary of unsupervised use
6. Education of physicians of all specialties, pharmacists, and lay public on the ills of misuse of topical steroids.

References

1. Sulzberger MB, Witten VH. The effect of topically applied compound F in selected dermatoses. J Invest Dermatol. 1952;19:101–2.
2. Rindani TH. Topical action of steroid hormones on inflammation. Arch Int Pharmacodyn Ther. 1954;99:467–73.

3. Epstein NN, Epstein WL, Epstein JH. Atrophic striae in patients with inguinal intertrigo. Arch Dermatol. 1963;87:450–7.
4. Burry JN. Topical drug addiction: adverse effects of fluorinated corticosteroid creams and ointments. Med J Aust. 1973;1:393–6.
5. Kligman AM, Frosch P. Steroid addiction. Int J Dermatol. 1979;18(1):23–31.
6. Kligman AM. Letter: Topical steroid addicts. JAMA. 1976;235:1550.
7. Rapaport MJ, Rapaport V. The red skin syndromes: corticosteroid addiction and withdrawal. Expert Rev. Dermatol. 2006;1:547–61.
8. Rathi S. Abuse of topical steroid as cosmetic cream: a social background of steroid dermatitis. Indian J Dermatol. 2006;51:154–5.
9. Rathi SK, Kumrah L. Topical corticosteroid-induced rosacea-like dermatitis: a clinical study of 110 cases. Indian J Dermatol Venereol Leprol. 2011;77:42–6.
10. Saraswat A, Lahiri K, Chatterjee M, et al. Topical corticosteroid abuse on the face: a prospective, multicenter study of dermatology outpatients. Indian J Dermatol Venereol Leprol. 2011;77:160–6.
11. Ambika H, Sujatha VC, Yadalla H, et al. Topical corticosteroid abuse on face: a prospective study on outpatients of dermatology. Our Dermatol Online. 2014;5:5–8.
12. Lahiri K, Coondoo A. Topical steroid damaged/dependent face (TSDF): an entity of cutaneous pharmacodependence. Indian J Dermatol. 2016;61:265–72.
13. Narang T, Kumaran MS, Dogra S, et al. Red scrotum syndrome: idiopathic neurovascular phenomenon or steroid addiction? Sex Health. 2013;10(5):452.
14. Xiao X, Xie H, Jian D, Deng Y, Chen X, Li J, et al. Rebounding triad (severe itching, dryness and burning) after facial corticosteroid discontinuation defines a specific class of corticosteroid-dependent dermatitis. J Dermatol. 2015;42:697–702.
15. Hajar T, Leshem YA, Hanifin JM, Nedorost ST, Lio PA, Paller AS, et al. A systematic review of topical corticosteroid withdrawal ("steroid addiction") in patients with atopic dermatitis and other dermatoses. J Am Acad Dermatol. 2015;72:541–549.e2.
16. Mooney E, Rademaker M, Dailey R. Adverse effects of topical corticosteroids in paediatric eczema: Australasian consensus statement. Australas J Dermatol. 2015;56:241–51.
17. The Lancet. Drug regulation in India—the time is ripe for change. Lancet. 2012;379(9829):1862.
18. Porter G, Grills N. Medication misuse in India: a major public health issue in India. J Public Health. 2015;38(2):e150–7.
19. Schedule H of DCA 1945. http://cdsco.nic.in/writere-addata/Notoifi.pdf. Retrieved 12 Feb 2017.
20. Minutes of meeting of DTAB. 13 May 2016. http://www.cdsco.nic.in/writereaddata/redtab71st.pdf. Retrieved 12 Feb 2017.
21. India. Dept of health and family welfare. Drugs and Cosmetics (Amendment) Rules, 2016. Government gazette (extraordinary) No. 562: G.S.R 790(E) 12 Aug.
22. Central drugs standards control organization, Directorate General of Health Services, Ministry of Health and family welfare, Govt of India (Office of the DCGI). No DCG(I)/Misc/2017(36) dated 31st March, 2017.
23. HYPERLINK "http://medicinman.net/author/ims-health/" IMS HEALTH OCTOBER 14, 2016. IMS Health Market Reflection Report for September 2016. Medicinman. Retrieved from http://medicinman.net/2016/10/ims-health-market-reflection-report-for-september-2016.
24. Verma SB, Vasani R. Male genital dermatophytosis–clinical features and the effects of the misuse of topical steroids and steroid combinations–an alarming problem in India. Mycoses. 2016;59(10):606–14.
25. Verma SB. Topical corticosteroid misuse in India is harmful and out of control. BMJ. 2015;351:h6079.
26. Government of India. Dept of health and family welfare. Government gazette (extraordinary) No. 608: PART II—Section 3—Sub-section (ii). March 10.
27. DPCO circular regarding betamethasone.
28. Mahé A, Ly F, Aymard G, Dangou JM. Skin diseases associated with the cosmetic use of bleaching products in women from Dakar, Senegal. Br J Dermatol. 2003;148(3):493–500.
29. Malangu N, Ogunbanjo GA. Predictors of topical steroid misuse among patrons of pharmacies in Pretoria. SA Fam Pract. 2006;48(1):14.
30. Maneli MH, Wiesner L, Tinguely C, et al. Combinations of potent topical steroids, mercury and hydroquinone are common in internationally manufactured skin-lightening products: a spectroscopic study. Clin Exp Dermatol. 2016;41(2):196–201.
31. Dlova NC, Hendricks NE, Martincgh BS. Skin-lightening creams used in Durban, South Africa. Int J Dermatol. 2012;51(Suppl 1):51–3.
32. Warnings against use of illegal cosmetics. 2012. Available at: http://www.iol.co.za/dailynews/news/warnings-against-use-of-illegal-cosmetics-1.1309747#.VPX2Rd5yaHt. Accessed 25 Feb 2015.
33. Commission Regulation (EU) No. 1223/2009 of the European Parliament and of the Council on cosmetic products Text with EEA relevance. Off J Eur Union. 2009;L 342:59–209.
34. Verma SB. Sales, status, prescriptions and regulatory problems with topical steroids in India. Indian J Dermatol Venereol Leprol. 2014;80:201–3.

Topical Corticosteroids: The Pharmacovigilance Perspective

32

Rishi Kumar, V. Kalaiselvan, and G.N. Singh

Abstract

Pharmacovigilance is the need of hour for use of topical steroids because the irrational use of topical steroids may harm the patients in long and short term; the outcome of such treatments can be assessed by using pharmacovigilance as a scientific tool to assess safety of medicine. Pharmacovigilance system of some developed countries is very strong, while in developing and poor countries, it is still in infancy state. The role of international bodies like ICH, CIOMS, WHO-UMC is very significant for harmonising the process of pharmacovigilance across the world. In this chapter, authors tries to establish the need of pharmacovigilance to ascertain frequency of rarely reported cases due to steroids and other drugs; an analysis of International ADR database is presented to show the culture of reporting across the world.

Keywords

Pharmacovigilance • Adverse drug reactions • ICH • Methods of pharmacovigilance • Spontaneous reporting

R. Kumar (✉)
Pharmacovigilance Division, Indian Pharmacopoeia Commission, National Coordination Centre, Pharmacovigilance Programme of India, Ministry of Health and Family Welfare, Government of India, Sec-23, Ghaziabad 201002, India
e-mail: tawar.rishi@gmail.com

V. Kalaiselvan
Principal Scientific Officer, Indian Pharmacopoeia Commission, National Coordination Centre- Pharmacovigilance Programme of India, Ministry of Health and Family Welfare, Government of India, Raj Nagar, Sec-23, Ghaziabad 201002, Uttar Pradesh, India

G.N. Singh
Secretary-cum-Scientific Director, Indian Pharmacopoeia Commission, National Coordination Centre- Pharmacovigilance Programme of India, Ministry of Health and Family Welfare, Government of India, Raj Nagar, Sec-23, Ghaziabad 201002, Uttar Pradesh, India

© Springer Nature Singapore Pte Ltd. 2018
K. Lahiri (ed.), *A Treatise on Topical Corticosteroids in Dermatology*,
DOI 10.1007/978-981-10-4609-4_32

Learning Points

1. What is pharmacovigilance
2. Need of pharmacovigilance
3. Terminology used in pharmacovigilance
4. Methods of pharmacovigilance
5. Organisations involved in pharmacovigilance across globe
6. Reporting requirement in special population
7. Classification of topical corticosteroids as per WHO Classification
8. Analysis of global data of corticosteroids from VigiBase®

32.1   Introduction

Pharmacovigilance is the science of detection, assessment, understanding and prevention of adverse drug reactions. The uses of topical steroids are abundant in humans. In recent times, the use of topical steroids has increased drastically. There are practices of using multiple steroids for topical ailments, which are sometimes not justified therapeutically. In this chapter, the authors would like to highlight the need of control on use of topical steroids, for which there is strong need of close monitoring of the populations who are using these steroids. There are a number of serious adverse drug reactions reported due to use of topical steroids. These includes atrophy, telangiectasia, periorificial dermatitis, facial erythema, thinning of skin, tinea incognito, comedonal acne, marked facial erythema, nodular acne with crusting, rosacea, striae rubra with associated hypopigmentation, perioral dermatitis, facial hypertrichosis, striae alba, striae secondary to steroid application for tinea corporis, diffuse hypopigmentation, bilateral hypopigmentation, bilateral mild hypopigmentation with erythema and labial hypertrichosis, perilesional diffuse hypopigmentation and diffuse scalp hypopigmentation [1–4].

32.2   Terminology of Pharmacovigilance

32.2.1   Adverse Event

Any untoward medical occurrence that may present during treatment with a pharmaceutical product but which does not necessarily have a causal relationship with this treatment.

32.2.2   Adverse (Drug) Reaction (ADR)

A response which is noxious and unintended and which occurs at doses normally used in humans for the prophylaxis, diagnosis, or therapy of disease or for the modification of physiological function (WHO, 1972) [5].

An adverse drug reaction, contrary to an adverse event, is characterised by the suspicion of a causal relationship between the drug and the occurrence, i.e. judged as being at least possibly related to treatment by the reporting or a reviewing health professional.

32.2.2.1   Side Effect

Any unintended effect of a pharmaceutical product occurring at normal dosage which is related to the pharmacological properties of the drug.

32.3   Methods of Pharmacovigilance

Adverse drug reactions can be monitored through two ways:

1. Active surveillance system
2. Passive surveillance system

Spontaneous or voluntary reporting of adverse event/adverse drug reaction is the type of passive surveillance. Active surveillance, in contrast to passive surveillance, requires a continuous pre-organised process. An example of active surveillance is cohort event monitoring.

32.3.1 Spontaneous Reporting

A spontaneous report is an unsolicited adverse event/adverse drug reaction report by healthcare professionals, pharmaceutical company and consumers to regulatory authority that describes one or more suspected adverse drug reactions in a patient due to therapeutic products.

32.3.2 Pharmacovigilance in Special Population

When we use drugs in special population like pregnant women, nursing mother, paediatrics and geriatrics for the treatment of various ailments, we require to monitor them closely because during clinical trials, these groups of special population are not always included, due to which the chances of adverse drug reactions in these groups are more. Especially in the case of topical steroids for nursing mothers and pregnant women, there is lack of scientific data which clearly states that topical steroids are safe for nursing mothers and pregnant women. Paediatrics and geriatrics group of population need to monitor closely for use of drugs for patient safety.

32.3.3 Pharmacovigilance System in Developed Countries [6]

32.3.3.1 US Pharmacovigilance System

It is controlled by the US Food and Drug Administration (USFDA). The MedWatch is the system used to collect spontaneous reports on adverse reactions associated with all types of medical products including prescription and over-the-counter drugs, biologics, medical devices, radiopharmaceuticals, etc.

32.3.3.2 Europe Pharmacovigilance System

In Europe, the European Medicines Agency (EMA) is responsible to carry out the pharmaco-vigilance activities. EudraVigilance system is the centralised computer database for adverse drug reaction reporting. The pharmacovigilance system of EMA is very robust and well managed across all member countries of European Union. In the UK, there is supportive pharmacovigilance system which includes Black Triangle Drugs and Yellow Card Scheme. The Black Triangle Drugs are those drugs which are newly launched in the market and are under intensive monitoring for pharmacovigilance. A black colour triangle is marked on the label of such new drugs. It also marks on label of such drugs which are newly approved for new indication and which may affect the benefit risk profile of the drugs. The Yellow Card Scheme is the system used for collecting information on adverse drug reaction in the UK which is administered by two government agencies: Medicines and Healthcare Products Regulatory Agency (MHRA) and Committee on the Safety of Medicines (CSM). This scheme was started in 1964 after the thalidomide disaster.

32.3.3.3 Japan

The pharmacovigilance system in Japan is regulated by Japanese regulatory authority Pharmaceuticals and Medical Devices Agency (PMDA). PMDA works under the aegis of Ministry of Health, Labour and Welfare. It works in line with ICH for pharmacovigilance. It has a unique system of Early Post-Marketing Phase Vigilance, and under this system, for every new medical product which is due for launch by any pharmaceutical company, the company representatives needs to visit all medical institutions which may use their products.

32.4 WHO Collaborating Centre for International Drug Monitoring: The Uppsala Monitoring Centre

The WHO is a specialised agency of the UN that is concerned with international public health. The UMC is an independent foundation and a centre for international service and scientific research.

UMC is a for-benefit foundation committed to innovative research and development in patient safety and to providing data, tools, and consultation and training resources to health professionals all over the world. The World Health Organization set up its international drug monitoring programme after the thalidomide disaster. Since 1978 the WHO Programme for International Drug Monitoring has been carried out by Uppsala Monitoring Centre (UMC) in Sweden. UMC is the custodian and manager of VigiBase, the WHO global database of more than 14 million reports of adverse reactions to medicines. (Official website: www.who-umc.org).

## 32.5	Council for International Organizations of Medical Sciences (CIOMS) [7]

CIOMS is an international organisation work in collaboration with the UN, WHO and UNESCO. It has many experts groups which work for drug safety and cover most of the drug-related issues. CIOMS has pool of experts from industries, academics and research, and these experts joined together to develop an acceptable guideline such as international reporting of adverse drug reactions (CIOMS-I), periodic safety update reports, core clinical safety information, etc. There are ten working groups working under CIOMS, and they have played a significant role in the development of pharmacovigilance. The recommendations of CIOMS working groups have been adopted by the ICH (International Council for Harmonisation of Technical Requirements for Pharmaceuticals for Human Use).

## 32.6	International Council for Harmonisation of Technical Requirements for Pharmaceuticals for Human Use (ICH) [8]

ICH guidelines are broadly described in four categories, namely, efficacy, safety, quality and multidisciplinary. The clinical safety guidelines are explained under the efficacy section of ICH. In total, there are eight clinical safety guidelines

that address the various aspects of drug safety. These are:

1. E1 – Clinical Safety of Drugs used in Long-Term Treatment
2. ICH E2A – Clinical Safety Data Management: Definitions and Standard for Expedited Reporting
3. ICH E2B – Clinical Safety Data Management: Data Elements for the Transmission of Individual Case Safety Reports
4. ICH E2C – Periodic Safety Update Reports for Marketed Drugs and Addendum to ICH E2C
5. ICH E2D – Post Approval Safety Data Management: Definitions and Standards for Expedited Reporting
6. ICH E2E – Pharmacovigilance Planning
7. ICH E2F – Development Safety Update Reports
8. ICH E14 – Clinical Evaluation of QT/QTc Interval Prolongation and Proarrhythmic Potential for Nonarrhythmic Drugs

The above guidelines are available online on the website of ICH.

### 32.6.1	Classification of Topical Corticosteroids [9]

The topical corticosteroids are classified based on their potency as follows:

Ultrahigh potent: Clobetasol propionate (cream, 0.05%), diflorasone diacetate (ointment, 0.05%)

Highly potent: amcinonide (ointment 0.1%), betamethasone dipropionate (ointment 0.05%), desoximetasone (ointment or cream 0.025%), fluocinonide (cream, ointment or gel 0.05%), halcinonide (cream 0.1%), betamethasone valerate (ointment 0.1%), diflorasone diacetate (cream 0.05%), triamcinolone acetonide (ointment 0.1%).

Moderately potent: desoximetasone (cream 0.05%), fluocinolone acetonide (ointment, 0.025%), fludroxycortide (ointment, 0.05%), hydrocortisone valerate (ointment, 0.2%), triamcinolone acetonide (cream 0.1%).

Low potent: betamethasone valerate (lotion 0.05%), desonide (cream 0.05%), fluocinolone (solution (0.01%), dexamethasone sodium phosphate (cream 0.1%), hydrocortisone acetate (cream 1%), methylprednisolone acetate (cream, 0.25%).

32.7 Analysis of International Adverse Drug Reaction Data from VigiBase [10]

VigiBase is the WHO international database of adverse drug reactions. The total no. of ICSRs reported to VigiBase is 14,476,200. An analysis of data was done till 22 January 2017, in which we found 94,579 ICSRs reported due to steroids. A total of 13 steroids substances were searched in VigiBase ADR database. The number of ADRs due to respective steroids substance is shown in Fig. 32.1. The age-wise distribution of ICSRs is shown in Fig. 32.2. The gender-wise distribution of ICSRs is shown in Fig. 32.3. The adverse drug reactions classifica-

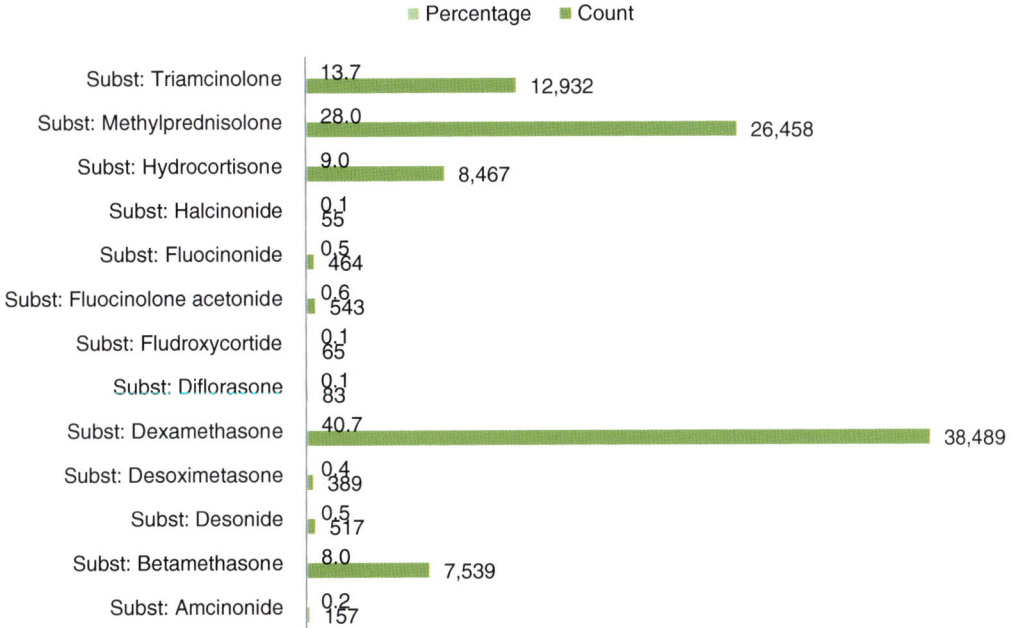

Fig. 32.1 The number of ICSRs due to steroid substances

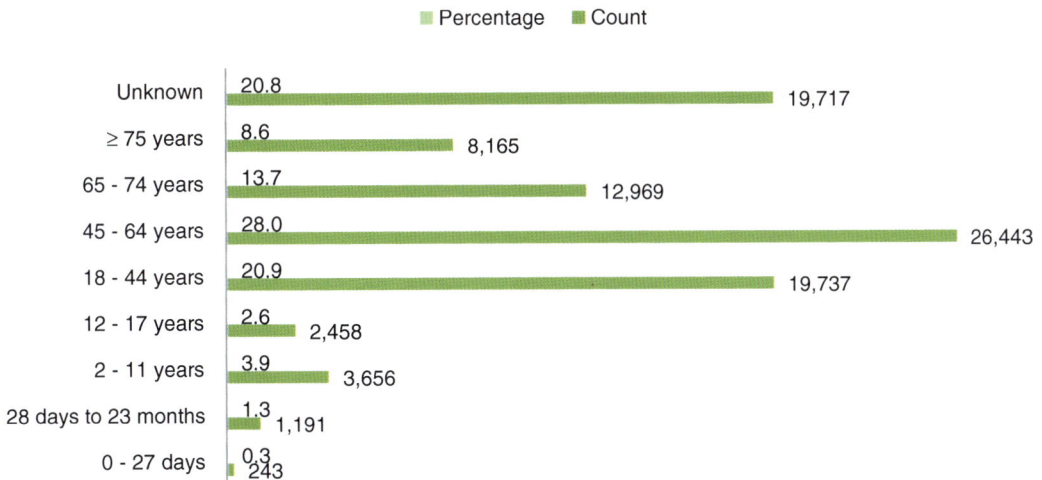

Fig. 32.2 Age-wise distribution of ICSRs due to steroids

Fig. 32.3 Gender-wise distribution of ICSRs

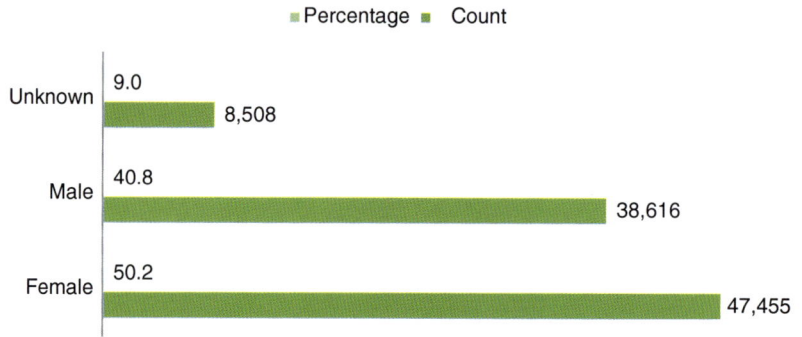

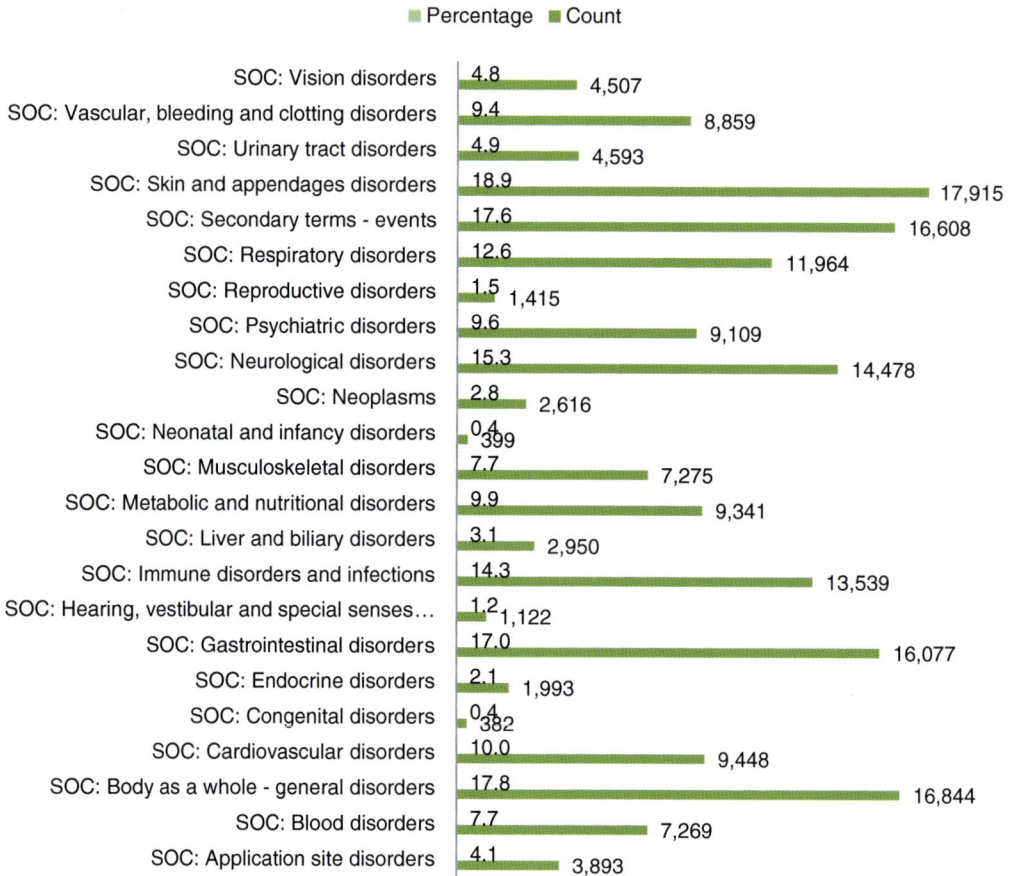

■ Percentage ■ Count

Unknown — 9.0 — 8,508

Male — 40.8 — 38,616

Female — 50.2 — 47,455

■ Percentage ■ Count

SOC: Vision disorders — 4.8 — 4,507
SOC: Vascular, bleeding and clotting disorders — 9.4 — 8,859
SOC: Urinary tract disorders — 4.9 — 4,593
SOC: Skin and appendages disorders — 18.9 — 17,915
SOC: Secondary terms - events — 17.6 — 16,608
SOC: Respiratory disorders — 12.6 — 11,964
SOC: Reproductive disorders — 1.5 — 1,415
SOC: Psychiatric disorders — 9.6 — 9,109
SOC: Neurological disorders — 15.3 — 14,478
SOC: Neoplasms — 2.8 — 2,616
SOC: Neonatal and infancy disorders — 0.4 — 399
SOC: Musculoskeletal disorders — 7.7 — 7,275
SOC: Metabolic and nutritional disorders — 9.9 — 9,341
SOC: Liver and biliary disorders — 3.1 — 2,950
SOC: Immune disorders and infections — 14.3 — 13,539
SOC: Hearing, vestibular and special senses… — 1.2 — 1,122
SOC: Gastrointestinal disorders — 17.0 — 16,077
SOC: Endocrine disorders — 2.1 — 1,993
SOC: Congenital disorders — 0.4 — 382
SOC: Cardiovascular disorders — 10.0 — 9,448
SOC: Body as a whole - general disorders — 17.8 — 16,844
SOC: Blood disorders — 7.7 — 7,269
SOC: Application site disorders — 4.1 — 3,893

Fig. 32.4 System organ class-wise distribution of ICSRs

tion as per system organ class is depicted in Fig. 32.4; in this figure, we can see that 19% of ADR are related to skin and appendages disorders. The top 20 preferred terms used during the reporting of these ICSRs are shown in Fig. 32.5.

The trends of ADR reporting due to steroids since 1968 are shown in Fig. 32.6.

However, UMC states that (1) regarding the source of the information (2) that the information comes from a variety of sources, and the likeli-

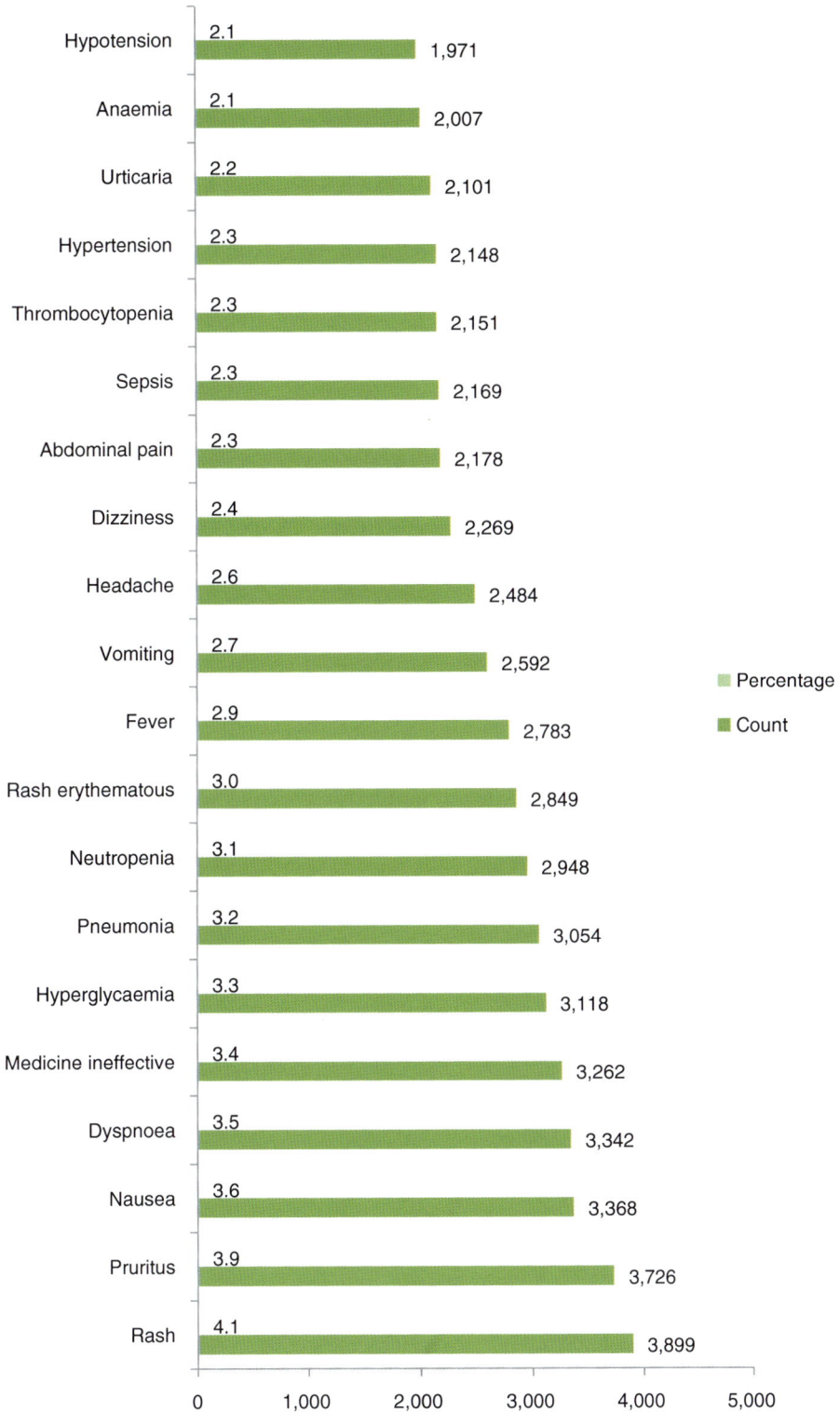

Fig. 32.5 Top 20 preferred terms (adverse drug reaction term) used during reporting of ICSRs due to steroids substances

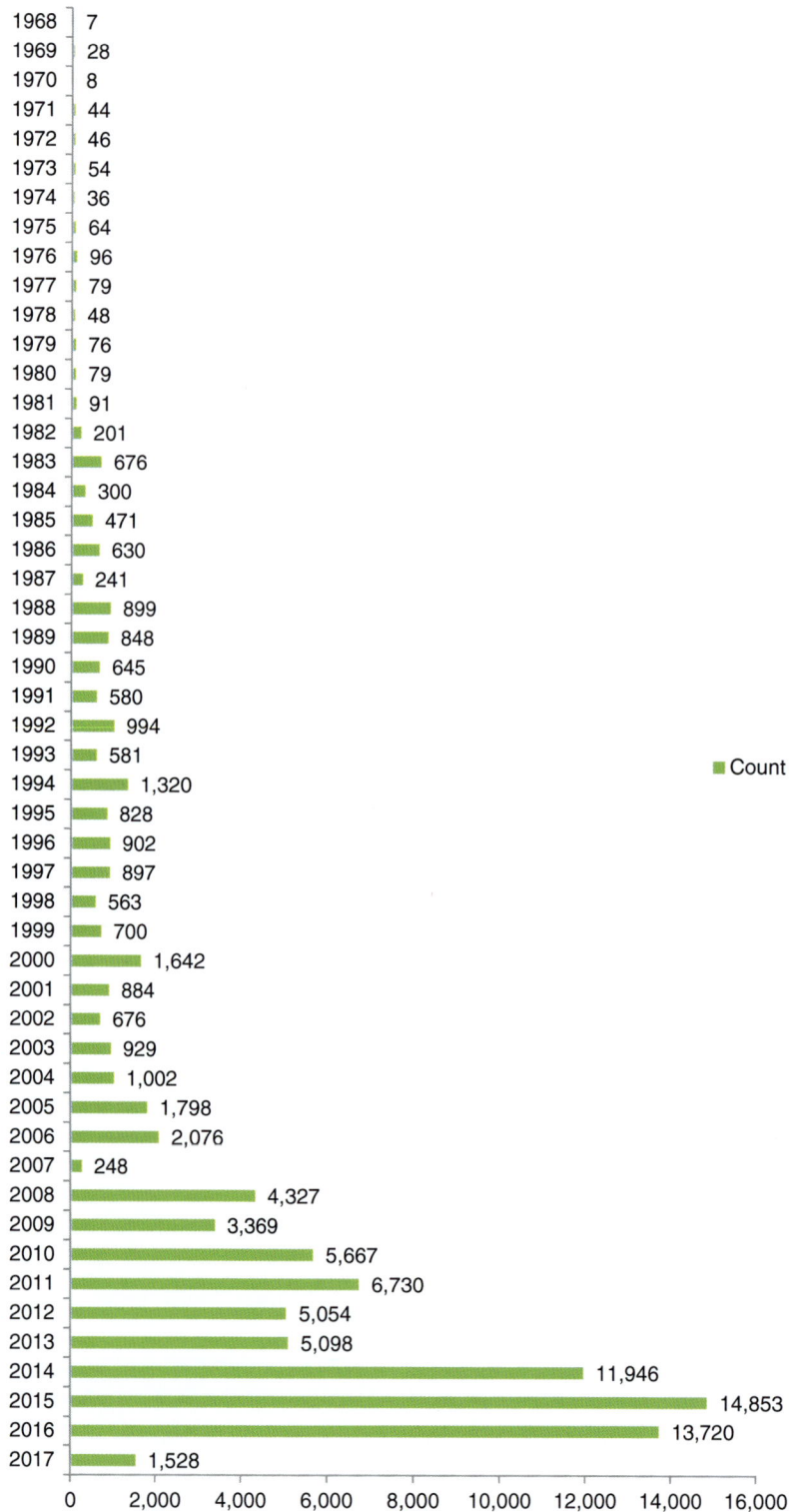

Fig. 32.6 The year-wise number of ICSRs received at UMC-Sweden due to steroids substances

hood that the suspected adverse reaction is drug-related is not the same in all cases, (3) that the information does not represent the opinion of the World Health Organization [11].

Conclusion

The present study revealed that topical steroids are associated with various serious and non-serious adverse events including rash, pruritis, atrophy, telangiectasia, periorificial dermatitis, etc. However, the present study could not assess the causal relationship because the drug may be abruptly stopped or the use of topical steroids may be irrational. Therefore, the author concludes that the steroids need to be prescribed rationally. If such adverse events occurred or came to the notice of healthcare professionals, they are encouraged to report known and unknown adverse events due to steroids to their respective countries pharmacovigilance system.

Acknowledgement The authors express their gratitude to Ministry of Health and Family Welfare, Government of India and World Health Organization–Uppsala Monitoring Centre for providing technical support in the preparation of this manuscript.

References

1. Kumar R, Kumar P, Kaur I, Kalaiselvan V, Singh GN. Best practices for improving quality of individual case safety reports in pharmacovigilance. Ther Innov Regul Sci. 2016;50(4):464–71.
2. Vivekanandan K, Arunabh T, Kumar R, Prasad T, Singh GN. Quantitative methods for identification of signals. Ther Innov Regul Sci. 2015;49(6):898–902.
3. Vivekanandan K, Kumar R, Prasad T, Arunabh T, Singh GN. Status of documentation grading and completeness score for Indian individual case safety reports. Indian J Pharmacol. 2015;47:325–7.
4. Coondoo A, Phiske M, Verma S, Lahiri K. Side effects of topical steroids: a long overdue revisit. Indian Dermatol Online J. 2014;5(4):416–25.
5. WHO, 1972. http://apps.who.int/medicinedocs/en/d/Js4893e/9.html. Assessed on 24th May 2017.
6. Arora D. Pharmacovigilance an industry perspective. 1st ed. Sonepat: Pharmapublisher; 2012.
7. URL: http://www.cioms.ch. Assessed 31 Jan 2017.
8. URL: http://www.ich.org/products/guidelines/efficacy/article/efficacy-guidelines.html. Assessed 31 Jan 2017.
9. URL: http://apps.who.int/medicinedocs/en/d/Jh2918e/32.html#Jh2918e.32.1. Assessed 22 Jan 2017.
10. URL: https://vigilyze.who-umc.org/#. Assessed 22 Jan 2017.
11. URL: https://www.who-umc.org/media/1417/umc_caveat_201605.pdf. Assessed 22 Jan 2017.

Combating Topical Corticosteroids Abuse at the Community Level

33

Venkataram Mysore and Gousia Sheikh

Abstract

- A concerted effort involving different agencies such as the government, industry, patients, public at large, dermatologists and physicians is needed to fight the menace
- Legislative means as well as administrative means need to be focused persistently
- Education of doctors to change attitudes in prescription practices is essential
- Community education through posters, videos and handouts need to be performed continuously

Keywords

Tpoical steroid abuse · Education · Legislation

33.1 Introduction

Topical steroid abuse has assumed menacing proportions as shown by several data [1–4]. The problem has reached epidemic proportions in India, aided and abetted by:

- Irrational combinations
- Tendency to use potent topical steroids by practitioners
- Misuse by pharmacists and beauticians

- Misconceptions amongst public aided by a fascination for fairness
- Hyped and misleading advertisements by industry
- Lack of commitment by dermatological community and governmental agencies
- Lack of commitment on the part of industry to address the issue

This has led to misuse of steroids as a fairness cream and as a panacea for all skin diseases including infections. It is obvious therefore that the menace has to be fought. However, a single-minded strategy, about how and how far it has to be fought, has been lacking. Differences arose within dermatologist community about its seriousness, whether it should be a priority and if

V. Mysore (✉) • G. Sheikh
Venkat Charmalaya, Centre for Advanced Dermatology and Postgraduate Training, Bangalore, India
e-mail: mnvenkataram@gmail.com

© Springer Nature Singapore Pte Ltd. 2018
K. Lahiri (ed.), *A Treatise on Topical Corticosteroids in Dermatology*,
DOI 10.1007/978-981-10-4609-4_33

publicity about steroid abuse will lead to steroid phobia [5]. These differences have slowed down the fight against the menace. Of late, however, a contour has emerged about the way to fight the menace, with some progress made, and this chapter will outline such a strategy.

33.2 Topical Steroid Abuse/ Topical Steroid Damaged/ Dependent Face (TSDF) and the Community

Questions have been raised whether this issue is big enough to be fought at the community level, particularly when there are bigger and larger issues such as leprosy, cancer, HIV, vitiligo, etc. Several dermatologists and those in the government feel valuable resources of time, effort and money need not be squandered on what seems to be a problem in urban areas, in a relatively nonlife-threatening field. There is also an opinion that too much emphasis on TSDF would lead to steroid phobia amongst patients and people, leading to underuse of steroid creams in diseases where the drug is indicated [5]. However, several publications have shown and highlighted the magnitude of the problem [1–4]. What seems to have turned to tide in its favour is the emergence of resistant fungal infections due to steroid abuse.

Amongst the most rampant abusers of topical corticosteroids (TCs) are the laymen both patients and non-patients [1].

1. Patients apply TCs on the advice of their friends, relatives and other laymen for varying periods of time before turning up at the doctor's clinic. Prescription repetition, whereby prescriptions issued by dermatologists are used to purchase medicines much beyond the prescribed period, is a regular phenomenon. Also, the patients may be applying the TCs in an inappropriate manner.
2. Patients use TC for the wrong indications particularly dermatophytosis—often due to misdiagnosis and other times in the hope to get a quick solution. While general practitioners

and alternative medicine specialists are to be blamed largely for misdiagnosis of dermatophytosis, it has to be said with certain sadness that even qualified dermatologists often use combinations with potent steroids in the hope of a quick cure for the patient.

3. Non-patients use TCs for various purposes, but principally for beautification as "fairness creams" [6]. In this, beauticians, saloons and spas are the major culprits. The fact that many of these creams are cheap due to drug control seems to aid their misuse.

33.3 The Fairness Craze [6, 7]

In India, with a population which is predominantly brown in skin colour (Fitzpatrick type 4–5), there is a fairness craze whereby fairness of skin is equated with beauty. This craze has been fanned by advertisements in the audio-visual, social, electronic and print media wherein women and men with lighter skin have been portrayed as people who are more beautiful, attractive, marriageable, confident and professionally successful.

Indian society has always had a fascination with colour. "Kallu" and "Kalia" have always been terms used with some sense of derogation for people who are black, despite the fact that predominant colour of Indians is brown-black. Except perhaps in the state of Tamil Nadu, this fascination has increased and turned into a near obsession—with even mothers bringing their 3-year-old children with a request to change the colour. This has been further fuelled by the advertisements on media, with film stars endorsing the products unashamedly. Hype surrounds such advertisements as they promise "fairness in 1 week".

The fairness craze is further fanned by the fact that advertisement of fairness creams is not controlled by the Drugs and Magic Remedies (Objectionable Advertisement) Act 1954. What is alarming is that advertisements include products such as Kligman's formula due to this loophole.

Additionally, pharmacists and beauticians have played in to the hands of patients, by promoting the steroid creams and depigmenting creams. The creams have a multiplier effect as they change hands.

According to AC Nielsen, the market for skin lightening is rising at the rate of 18% every year and is expected to reach $432 million (Rupees 28,000 crores) by the end of 2016 [7].

The cosmetic industry, realizing a vast business opportunity, has capitalized on this obsession by marketing these skin lightening fairness creams [8, 9]. The business of fairness creams started with the marketing of the first fairness cream in India in 1975.

According to the WHO, a drug is defined as "any substance or product that is intended to be used to modify physiological systems or pathological states for the benefit of the system". In 2015 a pharmaceutical company marketed a product containing a topical corticosteroid as a fairness cream in newspapers and was forced to withdraw it under legal pressure [10].

How to fight the menace?

As mentioned earlier, there are several stakeholders in the problem:

1. Dermatologists
2. Physicians and other practitioners
3. Alternative medicine practitioners and quacks
4. Paramedical workers—pharmacists, nurses and beauticians
5. Governmental agencies—drug controller at state and central levels
6. Industry—executives, distributors and manufacturers
7. Media
8. Lay public

Hence, any strategy will have to deal with these different levels as depicted in Table 33.1. However, how these have to be tackled at different levels has proved to be a challenge.

Table 33.1 Multilevel strategy for TSDF

Level	Issue involved	Action needed
Bureaucratic red tape	• Loopholes in schedule H permitting over-the-counter sale of TCs	Modify the schedule
	• Approval of irrational drug combinations containing TCs	Ban such combinations
	• Inability to stop indiscriminate sale of TCs as OTC products at chemists	Better supervision and check
Pharmaceuticals	• Marketing scientifically unethical combinations	Pressure to be brought to prevent manufacture of such combinations
	• Advertisement of TC containing products as fairness creams	Boycott of such rogue companies by doctor community
Prescribers	• Dermatologists: incomplete prescriptions or counselling	Education, lectures, meetings
	• Non-dermatologists: not aware of norms of TC use	Education
	• Quacks: no knowledge about TCs	Education and punitive action
Chemists	• All TCs are sold as OTC products	Education supervision by drug inspectors
	• Salesmen considered as medical advisors by patients	
	• Sell TCs of all potencies for wrong indications	
	• Promote TCs as fairness creams	
Patients	• Apply TCs on advice of friends, neighbours or relatives	Education through counselling, brochures, social, visual and print media
	• Apply TCs in diseases which are not steroid responsive or may be aggravated by TCs	
	• Repeat TC prescriptions indefinitely	
	• Apply potent TCs of all potencies for melasma	
Laymen other than patients	• Misuse of TCs as fairness creams	Education through brochures, social, visual and print media

33.3.1 Dermatologists

It is obvious that dermatologists are primary stakeholders. They prescribe the steroids maximum and they know the steroids and perhaps also abuse them. Surprisingly, this has proved to be a challenge, partly because of attitude and partly because of compulsions of practices. The reasons are as follows:

a. Many dermatologists don't think that this is an important area. They feel it is much ado about a small thing and there are different, more pressing areas such as leprosy, eczema, cancer, vitiligo, HIV infection, etc.
b. They find fixed drug combinations (FDCs) as useful tools in practice.
c. They feel, somewhat smugly, they can convince patients about rational use of these combinations.
d. They also feel that highlighting the issue will lead to steroid phobia.
e. Lastly, they feel they are the best judges of what they do and resent suggestions for change in practice styles.

Overcoming this can be done in different ways:

a. Information, education through scientific data and studies
b. Communication through group emails, website and posters
c. Discussions in conferences
d. Discussions in social media
e. Naming and shaming—though controversial, irrational prescriptions highlighted on social media may have some efficacy

So as a first step to fight this menace, in 2014, the Indian Association of Dermatologists, Venereologists and Leprologists (IADVL) formed a taskforce named IADVL Taskforce Against Topical Steroid Abuse (ITATSA) which has been sensitizing the government, the media and the industry on this issue. Through their efforts during the past 2 years, all TCs have now been included under Schedule H so that no TC can be sold as OTC without a doctor's prescription. This taskforce under the leadership of motivated and passionate dermatologists has led a movement in the association to educate, cajole and push the dermatologists, the society, the government and the industry. History was created when IADVL became a party to a legal battle against a rogue pharma company which had marketed Kligman's formula unashamedly as a fairness cream for men, UB fair [10].

33.3.2 Non-Dermatologists

Physicians, general practitioners, paediatricians and other specialists all prescribe topical steroids. While patients now seek dermatologist's consultation early, in rural areas, these doctors take care of skin problems for much longer time. Hence, concerted efforts are needed to target them through:

a. Information, education through scientific data and studies
b. Communication through society-based emails, website and posters
c. Discussions in conferences of these specialities
d. Articles and advertisements in medical journals
e. Discussions in social media

However, this effort is more difficult and has not been carried out in a significant way.

33.3.3 Paramedical Staff

Recent craze for fairness coupled with the craving for aesthetic procedures has led to a surfeit of beauty clinics, SPAs, etc. Since the effort in these centres is to provide quick results and enhance commercial survival, the tendency is to use TCs liberally and unethically.

33.3.4 Governmental Agencies

The most important agency is of course the drug controller of India both at centre and at states. The emphasis has been:

a. Rational policy on FDCs—some success has been met in this area as the agency is seized of the issue in a larger context of all FDCs. Recently, a ban has been issued on scores of FDC products. However, the pharma companies have obtained a stay from the courts to prevent its implementation.

b. Changing statues: A loophole in schedule H of drug control act, which excluded topical steroids from the schedule, allowed for over-the-counter sale of the TCs. Persistent efforts have led to modifications in schedule H to remove such ambiguity about topical steroid creams being non-prescription items.

While these have proved to be easier to handle, implementation of the act at local level has been a far tougher issue. This is done through state-level drug controllers and drug inspectors. They are understaffed and have a number of other issues for supervision such as opioid drugs, etc. Persistent effort through dermatologists at local level is needed to enforce proper implementation.

33.3.5 Industry

The position of industry on this issue has been ambiguous. Publicly, they have supported the ITATSA and have even funded some programs to communicate the message. However, they have not digressed from their policy of marketing the combinations, perhaps due to the commercial interests involved. This has led to a debate as to whether these companies are indeed serious about fighting the menace of topical steroid abuse. There have been differences of opinion as to what is the best way to confront the industry on this issue:

- Should they be banned by doctors?
- Should they be prevented from participating in congresses?
- Are these feasible?

However, it is somewhat heartening to note that slowly, some change is happening in this scenario, with some companies at least withdrawing combinations with potent steroid creams.

33.3.6 Patients and Public

Educating the patients and public needs sustained and continuous effort. Handouts, brochures, videos and articles in press all have to be done again, again and again. Social media has to be used effectively. A case in point was a blog by a YouTuber who openly advocated the use of betnovate cream to make the skin look good. Such was the pressure brought on by the dermatologist community that the video had to be withdrawn the very next day. It is the author's strategy to put a poster on the wall right behind his consulting chair and ask all patients to click the poster and then post it on their Facebook accounts. Some examples of posters used for educating public are shown in Figs. 1–3.

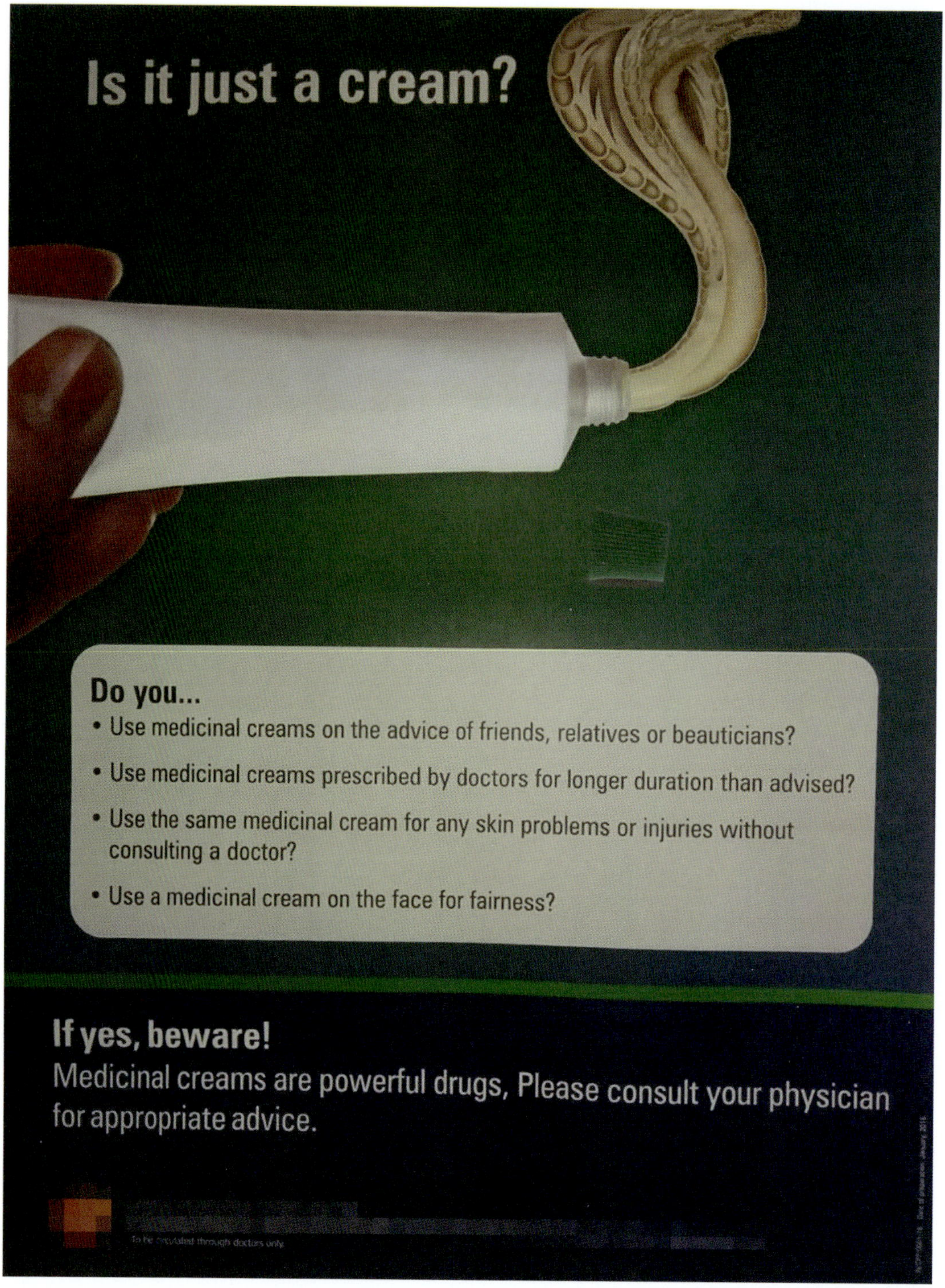
Is it just a cream?
Do you...
• Use medicinal creams on the advice of friends, relatives or beauticians?
• Use medicinal creams prescribed by doctors for longer duration than advised?
• Use the same medicinal cream for any skin problems or injuries without consulting a doctor?
• Use a medicinal cream on the face for fairness?
If yes, beware!
Medicinal creams are powerful drugs, Please consult your physician for appropriate advice.

आपकी सौन्दर्य (Beauty Cream) क्रीमों में त्वचा को खराब करने वाला जहर भी हो सकता है

- बैट्नोवेट (Betnovate C/N)
- टैनोवेट (Tenovate)
- लोबेट जी एम (Lobate GM)
- स्किन लाइट
- पैन्डर्म (Panderm)
- फोडर्म (Fourderm) आदि से सावधान रहें

चर्म रोग विशेषज्ञ डॉक्टर की सलाह के बिना अपने चेहरे पर लम्बे समय तक कोई भी क्रीम न लगाएं। इन सस्ती क्रीमों में स्टीरॉइड (Steroid) होता है जिससे

- चेहरे पर चमक आती है
- (Pimples) मुहांसे दब जाते है
- दाद/ छाजन की खुजली चली जाती है

परन्तु कोई भी बीमारी जड़ से नहीं जाती। लम्बे समय तक लगाने से यह त्वचा को हमेशा के लिए खराब कर देते है, जो फिर कभी ठीक नहीं हो सकती।

जब भी आप इन क्रीमों को बन्द करते है, तब चेहरे पर लाली आना, धूप में / गैस पर काम करने से चेहरा जलना, चेहरे पर बाल आना, मुहांसे की कीलें पड़ना एवं मुहांसे की गाँठे पड़ जाती है।

अत: चेहरे को ठीक होने में 6 से 12 महीने का समय लग सकता है।

Attention Please!!

Steroid creams are not beautifying products.

It will exacerbate skin conditions and cause early cataract formation, diabetes, hypertension and osteoporosis.

Hence, kindly consult a dermatologist and use them for specific skin conditions only.

"Stop steroid abuse to save your beautiful skin"

33.4   Summary

Topical steroid abuse is a challenge which needs serious attention at different levels of administration. It needs a multipronged focus, at government, association, industry and community levels.

References

1. Rathi S. Abuse of topical steroid as cosmetic cream: a social background of steroid dermatitis. Indian J Dermatol. 2006;51:154–5.
2. Bains P. Topical corticosteroid abuse on face: a clinical study of 100 patients. Int J Res Dermatol. 2016;2:40–5.
3. Jha AK, Sinha R, Prasad S. Misuse of topical corticosteroids on the face: a cross-sectional study among dermatology outpatients. Indian Dermatol Online J. 2016;7:259–63.
4. Ambika H, Sujatha VC, Yadalla H, et al. Topical corticosteroid abuse on the face: a prospective study on outpatients of dermatology. Our Dermatol Online. 2014;5(1):5–8.
5. Ghosh A, Sengupta S, Coondoo A, Jana A. Topical corticosteroid addiction and phobia. Indian J Dermatol. 2014;59:465–8.
6. Agarwal M, Roy V. Fairness creams in the Indian market: Issues to be resolved. Indian J Clin Pract. 2012;22:45–8. [Last accessed on 2016, October 5].
7. Durairaj L. The Indian whitening cream market is expanding at a rate of nearly 18% a year. Available from http://www.theweekendleader.com/cheers/1249/scare-and-sell.html [Last accessed 2016, Oct 5].
8. Majid I. Mometasone-based triple combination therapy in meliasma. Is it really safe? Indian J Dermatol. 2010;55:359–62.
9. Kumar S, Goyal A, Gupta YK. Abuse of topical corticosteroids in India: Concerns and the way forward. J Pharmacol Pharmacother. 2016;7:1–5.
10. Debroy S. Drug company faces heat over fairness cream. Available from http://timesofindia.indiatimes.com/city/mumbai/Drug-company-faces-heat-over-fairness-cream/articleshow/48644671.cms [Last accessed 2016, Oct 5].

Topical Corticosteroid Use and Misuse: Global Scenario and Role of International Topical Steroid Addiction Network (ITSAN)

34

Nidhi R. Sharma, JoAnne VanDyke, and Kathryn Z. Tullos

Abstract

Since their introduction, topical corticosteroids (TCs) have become a mainstay in treatment of many inflammatory and autoimmune conditions. Their clinical effects are mediated by anti-inflammatory, vasoconstrictive, antiproliferative, and immunosuppressive properties. These effects can also lead to multiple side effects if used non-judiciously.

Worldwide, their use for many non-approved indications by dermatologists, physicians, and non-registered practitioners has raised a great concern. They are advised inappropriately for skin conditions like acne, bacterial or fungal infections, and undiagnosed skin rash and especially as a fairness cream. They are available as fixed dose combination (FDC) in combination with antibacterial and antifungal agents to be used as a multipurpose cream. A number of studies have been published on this issue and related to the side effects. Globally many organizations and associations have come up against this sensitive issue.

Keywords

Topical corticosteroids misuse • Global scenario • Fixed drug combinations • International Topical Steroid Addiction Network

N.R. Sharma (✉)
Department of Dermatology, Venereology and Leprosy, Shaheed Hasan Khan Mewati Government Medical College, Nuh, Haryana, India
e-mail: drnidhirsharma@gmail.com

J. VanDyke • K.Z. Tullos
ITSAN, Palm Beach Gardens, FL 33410, USA
e-mail: jvandyke@itsan.org; ktullos@itsan.org

Learning Points

1. Topical corticosteroids used as FDC with antibacterial and antifungal agents are a major problem to this issue.
2. It has not only remained a clinical problem but has emerged as a social problem.

© Springer Nature Singapore Pte Ltd. 2018
K. Lahiri (ed.), *A Treatise on Topical Corticosteroids in Dermatology*,
DOI 10.1007/978-981-10-4609-4_34

3. We as dermatologists have to take the lead and make aware physicians, non-physicians, and general population regarding their proper use, misuse, and side effects and not allowing steroid phobia to set in which again can cause undertreatment of dermatosis.

34.1 Introduction

Topical corticosteroids (TCs) were first introduced by Sulzberger and Witten in 1952 [1]. It was marked as a significant milestone in dermatological therapy because of their prompt anti-inflammatory action, thus giving quick results in various dermatoses [2].

Compound F (hydrocortisone) was the first to be introduced. With modifications in this basic structure, other topical corticosteroid molecules were developed [1]. Different topical steroids have different potency ranging from mild to very potent topical steroids. Different potency of TCs is advised in different responsive dermatosis considering the first and foremost age of the patient, severity of the disease, and anatomic area of application along with duration of the treatment [3].

TCs are considered as double-edged weapon; if they are used judiciously, they do wonders, but if they are misused or abused, they can lead to a number of local, systemic, and psychological side effects [4, 5].

The use of TC has become ubiquitous with dermatologists and other non-dermatologists which has raised concerns regarding its misuse for non-labeled indications.

34.2 Global Scenario of TC Misuse

TCs are misused at various levels starting from pharmaceutical companies by making irrational fixed drug combinations, then the doctors or quacks prescribing wrong potency TCs for a wrong period of time, and then by the patients or chemists where they use or advise without proper guidance [6]. It has not remained a clinical problem but has become a major social problem.

In India, the annual sales figure of TCs was 14 billion rupees in 2013, which accounts for almost 82% of total dermatological product sale in the country [7]. There are a number of fixed drug combinations with steroids which are used rampantly by dermatologists and other nonqualified personnel [8, 9]. They have further led to resistance problems in the various infective dermatoses and irreversible side effects in others [10, 11]. Most of these combinations are irrational and nonscientific.

Incidentally, in India two of such irrational FDC of corticosteroids, antibacterial and antifungal agents, were the top selling formulations of TCs in 2013 [7]. However, such FDCs are uncommon in USA or other western countries and are neither provided without a presciption [12].

Worldwide across the pharmacies, hundreds of branded generic versions of FDCs of TCs are available as over-the-counter (OTC) drugs. This is well understood by the case reports and various studies published in the literature.

In 2014, Hajar et al. did a systematic review on topical corticosteroids withdrawal ("topical corticosteroids addiction") taking into consideration 34 studies related to topical steroids abuse leading to its addiction [13]. They concluded that TC withdrawal was reported mostly on the face and genital area (99.3%) of women (81.0%) mainly using potent TCs inappropriately for a long term. Majority of these patients (65.5%) had symptoms of burning and stinging, while erythema was the most common sign seen in 92.3% of patients. Furthermore, TC withdrawal can be broadly classified as papulopustular and erythemoedematous.

We have taken account of few of the studies related to TC withdrawal. These studies give us the insight into how the TCs have been used and misused worldwide. We will discuss them in a table shown below (Table 34.1).

A number of studies on this issue have been published from India which are discussed in the

Table 34.1 Data depicting studies conducted on topical corticosteroids misuse or abuse and their side effects

Year	Country	Sample size	Findings/conclusion	Type of study	Reference
1969	England	14 cases	The fluorinated topical steroids should not be used in the treatment of rosacea, though the less potent hydrocortisone preparations appear harmless	Case series	[14]
1969	England	1 case	TCS may worsen the condition of Rosacea, but at times, it may be the cause of it	Case report	[15]
1972	Germany	8 cases	Rosacea-like dermatitis is to be regarded as a result of intolerance reaction of seborrhoeic skin to topically applied strong corticosteroids, such as betamethasone valerate and fluocinolone acetonide	Case series	[16]
1974	Philadelphia	10 cases	Regular use of topically applied fluorinated steroids produced a distinctive eruption consisting of persistent erythema, telangiectasia, atrophy, and occasional papules and pustules	Case series	[17]
1974	San Francisco	1 case	Prolonged use of potent TCs on the face can lead to long-term and disfiguring side effects	Case report	[18]
1976	Philadelphia	3 cases	Long-term application of fluorinated steroids to the face produces persistent disorders such as rosacea-like syndromes and acne. The genitalia are another off-limits area for dispensation of potent steroids	Case series	[19]
1976	Japan	25 cases	Hydrocortisone 17-butyrate was more useful as a topical medication than hydrocortisone acetate but gave rise to withdrawal rebound eruptions in some cases. And about 1 year was required to recover from atrophy and telangiectasias	Case series	[20]
1979	United Kingdom	259 cases	Out of 259 patients, all but nine of the patients acknowledged the use of potent TCs over long periods; in many cases, these were self-administered	Cross-sectional study	[21]
1979	United States	4 cases	Fluorinated gluco-corticosteroids should not be used on the face of infants and children	Case series	[22]
1991	Taiwan	23 cases	The diminution in stratum corneum lipids and pro-fillagrin and fillagrin in steroid-treated skin may play an important role in the clinical manifestations of scaling and dryness of the skin in patients suffering from the rebound phenomenon after stopping TCs	Case series	[23]
1999 Rapaport	California and Pennsylvania	100 cases	Complete stoppage is the only treatment of topical corticosteroid addiction. No additional treatment is required once the complete remission has been obtained after TC abuse	Case series	[24]
1999 Rapaport	California and Pennsylvania	12 cases	TC preparations when used postoperatively in patients experiencing peeling and resurfacing can cause prolonged erythema, dermatitis, burning, and telangiectasias, due to vasoconstriction/vasodilatation secondary to the corticosteroids through a non-intact barrier	Case series	[25]
2006	India	5 cases	The development of steroid dermatitis due to self-use of local steroid as cosmetic cream is frequent, and this is not only merely a medical problem but also a social problem	Case series	[26]

(continued)

Table 34.1 (continued)

Year	Country	Sample size	Findings/conclusion	Type of study	Reference
2006	South Africa	66 TCs selling vendors	There is extensive sale of illegal and unregistered topical corticosteroid creams on the KwaZulu-Natal street markets. Furthermore, these products are being stored incorrectly leading to a decrease in the active ingredient and emergence of a degradation product	Cross-sectional study	[27]
2006	Iraq	1780 cases	140 (7.9%) had misused topical corticosteroids. The main burden of responsibility for the misuse of topical corticosteroids was put on paramedical personnel and the patient (plus friends or family)	Cross-sectional study	[28]
2011	India	200 cases	Majority of patients were using potent (class II) topical steroids for trivial facial dermatoses. The common adverse effects were erythema, telangiectasia, xerosis, hyperpigmentation, photosensitivity, and rebound phenomenon	Cross-sectional study	[29]

previous chapters pertaining to Indian Scenario of TC abuse. A prospective, multicentric study from India concluded that in patients with TC abuse, facial dermatosis was very common and TCs are mainly abused as a fairness cream [30].

There are many single case reports on varied side effects of TC misuse depicting various side effects of them.

Cushing syndrome and adrenocortical insufficiency have been reported in literature with long-term use of potent TCs [31, 32]. Prolonged application of topical steroids transiently suppresses the hypothalamic-pituitary-adrenal axis (HPA) leading to generalized infections and hepatosteatosis. Therefore, less potent steroids should be prescribed in infancy, and the adverse effects should be known to physicians and the parents. There has been another side to this issue, that people have developed phobias to TC treatment which has led to non-adherence and treatment failure in conditions like atopic dermatitis, where TCs are still the gold standard for treatment [33].

In China, 999 abuse—a misuse of topical cream called "999" containing dexamethasone acetate—has been reported. Parents were unaware of the potential contents of this topical and over used it in children, wherein one patient resulted in necrotizing fasciitis due to inappropriate use on ulcer [34].

A literature from China showed that the uncontrolled use of topical steroids over the face has led to various symptoms like dermatitis, acne rosacea, angiotelectasia, and dermotrophia/hyperpigmentation constitutively termed as facial corticosteroid addictive dermatitis (FCAD) [35].

Furthermore, neuropsychiatric manifestations have been reported due to misuse of clobetasol propionate [36].

34.3 About ITSAN and Various Organizations Against TC Misuse

Globally, a number of organizations have come up to tackle this sensitive issue of TC misuse and abuse.

From India, the IADVL Task Force Against Topical Steroid Abuse (ITATSA) has come up strongly against this problem [37]. ITATSA is a special task force created by the Indian Association of Dermatologists, Venereologists and Leprologists (IADVL) to look into issues related to TC abuse. It has raised the issue of TC misuse at various fronts including physicians, manufactures, pharmaceutical companies, and regulators.

There are few more associations working on it like National Eczema Association [38], Eczema

Association of UK [39], Eczema Association of New Zealand [40], and Eczema Association of Australasia [41].

A very promising and effective network has been formed internationally against this issue, named as International Topical Steroid Addiction Network (ITSAN) [42]. We will be learning about ITSAN in detail.

34.3.1 Brief Profile of ITSAN

The International Topical Steroid Addiction Network (ITSAN) is a nonprofit charity based in the United States and formed to raise awareness about a condition called Red Skin Syndrome (RSS), also known as Topical Steroid Addiction or Topical Steroid Withdrawal Syndrome.

In July 2009, Red Skin Syndrome sufferer Kelly Palace created the website "AddictedSkin. com" based on her own topical steroid withdrawal experience. The website featured her story with photos, as well as peer-reviewed, scholarly journal articles about topical steroid addiction and withdrawal. This website quickly evolved into an online support community.

In January 2012, Palace changed AddictedSkin. com to ITSAN.org and filed for nonprofit charity status with her former dermatologist, Dr. Marvin Rapaport, as cofounder. The International Topical Steroid Addiction Network was granted 501 c 3 nonprofit status in the United States on February 3, 2012. Dr. Rapaport left ITSAN in June 2013, and Palace continued as ITSAN president until January 2015. JoAnne VanDyke then took over as the current president of ITSAN, joined by a volunteer board of directors.

ITSAN Red Skin Syndrome Support has since expanded into a vast network of RSS sufferers from all over the world, communicating in the online forum and Facebook groups, as well as corresponding via email. ITSAN also holds patient conferences where caregivers, sufferers, and family members meet together to gain support in person.

ITSAN board members volunteer many hours creating educational materials, networking with healthcare providers, connecting with fellow patient advocacy organizations, traveling to conferences, and offering support to members suffering from Red Skin Syndrome.

34.3.2 Mission of This Network

The mission of ITSAN is to raise awareness of Red Skin Syndrome and support all affected individuals. From the sufferer to the caregiver to family members, ITSAN provides scholarly information, resources, support, and a safe place to share experiences.

The short-term goal of ITSAN is recognition of Red Skin Syndrome within the medical community. Members of ITSAN support groups report having difficulty getting a diagnosis—either due to their doctors being completely unaware of the diagnosis of Red Skin Syndrome or due their doctors being resistant to acknowledging this diagnosis. Many doctors simply do not believe that topical steroids could have caused such a severe, protracted issue.

The long-term goals of ITSAN are prevention, early detection, accurate diagnosis, and proper treatment of RSS. Many of our members report having been misdiagnosed for years prior to diagnosis of Red Skin Syndrome and therefore not receiving appropriate or timely care. Other members report that they hadn't been taught by their physicians how to use topical steroids according to guidelines or were instructed to use "off label" despite warning labels. Patients should be educated about the risks associated with topical steroid therapy and the warning signs of RSS. If the physician is aware of the potential for Red Skin Syndrome, they will be better able to prevent it by educating and monitoring their patients.

34.3.3 Associations of ITSAN

ITSAN has been a Member in Good Standing of the Coalition of Skin Diseases (CSD) since 2014. The CSD works closely with the American Academy of Dermatology (AAD) to advocate for patients with skin diseases. For more about this partnership, please see the Patient Advocate

Resource Center on the AAD website (https://www.aad.org/about/affiliate/patient_advocates) or visit the CSD website (http://coalitionofskindiseases.org/).

Though ITSAN is based in the USA, ITSAN. org serves an international population as an informational resource for the individual, the caregiver, and the healthcare provider. Our volunteer board of directors have all had direct experience with Red Skin Syndrome either personally, as a caregiver, or with a member of their family. They want to raise awareness so that this condition can be prevented altogether or diagnosed as soon as possible. ITSAN board of directors come from varying backgrounds—including medical and nonmedical professions—but share this in common: (1) a sincere desire to prevent the devastating effects of this iatrogenic condition from happening to others and (2) a commitment to supporting those already suffering with RSS.

Currently, there are over 3700 members in the ITSAN forum and approximately 2300 in the ITSAN Red Skin Syndrome Support Facebook group. ITSAN also keeps in contact with its members via email and has nearly 3000 subscribers to its newsletter.

For information about members of the ITSAN board, please visit http://itsan.org/about-itsan/. ITSAN provides information first and foremost. ITSAN.org was created to help topical steroid users, as well as medical professionals, recognize what topical steroid addiction is, what it looks and feels like, and how to treat it.

Each tab on ITSAN.org is meant to be used as a tool to open up dialogue between the patient and doctor. None of the information is meant to take the place of a physician or medical advice.

The "What is RSS tab" is a high-level, brief overview of Red Skin Syndrome for the layperson to learn quickly and basically what RSS is, what causes it, common symptoms, and what can help treat the condition. There are links to definitions, answers to questions, explanations of symptoms, and pictures to help anyone who lands on the site gain a better understanding and a basic knowledge of RSS.

For those who may be unsure of what topical steroids are and what they do, the "Topical Steroids 101" tab serves to educate and inform. Some people are unaware that the over-the-counter or prescription creams they are using are actually steroid-containing creams. Steroid addiction is much less likely if people are aware of what they are applying to their skin and understand the basics, such as potency, absorption rates on different parts of the body, use of occlusion, and so forth.

The core of treatment is ceasing topical steroid therapy, which causes a lengthy, uncomfortable withdrawal phase. But there are many options to treat the symptoms of RSS during the extended withdrawal period. Some of these options are medical interventions. Some of these are comfort measures, shared from one member to another, under the "Coping with RSS" tab.

The "Resources" tab on ITSAN.org provides relevant journal articles, videos, a symptom checklist, an informational brochure, and a member survey to evaluate corticosteroid exposure as it relates to the withdrawal/recovery process. The data collected from the survey is being compiled and reviewed for presentation at the 2017 Annual American Academy of Dermatology conference. These are all tools to assist the patient, caregiver, and physician in recognizing this condition.

The "Stories and Photos" tab gives a snapshot of what RSS physically looks like, as well as what recovery looks like, and approximately how long recovery takes. These are all member-reported testimonies and are not case studies, per se.

ITSAN moderates the ITSAN forum and Facebook support group to ensure it is a safe, healing space for all members. Members can share tips, vent frustrations, and provide support for one another. ITSAN shares new information from publications as they become available, but does not medically advise. ITSAN encourages members to be under a doctor's care.

34.3.4 ITSAN Newsletter

ITSAN has sent out newsletters since its founding in 2012. As of January 2017, there are nearly 3000 subscribers to the ITSAN newsletter. The newsletters communicate how ITSAN is advocating for Red Skin Syndrome awareness, understanding, and legitimacy, as well as how members can help ITSAN with its mission. The newsletters update members about ITSAN board members attending conferences such as the American Academy of Dermatology's Annual Meeting, Coalition of Skin Diseases Annual Meeting, American Academy of Dermatology Association's Legislative Conference in Washington, D.C., etc. In addition, the newsletters provide information about supportive doctors, relevant journal articles, recovery stories, and ITSAN fundraisers.

ITSAN is largely a volunteer run network, so we invite anyone who would like to volunteer their time, skills, or services to contact us via email at info@itsan.org for more information.

As with any nonprofit charity, making a donation is a wonderful way to contribute to ITSAN. Our volunteer board uses funds to pay for the incidentals of running a nonprofit, travel and lodging to attend conferences, membership dues to professional organizations, website upkeep, bookkeeping, contract work, and printed materials. Much can be done by volunteers, but financial backing is also necessary to continue this work.

The most important way to contribute to ITSAN is to simply share the expert articles and information found on ITSAN.org to educate doctors, patients, and caregivers about Red Skin Syndrome. Raising awareness takes time and dedication, but is accomplished by everyone working together.

References

1. Sulzberger MB, Witten VH. The effect of topically applied compound F in selected dermatoses. J Invest Dermatol. 1952;19(2):101–2.
2. Lagos BR, Maibach HI. Topical corticosteroids: unapproved uses, dosages, or indications. Clin Dermatol. 2002;20:490–2.
3. Stoughton RB. Vasoconstrictor activity and percutaneous absorption of glucocorticosteroids. A direct comparison. Arch Dermatol. 1969;99(6):753.
4. Wolverton SE. Topical corticosteroids. In: Comprehensive dermatologic drug therapy. 2nd ed. Philadelphia, PA: Saunders Elsevier; 2007. p. 595–624.
5. Hengge UR, Ruzicka T, Schwartz RA, Cork MJ. Adverse effects of topical glucocorticosteroids. J Am Acad Dermatol. 2006;54:1–15.
6. Coondoo A. Topical corticosteroid misuse: the Indian scenario. Indian J Dermatol. 2014;59(5):451–5.
7. Verma SB. Sales, status, prescriptions and regulatory problems with topical steroids in India. Indian J Dermatol Venereol Leprol. 2014;80(3):201.
8. Rathod SS, Motghare VM, Deshmukh VS, Deshpande RP, Bhamare CG, Patil JR. Prescribing practices of topical corticosteroids in the outpatient dermatology department of a rural tertiary care teaching hospital. Indian J Dermatol. 2013;58:342–5.
9. Jha AK, Sinha R, Prasad S. Misuse of topical corticosteroids on the face: a cross-sectional study among dermatology outpatients. Indian Dermatol Online J. 2016;7(4):259–63.
10. Coondoo A, Phiske M, Verma S, Lahiri K. Side-effects of topical steroids: a long overdue revisit. Indian Dermatol Online J. 2014;5:416–25.
11. Fisher DA. Adverse effects of topical corticosteroid use. West J Med. 1995;162:123–6.
12. Monthly Index of Medical Specialities—Online version, USA. Available from: https://www.mims.com/USA/home/Index. [Last accessed on Dec 2016].
13. Hajar T, Leshem YA, Hanifin JM, et al. A systematic review of topical corticosteroid withdrawal ("steroid addiction") in patients with atopic dermatitis and other dermatoses. J Am Acad Dermatol. 2015;72(3):541–9.
14. Sneddon I. Adverse effect of topical fluorinated corticosteroids in rosacea. Br Med J. 1969;1:671–3.
15. Sneddon I. Iatrogenic dermatitis. Br Med J. 1969;4:49.
16. Weber G. Rosacea-like dermatitis: contraindication or intolerance reaction to strong steroids. Br J Dermatol. 1972;86:253–9.
17. Leyden JJ, Thew M, Kligman AM. Steroid rosacea. Arch Dermatol. 1974;110:619–22.
18. Stegman SJ. Pustular dermatosis on withdrawal of topically applied steroids [letter]. Arch Dermatol. 1974;109:100.
19. Kligman AM. Topical steroid addicts [letter]. J Am Med Assoc. 1976;235:1550.
20. Urabe H, Koda H. Perioral dermatitis and rosacea like dermatitis: clinical features and treatment. Dermatologica. 1976;152(1):155–60.
21. Wilkinson DS, Kirton V, Wilkinson JD. Perioral dermatitis: a 12-year review. Br J Dermatol. 1979;101:245–57.
22. Franco HL, Weston WL. Steroid rosacea in children. Pediatrics. 1979;64:36–8.
23. Sheu HM, Chang CH. Alterations in water content of the stratum corneum following long-term topical corticosteroids. J Formos Med Assoc. 1991;90:664–9.
24. Rapaport MJ, Rapaport V. Eyelid dermatitis to red face syndrome to cure: clinical experience in 100 cases. J Am Acad Dermatol. 1999;41:435–42.
25. Rapaport MJ, Rapaport V. Prolonged erythema after facial laser resurfacing or phenol peel secondary to corticosteroid addiction. Dermatol Surg. 1999;25:781–5.

26. Rathi S. Abuse of topical steroid as cosmetic cream: a social background of steroid dermatitis. Indian J Dermatol. 2006;51:154–5.

27. Lutchman D, Naidoo P. Ilegal topical corticosteroids in KwaZulu-Natal-abuse continues. S Afr Med J. 2006;96(4):284–6.

28. Dhalimi MA, Aljawahiry N. Misuse of topical corticosteroids: a clinical study in an Iraqi hospital. East Mediterr Health J. 2006;12(6):847–52.

29. Bhat YJ, Manzoor S, Qayoom S. Steroid-induced rosacea: a clinical study of 200 patients. Indian J Dermatol. 2011;56(1):30–2.

30. Saraswat A, Lahiri K, Chatterjee M, Barua S, Coondoo A, Mittal A, et al. Topical corticosteroid abuse on the face: a prospective, multicenter study of dermatology outpatients. Indian J Dermatol Venereol Leprol. 2011;77:160–6.

31. Güven A, Gülümser O, Ozgen T. Cushing's syndrome and adrenocortical insufficiency caused by topical steroids: misuse or abuse? J Pediatr Endocrinol Metab. 2007;20(11):1173–82.

32. Tempark T, Phatarakijnirund V, et al. Exogenous Cushing's syndrome due to topical corticosteroid application: case report and review literature. Endocrine. 2010;38(3):328–34.

33. Gustavsen HE, Gjersvik P. Topical corticosteroid phobia among parents of children with atopic dermatitis in a semirural area of Norway. J Eur Acad Dermatol Venereol. 2016;30(1):168.

34. Hon KL, Burd A. 999 abuse: do mothers know what they are using? J Dermatolog Treat. 2008;19(4):241–5.

35. Lu H, Xiao T, et al. Facial corticosteroid addictive dermatitis in Guiyang City, China. Clin Exp Dermatol. 2010;35(6):618–21.

36. Lawrence M, Claire P, et al. Misuse of clobetasol propionate and neuropsychiatric manifestations. Therapy. 2013;68(3):179–81.

37. Petitioning the Drug Controller of India-Stop indiscriminate OTC sale of topical steroid without prescription, most are Schedule H drugs. Available from: http://www.change.org/p.

38. https://nationaleczema.org/education-announcement-topical-corticosteroids-eczema.

39. http://www.eczema.org.

40. http://eczema.org.nz.

41. http://www.eaaci.org.

42. http://itsan.org.

Topical Corticosteroid Awareness Among General Population and Dermatology Outpatients

35

T.S. Nagesh

Abstract

Topical steroids are one of the most commonly abused drugs. There are few studies available which have highlighted the severity of this problem in India. However, these studies have concentrated mainly on the topical steroid abuse and its side effects over the face.

In this chapter we have tried to highlight about the awareness among the people about various commonly available topical steroids and its combinations irrespective of its usage and also the extent of misuse of these drugs. Along with this we also tried to find the source of recommendation of these medicines which will help to sensitize people about this menace.

Conclusion: Misuse of topical steroids as a general purpose skin cream or fairness cream is common not just over the face, but also on other parts of the body. It is most often recommended by general practitioners or pharmacists. Hence it is important to sensitize these people about the possible complications of these drugs and the extent of problem the society is facing because of irrational and unregulated use of these drugs.

Keywords

Awareness • Topical steroid abuse

Learning Points
1. Awareness about topical steroids is poor in general population.
2. It is important to sensitize general practitioners and pharmacists regarding the uses and misuse of topical steroids.

T.S. Nagesh
Department of Dermatology, Venereology and Leprosy, Sapthagiri Institute of Medical Sciences and Research Center, Bangalore, India
e-mail: drnageshts@gmail.com

35.1   Introduction

Topical steroids are commonly used drugs in dermatology. They are used for various indications like psoriasis, lichen planus, eczema, lichen simplex chronicus, and other steroid-responsive dermatoses. However, because of their property of lightening of skin and reducing inflammation, they have been misused frequently. Acne, pigmentation, fungal infection, and pruritus are the common conditions for which topical steroids are misused, and also they have been used as a cosmetic or a skin cream for any type of rash. The free availability of these creams as an over the counter medication is one of the main reason for such misuse in our country. Also availability of various irrational combinations of topical steroids which cause more damage to the skin adds to the existing menace. There is a lack of awareness among general practitioners who regularly prescribe these creams as general skin creams for conditions varying from tinea to acne and as fairness creams. Various studies have tried to highlight the side effects and harm caused by misuse of topical steroids and its combinations. These studies have tried to bring to the notice of regulatory authorities about the damage caused by free availability of these creams. In this chapter we will try to discuss regarding the awareness among patients about these drugs and its side effects.

35.2   Awareness About Topical Steroids

In 1952, Sulzberger and Witten were the first to use topical steroids in dermatology [1]. Followed by this, topical steroids of different potencies and formulations were introduced which revolutionized the treatment of various steroid-responsive dermatoses. The availability of topical steroids has immensely contributed to the dermatologist's ability to effectively treat several difficult dermatoses [2]. They became popular rapidly and were considered as a panacea for all ills by both physicians and patients [3]. Topical steroids are one of the most commonly used drugs by dermatologists worldwide [4–6]. In India, the annual sales

figure of TCs was 14 billion rupees in 2013, which accounts for almost 82% of total dermatological product sale in the country [7].

The misuse and abuse of these drugs by both non-dermatologists and patients is mainly because of the immediate and dramatic symptomatic relief from these creams. They are also used as fairness or cosmetic creams [8, 9]. Various side effects, both cutaneous and systemic, have been noticed because of the rampant misuse and abuse of these medicines [9–12].

Various studies have tried to highlight the menace caused by the use of topical steroids [13–17]. A multicentric study by Saraswat et al. has taken 2296 patients with facial dermatoses of which 433 patients were using topical steroids [13]. These studies have highlighted the various side effects encountered by the patients who were using topical steroid, and the patients who already had developed the side effects were included. Most of the patients in the study were not aware if the side effects they developed were because of the creams they had used.

We conducted a study to check for the awareness among people about the use of topical steroids [18]. Our study includes 1000 patients attending the dermatology outpatient department irrespective of their skin complaints. This was a questionnaire-based study to find out their awareness about the common topical steroid available over the counter in our area. The source of recommendation/knowledge about these creams, usage duration, and their awareness about the side effects of these creams were also assessed.

In our study, 809 patients (80.9%) had heard of at least one of the topical steroid or its combinations and 612 (61.2%) patients had used one of the steroid or steroid combination. The duration of usage varied from1 day to 10 years. Acne, fairness (as cosmetic), pigmentation, and allergy were the common indications for which these creams were applied. Also many of the patients thought these creams were general-purpose skin creams and fairness creams. Similar findings were seen in other studies [13–17].

In our study, doctors had prescribed this cream in 302 (49.5%) patients. This finding was almost similar to the study by Saraswat et al. where 41% of the patients had received the recommendation from a doctor [13]. General practitioners and doctors from alternative medicine had prescribed these medicines in most of the patients. This again shows the lack of awareness about topical steroids and its side effects among non-dermatologists and general practitioners.

Pharmacists, friends, and relatives had recommended these creams in 301 (49%) patients, which shows the lack of implementation of regulations in the sale of these creams though it comes under schedule H category [6]. General practitioners and pharmacists are often the first point of contact for most of the patients. Topical steroid abuse and its side effects can be reduced by training and creating awareness among general practitioners and pharmacists.

Acne, pigmentation, redness, itching, burning sensation, striae, and aggravation of existing skin problem were the common side effects noticed in our study. The duration of use of topical steroid correlated with the nature of side effect. However many of our patients were not aware of the fact that the problems they were facing were due to the long-term use of steroids.

A study done by Kim et al. to assess the awareness, knowledge, and behavior of topical steroid use in dermatological outpatients has shown that 53.8% bought topical steroids with a dermatologist's prescription, whereas 33.6% obtained their topical steroids without prescription [19]. Also almost 20% of the patients were applying topical steroids more than 5 times a day and for more than 16 weeks. They concluded by mentioning that topical steroids have been used without sufficient information and guidelines. Also they suggest that dermatologists should more thoroughly explain the therapeutic effects, indications, and side effects of topical steroids to their patients [19].

Conclusion

Awareness about topical steroid and its side effects is very less in our population. There is a rampant abuse of topical steroid cream for fairness and acne and as a general-purpose skin cream. The various reasons for such misuse/abuse include wrong prescription, dubious marketing by pharmaceutical companies, free availability of these medicines as OTC drugs, and lack of regulations regarding the manufacturing of irrational combinations. It is very important to create awareness among general practitioners and pharmacists about the possible complications of these drugs and the extent of problem the society is facing because of irrational and unregulated use of these drugs as they are recommending these products in majority of cases. Even the dermatologists should clearly explain to the patients about dose, duration, and the importance of using the topical steroids properly. Meanwhile we should also need to take care not to create a steroid phobia among the patients as topical steroids are one of the main drugs in dermatologist's armamentarium to treat various steroid-responsive dermatoses.

References

1. Sulzberger MB, Witten VH. The effect of topically applied compound F in selected dermatoses. J Invest Dermatol. 1952;19:101–2.
2. Rathi SK, D'Souza P. Rational and ethical use of topical corticosteroids based on safety and efficacy. Indian J Dermatol. 2012;57(4):251.
3. Coondoo A. Topical corticosteroid misuse: the Indian scenario. Indian J Dermatol. 2014;59(5):451.
4. Stern R. The pattern of topical corticosteroid prescribing in the United States 1989–1991. J Am Acad Dermatol. 1996;35:183–96.
5. Kumar AM, Noushad PP, Shailaja K, Jayasutha J, Ramasamy C. A study on drug prescribing pattern and use of corticosteroids in dermatological conditions at tertiary care teaching hospital. Int J Pharm Sci Rev Res. 2011;9:132–5.
6. Kumar S, Goyal A, Gupta YK. Abuse of topical corticosteroids in India: concerns and the way forward. J Pharmacol Pharmacother. 2016;7(1):1.
7. Verma SB. Sales, status, prescriptions and regulatory problems with topical steroids in India. Indian J Dermatol Venereol Leprol. 2014;80:201–3.
8. Nnoruka E, Okoye O. Topical steroid abuse: its use as a depigmenting agent. J Natl Med Assoc. 2006; 98(6):934.
9. Rathi S. Abuse of topical steroid as cosmetic cream: a social background of steroid dermatitis. Indian J Dermatol. 2006;51:154–5.
10. Hengge UR, Ruzicka T, Schwartz RA, Cork MJ. Adverse effects of topical glucocorticosteroids. J Am Acad Dermatol. 2006;54:1–18.

11. Dhar S, Seth J, Parikh D. Systemic side-effects of topical corticosteroids. Indian J Dermatol. 2014;59(5): 460.

12. Coondoo A, Phiske M, Verma S, Lahiri K. Side-effects of topical steroids: a long overdue revisit. Indian Dermatol Online J. 2014;5(4):416.

13. Saraswat A, Lahiri K, Chatterjee M, Barua S, Coondoo A, Mittal A, et al. Topical corticosteroid abuse on the face: a prospective, multicenter study of dermatology outpatients. Indian J Dermatol Venereol Leprol. 2011;77:160–6.

14. Dey VK. Misuse of topical corticosteroids: a clinical study of adverse effects. Indian Dermatol Online J. 2014;5(4):436.

15. Ambika H, Vinod CS, Yadalla H, Nithya R, Babu AR. Topical corticosteroid abuse on the face: a prospective, study on outpatients of dermatology. Our Dermatol Online. 2014;5:5–8.

16. Kumar A, Neupane S, Shrestha PR, Pun J, Thapa P, Manandhar M, et al. Pattern and predictors of topical corticosteroid abuse on face: a study from Western Nepal. Res J Pharm Biol Chem Sci. 2015;6(3):1154–9.

17. Al-Dhalimi MA, Aljawahiri N. Misuse of topical corticosteroids: a clinical study from an Iraqi hospital. East Mediterr Health J. 2006;12:847–52.

18. Nagesh TS, Akhilesh A. Topical steroid awareness and abuse: a prospective study among dermatology outpatients. Indian J Dermatol. 2016;61:618–21.

19. Kim SY, Lee SD, Kim HO, Park YM. A survey of the awareness, knowledge, and behavior of topical steroid use in dermatologic outpatients of the university hospital. Kor J Dermatol. 2008;46(4):473–9.

A Pictorial Album on Topical Corticosteroid Abuse

36

Abir Saraswat

Abstract

This is a representative collection of photographs that show the adverse effects of topical corticosteroids.

Most if not all occurred due to egregious misuse or overuse.

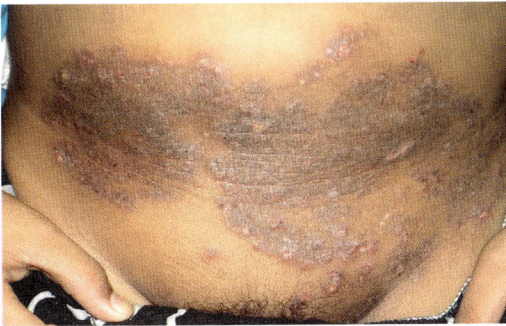

Majocchi's granuloma of the lower abdomen. The patient had applied clobetasol-salicylic acid cream for 6 months on the area

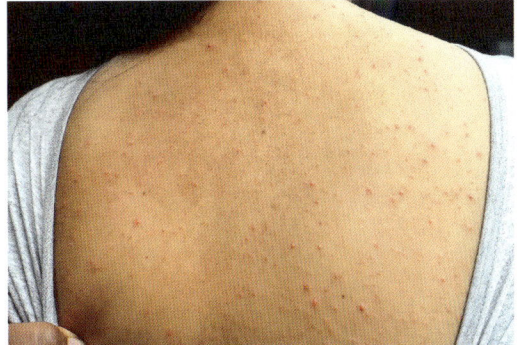

Malassezia folliculitis on a 40-year-old woman's back. She had applied mometasone cream on her back for 1 year to make it fairer

A. Saraswat
Indushree Skin Clinic, Indiranagar, Lucknow, India
e-mail: abirsaraswat@yahoo.com

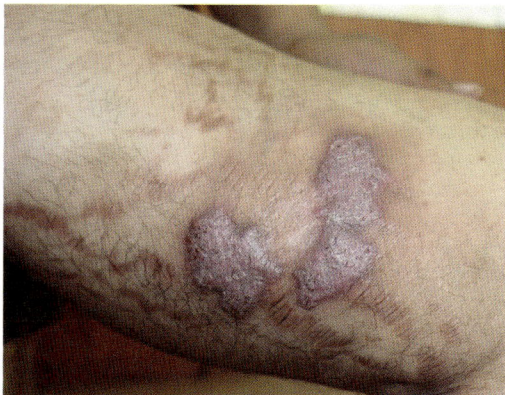

Lupus vulgaris with surrounding striae on the arm of a 26-year-old man. He had applied a clobetasol-ornidazole--ofloxacin-terbinafine combination cream for 2 years on the prescription of a general practitioner

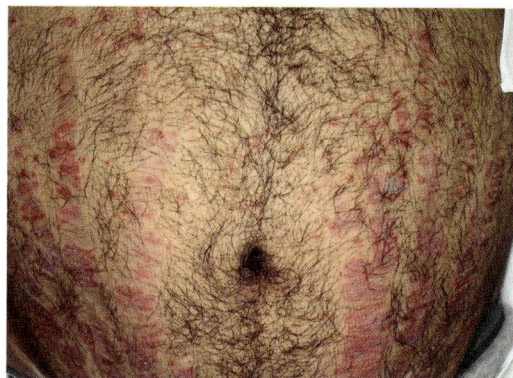

A patient with psoriasis Koebnerizing onto broad topical steroid-induced striae

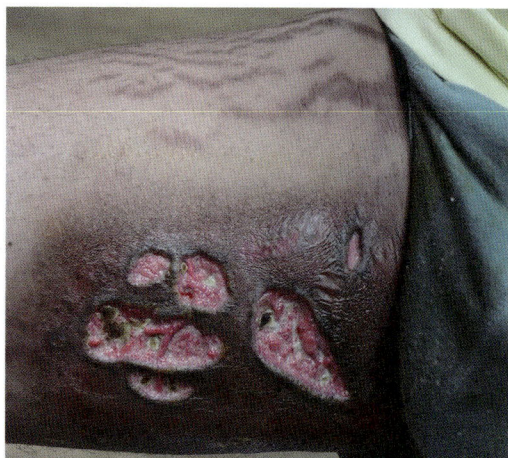

Deep ulcers on the striae on the thighs of a 30-year-old pharmacist. He was self-treating his tinea with clobetasol-gentamicin-miconazole combination cream, occluded with a sanitary napkin. When the striae broke down, he applied more of the same cream on them under occlusion

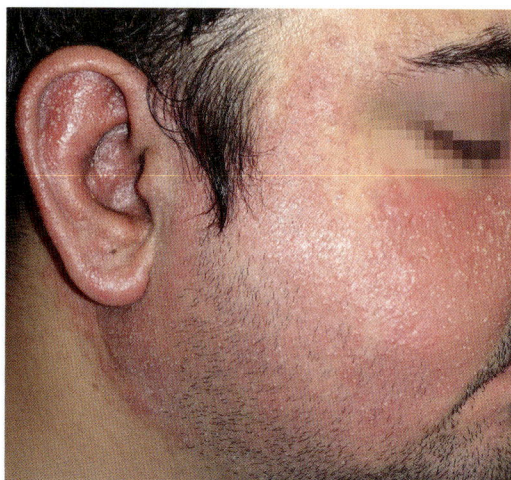

Tinea faciei superimposed on steroid rosacea. This man was applying a clobetasol-salicylic acid cream on the face for more than 2 years to become fairer. Note the classical edge of the lesion in the retro-auricular area

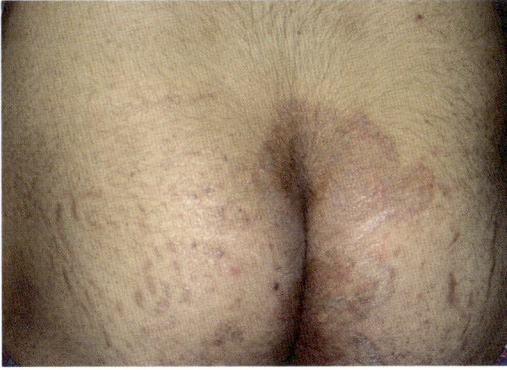

Tinea surrounded by topical steroid-induced striae

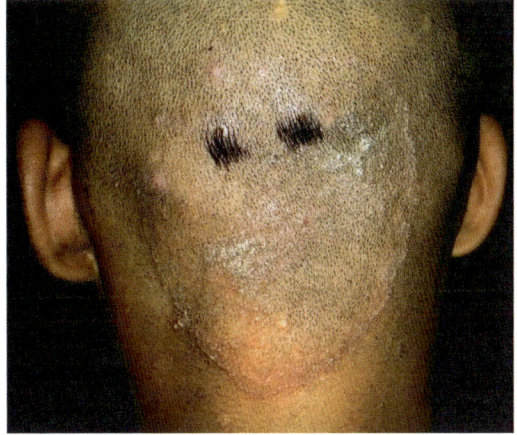

Tinea corporis of the scalp. Clobetasol-miconazole--gentamicin used for 4 months

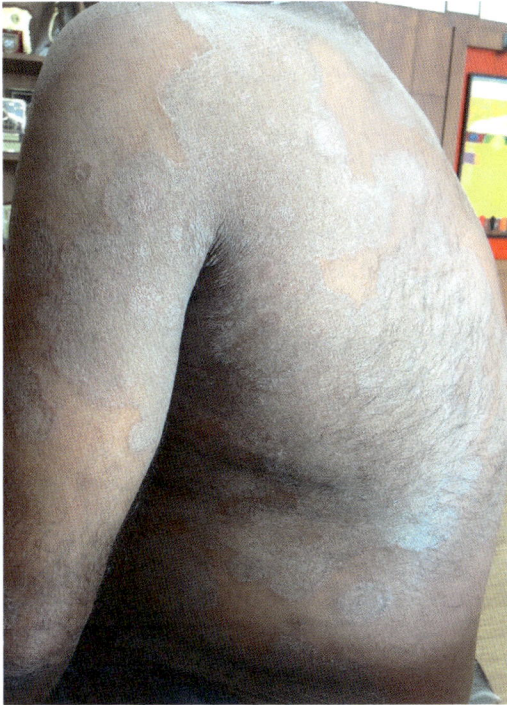

Widespread tinea on the trunk due to application of mometasone-eberconazole cream for 6 months

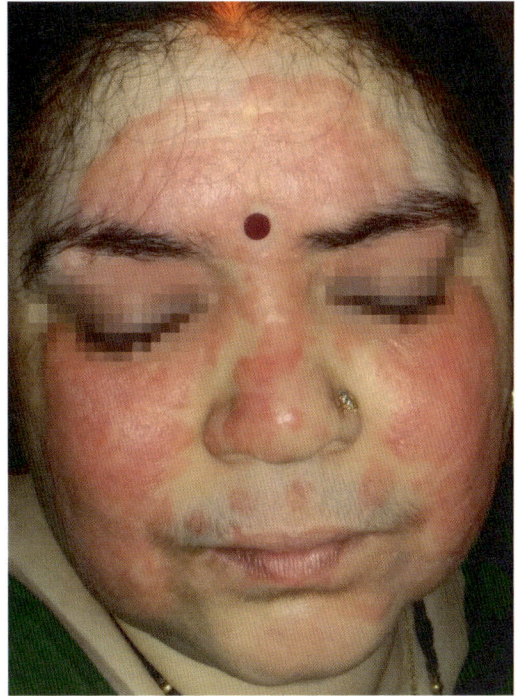

Tinea faciei. Mometasone-hydroquinone-tretinoin used for 2 years

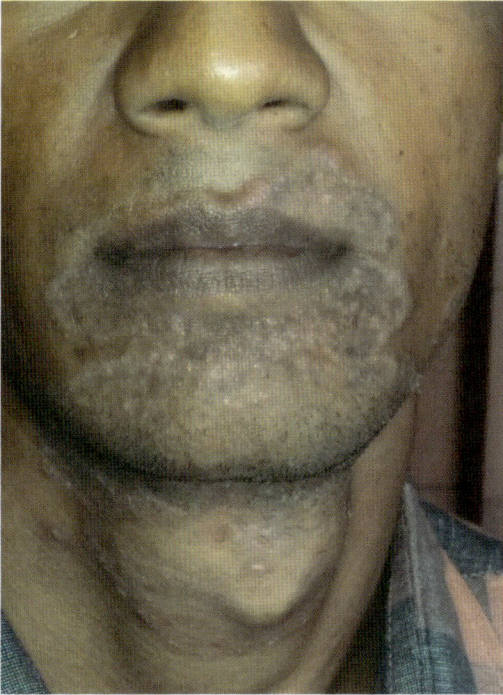

Majocchi's granulomas on the face. Clobetasol-salicylic acid ointment used for 6 months

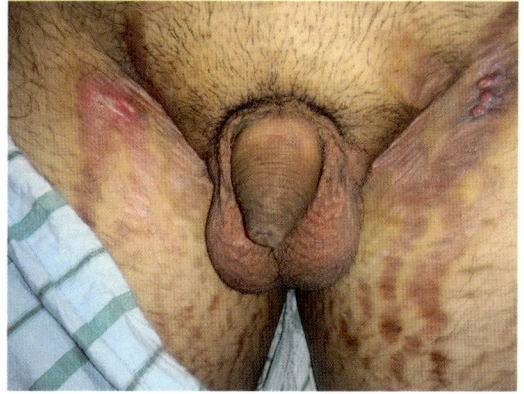

Early ulceration on the steroid-antibiotic striae on the thighs of a 40-year-old man. He was applying clobetasol-ornidazole-ofloxacin-terbinafine combination cream for 1 year

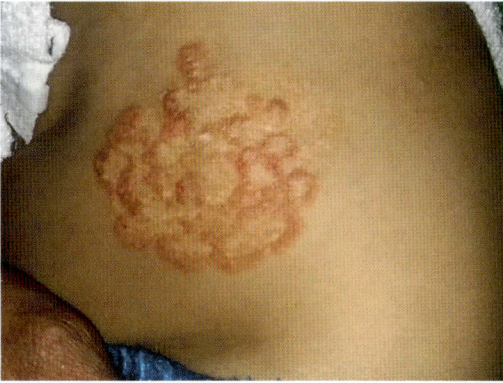

Geographic, imbricated tinea on the abdomen of a 3-year-old child. The whole family was affected. All were applying clobetasol-ornidazole-ofloxacin-terbinafine combination cream

Index

Printed in Great Britain
by Amazon